WD

THE ENCYCLOPEDIA OF

DEAFNESS
AND
HEARING DISORDERS

Second Edition, Updated

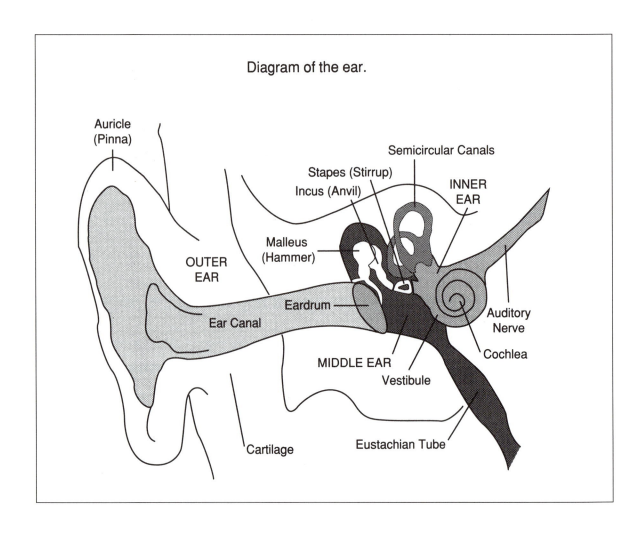

Diagram of the ear.

THE ENCYCLOPEDIA OF

DEAFNESS AND HEARING DISORDERS

Second Edition, Updated

Carol Turkington
and
Allen E. Sussman, Ph.D.

Facts On File, Inc.

The Encyclopedia of Deafness and Hearing Disorders, Second Edition, Updated

Copyright © 2004, 2000, 1992 by Carol Turkington

Facts On File, Inc.
132 West 31st Street
New York NY 10001

The Library of Congress Cataloging-in-Publication Data

Turkington, Carol.
The encyclopedia of deafness and hearing disorders / Carol Turkington and
Allen E Sussman.—2nd ed. [updated]
p.   cm.
Includes bibliographical references and index.
ISBN 0-8160-5615-3 (hc: alk. paper)
1. Deafness—Encyclopedias. 2. Ear—Diseases—Encyclopedias. I. Sussman, Allen E. II. Title.
RF290.T93 2003   617.8´003—dc22
2003049358

Text and cover design by Cathy Rincon

Printed in the United States of America

VB FOF 10 9 8 7 6 5 4 3 2 1

This book is printed on acid-free paper.

CONTENTS

ACKNOWLEDGMENTS

The authors would like to thank the staff members at Gallaudet University who so generously offered their time during this project. In particular, we wish to thank the staffs at the university's library, public relations office, university press, information center and law center.

In addition, we appreciate the efforts of countless people from national organizations, services and government agencies concerned with deaf and hard-of-hearing people who offered a great deal of helpful information, statistics and support.

Thanks also to Elca Swigart, Ph.D., director of the Speech and Hearing Center at Reading Hospital and Medical Center, and audiologist Robert Gance for their valuable technical assistance and review; and to staffers at the National Library of Medicine and the medical libraries of Hershey Medical Center, the University of Pennsylvania Medical Center and Reading Medical Center. Hats off as well to public relations personnel at the National Institute of Mental Health and the National Institutes of Health.

We would also like to thank our editor at Facts On File, James Chambers, for his thoughtful suggestions and editorial guidance. We are also grateful to Bert Holtje and Gene Brissie of James Peter Associates for their valuable support.

Finally, thanks to friends and family for their patience and understanding. And a very special thank you to Michael and Kara.

PREFACE

One out of 10 Americans has some degree of hearing loss, and one out of every 400 is profoundly deaf. Yet many hard-of-hearing and deaf people in this country do not consider themselves handicapped, at a disadvantage or lacking in any way. They do not believe their hearing loss makes them less—just different—and they look upon the deaf community as a separate culture, as rich and diverse as that of the hearing world.

The Encyclopedia of Deafness and Hearing Disorders reflects the continuing struggle within the deaf community to maintain its integrity following years of segregation and misunderstanding. Although educators, linguists, experts in the field of deafness, and deaf and hard-of-hearing people have come a long way toward replacing antagonism with cooperation, there still remain areas of controversy.

Where there are conflicting philosophies on a particular point, we have tried to identify and explain all sides. An extensive bibliography at the end of the book will assist anyone who wishes to explore any specific topic in further depth.

In addition, we made a great effort to include comprehensive appendixes that reflect the diverse range of organizations and support services available to deaf and hard-of-hearing people. We have tried to list as many of these special groups and services as we could find, with current addresses, websites and phone/TDD numbers.

Entries include all facets of deafness and hearing disorders: physiology of the ear, experts in education, science, linguistics and communication, famous deaf individuals, organizations and groups for deaf people, brief outlines of deaf culture in foreign countries, and more. All entries are cross-referenced to related subjects.

Although information presented in this book comes from the most recent sources available, readers should keep in mind that changes can occur very rapidly in medicine and technology. The very latest technical information on hearing aids and on assistive and telecommunications devices should be obtained from specialists. The authors would also like to stress that information in any medical entry should not be substituted for prompt medical attention.

—Carol Turkington
Cumru, PA
Allen E. Sussman, Ph.D.
Washington, DC

ABLEDATA An information and referral project that maintains a database of more than 25,000 assistive technology products. The project also produces fact sheets on types of devices and other aspects of assistive technology. See Appendix II.

Academy of Dispensing Audiologists A professional association formed in 1977 to support the dispensing of hearing aids by AUDIOLOGISTS with advanced degrees in rehabilitative practice. The ADA holds an annual meeting in the fall together with seminars providing information on all aspects of hearing aid dispensing. They publish a quarterly magazine (*Feedback*) for professionals but do not offer information for consumers.

acoupedic method See AUDITORY-ORAL METHOD.

Acoustical Society of America The premier scientific society in acoustics, dedicated to increasing the knowledge of acoustics and its practical applications. Founded in 1929, this group holds regular meetings to discuss research, and publishes the *Journal of the Acoustical Society of America*. The society holds two meetings a year to discuss current research.

acoustic immitance The measure of acoustic immitance can be defined as either acoustic admittance (how easily energy flows through a system) or ACOUSTIC IMPEDANCE (the opposition to the flow of energy). A system with high acoustic impedance to the flow of sound will have low acoustic admittance.

Acoustic-immitance tests are used together with hearing tests because a patient may have a significant ear disease with little hearing loss. Although most hearing tests can uncover the type and degree of hearing loss, they may not reveal specific ear diseases.

Unlike most hearing exams, acoustic immitance tests can reveal middle ear disorders without requiring any active participation by the patient. This is particularly helpful in the testing of young children. See also AUDIOMETRY.

acoustic impedance Some sounds that enter the ear canal and reach the EARDRUM are reflected, while others are absorbed and eventually reach the inner ear. The tendency of the ear to reflect the passage of sound is called its acoustic impedance. How great the acoustic impedance will be depends on the size and stiffness of the eardrum membrane and the OSSICLES.

Testing a person's acoustic impedance gives important information about the health of the middle ear. This is because a person may have an ear disease with very little hearing loss. Unlike more routine hearing tests, impedance tests can detect both the presence and characteristics of MIDDLE-EAR DISEASES. See also ACOUSTIC IMMITANCE; AUDIOMETRY.

acoustic nerve See AUDITORY NERVE.

acoustic neuroma A rare benign tumor (also called an auditory nerve tumor or Schwannoma) arising from the Schwann cell sheath of cranial or spinal nerve roots usually involving the hearing nerve. This type of slow-growing tumor can cause HEARING LOSS on the affected side. About 5 percent to 7 percent of brain tumors fall into this type, which occur more often in women between ages 40 and 60.

Almost all are located within the internal auditory canal and originate from the vestibular division of the AUDITORY NERVE, although occasionally these tumors arise from the cochlear division of the nerve.

Symptoms begin with TINNITUS in one ear with a progressive high-frequency hearing loss. There is often a loss of speech discrimination out of proportion with the hearing loss, probably due to the lessened ability of the cochlear nerve to conduct sound because of the tumor's pressure. Compression of the blood vessels within the internal auditory canal also may cause hearing loss because of the reduced blood flow to and from the COCHLEA.

As it enlarges, the tumor may press on the brainstem and cerebellum, causing lack of coordination. Eventually it may press on the fifth cranial nerve (causing pain in the face) or the sixth cranial nerve (causing double vision). As the vestibular nerve cells within the internal auditory canal degenerate, unsteadiness or VERTIGO can result.

Tumors in both ears are caused by a genetic problem called central neurofibromatosis (elephant man's disease).

Diagnosis is confirmed by hearing and balance tests, AUDITORY BRAINSTEM RESPONSE TEST, and by brain scans. (Most acoustic neuromas affect the size and shape of the internal auditory canal by eroding the bone, which can be detected through scanning.)

While these tumors rarely become malignant, it's important to diagnose the problem early because hearing may be spared with early intervention. (See also AUDITORY NERVE TUMORS.)

Today it is possible to identify even small acoustic neuromas. If routine auditory tests reveal loss of hearing and speech discrimination (hearing sound in that ear, but not understanding what is being said), an AUDITORY BRAINSTEM RESPONSE TEST may be done. This test provides information on how sound passes along the path from the ear to the brain. A detailed "imaging scan" is usually ordered if there is an abnormality in the ABR test, which suggests the presence of an acoustic neuroma.

The CT scan is a powerful tool in locating acoustic neuromas. Although small tumors still confined to the internal auditory canal may not show up on a simple CT scan, a scan using contrast dye will enhance the image of the tumor.

Magnetic resonance imaging (MRI) is a newer diagnostic test that is very effective in identifying acoustic neuromas. MRI combines modern computer technology with harmless magnetic pulses and radio frequency waves passed through the portion of the body being studied. The image that is formed clearly defines any acoustic neuroma. A contrast material is required to enhance the tumor, making it easier to see. Currently, an MRI with gadolinium contrast is the preferred study for diagnosing an acoustic neuroma.

At this time, the only treatment that can totally eradicate the tumor is microsurgical removal, which is the treatment of choice for acoustic neuromas.

Within the last three decades, microsurgical techniques have been refined so that the risk of total tumor removal has been greatly reduced. Microsurgical instruments and the operating microscope are routinely used, and damage to the surrounding nerve tissue has been markedly decreased. The death rate is extremely low.

In addition, facial nerve function is routinely monitored during surgery, which has reduced the frequency and severity of facial nerve injury. The surgeon will also monitor the cochlear nerve when it appears feasible to preserve hearing. According to the National Institutes of Health, patients do best if they are treated at medical centers with surgeons who have a specific interest in these tumors and sufficient continuing experience to develop, refine, and maintain proficiency.

After the surgery, the patient is carefully observed in the intensive care unit for one or two days. Possible postsurgical problems include headache, nausea, vomiting, decreased mental alertness, cerebrospinal fluid leak and meningitis. Patients usually stay in the hospital between four to seven days and recover at home for between four to six weeks. In the hands of an experienced microsurgeon, regrowth rates after microsurgery are less than 5 percent.

Alternatively, some patients have radiation instead of microsurgery. Conventional radiation of most tumors involves multiple doses of radiation delivered over three to six weeks. The treatment team usually consists of a neurosurgeon, a radio-physicist and a radiation oncologist working together to develop a treatment plan based on the size and shape of the tumor.

Radiation, even at relatively high doses, does not kill or injure cells immediately. Following radiation, some tumor cells die in a matter of weeks, but others die more gradually, generally six to 18 months after treatment. This treatment usually stops the growth of the tumor and some tumors will shrink, but the tumor does not disappear.

Follow-up studies are important because 5 percent to 10 percent of tumors will continue to grow after this treatment or at some time in the future. It appears that the tumor will be controlled throughout life following radiation treatment in at least 90 percent of patients. A tumor which has been irradiated and grows may be more difficult to remove than an unradiated tumor, just as a tumor which recurs after microsurgery may be more difficult to remove.

Symptoms such as dizziness and disturbances of balance get better quicker after microsurgical treatment than after radiation because recovery from the effects of radiation may require up to 18 months. Many patients have some residual dizziness and disturbed balance after either radiation or microsurgical treatment, but this is commonly less after microsurgical treatment.

In patients with useful hearing before radiation, about 50 percent will still have useful hearing two years later. Among patients with normal facial movement and sensation before treatment, 10 percent will develop some degree of facial weakness or numbness that usually recovers in several months. These early statistics compare very favorably with microsurgical tumor removal.

In the short term, radiation is less expensive than microsurgery. Most patients are treated on an outpatient basis; many patients return home several hours after treatment is complete and they can return to work within a few days. A few patients experience headaches, nausea and tiredness, but these side effects are considerably less than after microsurgical tumor removal. Patients treated with radiation are usually able to return to their job within a matter of days. Radiation requires follow-up MRIs over the years and there is the potential

for additional treatment in cases of continued growth or later regrowth. Microsurgery is initially more expensive, with follow-up MRIs suggested at one and five years if the tumor has been completely removed.

Radiation was originally restricted to selected patients in whom the risk of surgery was high because of age or preexisting health problems, patients whose tumors were small to moderate in size or patients who had tumors in both ears or tumors in their only hearing ear. Radiation is now being offered in some facilities to all patients who are unable or unwilling to undergo microsurgery. The National Institutes of Health recommends that radiation therapy is a treatment option limited to patients unable or unwilling to undergo otherwise indicated surgery.

In small tumors (usually up to an inch), it may be possible to save some hearing. In larger tumors (those that protrude from the internal auditory canal into the brainstem), the hearing usually has been partially or totally lost and cannot be restored. This loss means that problems locating the direction of sound, hearing a person speaking softly on the deaf side and understanding speech over a high level of background noise will continue. For some, a CROS hearing aid will be helpful.

Because the facial nerve, which controls muscles of facial expression, is in close contact with acoustic neuromas, it is usually necessary for the surgeon to manipulate and sometimes to remove portions of this nerve. In some instances nerve damage or swelling may cause facial paralysis. This paralysis resolves with time, but some permanent weakness may persist.

Nerve regeneration is a slow process, and it may take up to a year for recovery. If facial paralysis doesn't improve, a second operation may be performed to connect the healthy portion of the facial nerve to a nerve in the neck.

Studies show that long-term eye discomfort and other eye problems affect at least half of those who have had an acoustic neuroma removed, particularly if the tumor was medium or large. It is important to be under the care of an eye specialist if problems occur. Loss of eyelid function or altered tear production causes much of the scratchiness and irritation because the eye becomes dry and is unprotected. A few patients may experience double vision due to pressure on one of the cranial nerves (usually the sixth) which controls muscles that move the eyes. Others may have temporary problems with tiredness, headache, voice or balance.

Acoustic Neuroma Association A professional association that provides information and support to patients with an ACOUSTIC NEUROMA or other problems affecting the cranial nerves. Founded by a patient in 1981, the nonprofit group provides information on patient rehabilitation to health care professionals, promotes research on acoustic neuroma and provides information to the public on symptoms, diagnosis and treatment.

The association publishes a quarterly newsletter, distributes a patient information booklet, presents a twice-yearly national symposium, provides access to a network of local support groups, compiles a registry of statistical data on acoustic neuroma treatment and maintains a website for patient information and discussion. See also Appendix II.

acoustic reflex A reflex contraction of a small muscle in the middle ear that stiffens the chain of OSSICLES (hammer, anvil, stirrup) to protect the inner ear.

acoustics The science concerning the properties, production, control, transmission, reception and effects of sound. This subdivision of physics has two major branches: architectural acoustics and environmental acoustics.

Architectural acoustics involves the study of how sound waves operate in closed spaces and how to create the best acoustical conditions for a variety of purposes (such as sound transmission in concert halls and theaters). Environmental acoustics focuses on noise pollution and its control, including improved insulation, room partitions and so forth.

Other minor branches include musical acoustics (the operation and design of musical instruments and the study of how musical sounds affect listeners), engineering acoustics (development of high-fidelity sound recording and reproduction), ultrasonics (acoustical phenomena with vibration rates above the audible range of 20,000 hertz),

underwater sound, mechanical vibration and shock and speech communication.

acoustic spectrum The distribution of the intensity levels of various frequency components of a sound.

acoustic trauma Ear damage resulting from a sudden, intense noise (such as a gunshot) including an immediate sense of fullness, TINNITUS and HEARING LOSS. If the noise is loud enough, it can rupture the EARDRUM and disrupt the ossicular chain (hammer, anvil, stirrup), causing a CONDUCTIVE HEARING LOSS without much accompanying nerve damage because the middle ear defect now protects the inner ear.

Generally, the tinnitus and feeling of fullness subside after the injury, and hearing improves—although there may be a degree of permanent hearing loss. The amount of the loss depends on the intensity and duration of the noise and the sensitivity of the ear. In milder cases, the hearing loss occurs only in the ear closest to the noise.

Hearing loss from damage to the middle ear can sometimes be corrected; a ruptured eardrum can heal by itself in time, and the small bones of the ear may be repaired or replaced.

Normally, permanent loss is mild (a high tone dip between 3,000 to 6,000 hertz), although the loss may be greater if the ear is very sensitive or the noise was quite loud. Because there is almost always some amount of temporary hearing loss following acoustic trauma, some time must pass before the amount of permanent damage can be measured.

In addition, the body may sustain other types of damage from excess noise: Since the body's equilibrium is partly controlled by inner structures, intense sound can cause motion sickness, dizziness and disorientation. See also NOISE; OCCUPATIONAL HEARING LOSS.

acupuncture Acupuncture has been used to treat SENSORINEURAL HEARING LOSS and MÉNIÈRE'S DISEASE.

adenoidectomy The surgical removal of the ADENOIDS, the twin lymph nodes at the back of the nose above the tonsils. This operation is usually performed on a child with abnormally large adenoids that are causing recurrent middle ear or sinus infections that could lead to hearing loss. Often, an adenoidectomy is performed at the same time as a tonsillectomy.

There are few aftereffects of the operation, and the patient can usually begin to eat normal meals one day afterward.

adenoids The two lymph nodes above the tonsils at the back of the nose that are partly responsible for protecting the body's upper respiratory tract against infection. Although they tend to enlarge during childhood when these types of infections are common, adenoids usually shrink after about age five and disappear by adolescence.

However, they sometimes continue to grow, obstructing the eustachian tube and causing hearing problems. In addition, secretions behind the nose that are obstructed by oversized adenoids can lead to infections of the nose (rhinitis) that can spread to the middle ear.

Occasional infections can be treated with antibiotics, but surgery to remove the adenoids (ADENOIDECTOMY) may be needed if infections become chronic.

adhesive otitis media A chronic middle ear infection that scars the EARDRUM. The eardrum collapses and adheres to the OSSICLES (hammer, anvil, stirrup) and middle-ear promontory, causing HEARING LOSS. A chronic infection such as this also can cause new bone to form in the middle ear lining. Treatment involves drainage and antibiotics. See also OTITIS MEDIA.

adventitious deafness Also called acquired deafness, this term refers to hearing loss that occurs later in life. See also HEARING LOSS.

aero-otitis media Also called barotrauma, this is a temporary yet painful inflammatory reaction of the MIDDLE EAR caused by a difference in pressure between the gas in the middle ear and the surrounding atmosphere. It is usually caused by rapid descent in a poorly-pressurized airplane when swollen sinus membranes do not allow normal equalization of air pressure in the ear. The symptoms may include severe pain, inflammation, bleeding and rupture of the eardrum membrane. Underwater divers and airplane pilots are also susceptible to this problem.

The middle ear (located behind the eardrum) is connected to the nasal cavity by the EUSTACHIAN TUBE. Normally, when the external air pressure rises or falls, air from the nose goes through the eustachian tube and equalizes pressure in the middle ear cavity. Air pressure also can be equalized by periodically opening the eustachian tube by swallowing or yawning. But fluids from head colds, tumors or enlarged tonsils can block the eustachian tube and interfere with the equalization process.

In a descending airplane, the external air pressure increases and in order to equalize pressure in the middle ear, air must pass from the eustachian tubes to the middle ear. In an ascending airplane, air in the middle ear expands as external air pressure falls; if the eustachian tube is blocked, the expanding air in the middle ear has nowhere to go and presses against the eardrum, bulging it outward.

It is usually harder to equalize pressure when descending rather than ascending in a plane, as the increasing external pressure creates a vacuum in the middle ear that seals the eustachian tubes.

As pressure in the ear equalizes, the pain subsides unless the eardrum has already been damaged. Although the eardrum membrane can rupture because of the difference in pressure on its two sides, most often the pain continues until the middle ear fills with fluid.

Rupture of an eardrum membrane relieves the pain and pressure, but it can cause dizziness, partial hearing loss and middle ear infections. Usually, pain and hearing loss produced during a flight under these conditions is temporary and disappears by itself. If there are no complications, a ruptured eardrum heals itself in about a month.

Deep sea divers encounter the same problem: Every 10 to 15 feet as they descend in the water, they must equalize the pressure in their ears to the external pressure of the sea.

aging and hearing loss A certain amount of hearing loss is the natural result of aging. About 12 million Americans experience some form of hearing loss as they age, including half of those over age 75. These late-deafened older Americans are usually not profoundly deaf and are not likely to know sign language or consider themselves a part of the deaf community.

Hearing loss among the elderly is much more prevalent among men than women, whites than blacks, people earning less than $7,000 per year and who did not graduate from high school. One explanation for some of these characteristics could be that those in lower economic brackets are likely to become ill more often, and chronic health conditions can lead to or exacerbate hearing problems. If ignored and left untreated, the hearing problems among this country's elderly interfere with communication, curtailing social activities and unnecessarily limiting an older person's circle of friends.

Causes

Hearing loss among the elderly can be caused by a variety of things, including infections of the outer, middle or inner ear; blood clots; loud noises; hereditary conditions; bony growths in the middle ear; and adverse reactions to drugs or medication.

However, the most common cause of deafness in the elderly is PRESBYCUSIS—a progressive deterioration of the hearing organ leading to an intolerance for loud noises but not total deafness. Although presbycusis is usually blamed on old age, not every senior citizen is affected. The loss of hearing sensitivity may be caused by chemical and mechanical changes in the inner ear and breakdown of these structures, or by complex degenerative changes along the nerve pathways leading to the brain. These changes slow the signals traveling from the ear to the brain. Although these breakdowns also happen in the outer and middle ear, the most significant changes occur in the inner ear.

Researchers do not definitely know what causes presbycusis, but there are several things that may contribute to it: prolonged exposure to loud noise, reduced blood flow to the inner ear and atherosclerosis.

Damage to the outer or middle ear causes CONDUCTIVE HEARING LOSS, which involves the blocking or impairment of movement in the outer or middle ear so that sound waves can't travel through it. With this type of hearing loss, sounds are perceived as soft and muted. Talking louder often helps a person with this type of loss, and HEARING AIDS may help people with this problem. Conductive loss is usually caused by IMPACTED EARWAX, extra fluid, abnormal bone growth in the ear or infection.

Central deafness, which is quite rare among the elderly, is caused by damage to the hearing nerve centers inside the brain. It affects not the perception of sound but the understanding of language. Causes range from an extended illness with high fever, to head injuries, circulation problems or tumors.

Damage to the inner ear or auditory nerve causes a SENSORINEURAL HEARING LOSS in which perception of pitch and loudness may be affected. People with this type of loss can often hear sounds but cannot understand words (for example, "hem" for "hen," "pin" for "tin.") Hearing aids may help, but they will not eliminate the distortions associated with sensorineural hearing loss.

Many older people experience hearing loss, but they don't all experience loss in the same way; the kind of hearing loss depends on where the damage in the ear has occurred and the severity may range from mild to profound. For example, some older persons have high frequency losses, which means they have trouble hearing high-pitched sounds. Thus, the higher-pitched voices of women and children may be more difficult for them to understand.

Warning Signs

A hearing loss may be suspected if there is a history of ear infections and the person experiences TINNITUS (ringing in the ear) and starts talking loudly, increasing the TV or radio volume, complaining that others are mumbling, and confusing words that have similar sounds. The person may also be unable to hear soft or high-pitched sounds.

Diagnosis

The early signs of hearing loss may be very slight, but the earlier the problem is diagnosed, the better chance there is of successful management. The important first step is a correct diagnosis by a physician who specializes in the ear and evaluation by an

AUDIOLOGIST to identify the degree and type of hearing loss. Audiologists can also design a rehabilitation program and offer hearing aid evaluation and orientation, together with training in speechreading techniques and speech.

Services for Senior Citizens

Senior citizens who begin to experience hearing loss may find particular help from SELF HELP FOR HARD OF HEARING PEOPLE (SHHH), which is primarily designed for the needs of late-deafened people. Founded in the early 1980s by a former senior officer in the Central Intelligence Agency, the group stresses self-assertiveness and advocacy.

Other special services for senior citizens with hearing problems include the GALLAUDET UNIVERSITY summer program "Elder-hostel" designed for late-deafened adults and a special section for late-deafened adults as part of the ALEXANDER GRAHAM BELL ASSOCIATION FOR THE DEAF.

AIDS and hearing loss Both AIDS and AIDS-related complex (ARC) are associated with neurological complications that include hearing loss. An estimated 75 percent of adult AIDS patients and 50 percent of all ARC patients have auditory system abnormalities.

Why this happens is unknown, although direct infection of the nervous system by the AIDS virus is well documented. Hearing disorders in AIDS could be caused directly by infection of the cochlea or the central auditory system.

On the other hand, many AIDS complications are the result of opportunistic infections rather than the virus itself—the most prevalent infection, CYTOMEGALOVIRUS (CMV), is known to damage the auditory system in congenital infections. More than 90 percent of AIDS patients have CMV.

AIDS.Net A special computer bulletin board established by DEAFTEK.USA, a nonprofit group providing electronic mail service for deaf and hard-of-hearing people. AIDS.Net is an information-sharing network about AIDS established after a conference on AIDS and deafness held in 1988 in Toronto.

Information for the bulletin is provided by the National Information Clearinghouse on AIDS, together with agencies and professionals serving deaf people. Currently, members in the United States, Canada and England are participating in AIDS.Net. Subscribers are also free to ask questions of experts provided by the bulletin board.

air bags and hearing loss The sudden impact of an air bag hitting a passenger's face may cause hearing problems. According to a team of British researchers, the sound of an air bag inflating can be as loud as 150 to 170 decibels, lasting about 0.1 seconds, a sound that scientists believe may damage hearing in humans.

Researchers base their conclusions on two cases in which drivers suffered hearing loss and ringing of the ears (TINNITUS) in low-speed accidents. Ear problems following air bag inflation may be underreported because passengers often don't remember the noise of the inflation and attribute their loss to injuries suffered in the accident itself.

air bone gap The difference between air- and bone-conduction thresholds. See also AUDIOMETRY.

air conduction Transmission of sound to the inner ear via the ear canal and middle ear.

air conduction audiometry A subjective method of estimating hearing sensitivity by evoking responses of the patient to air-conducted pure tones. See also AUDIOMETRY.

air conduction test, pure tone See AUDIOMETRY.

alarms, sound sensitive See ALERTING DEVICES; WAKE-UP ALARMS.

alarms, visual See ALERTING DEVICES; WAKE-UP ALARMS.

Alberti, Salomon (1540–1600) This 16th-century German physician and professor at the University of Wittenborg was the first to call attention to hard-of-hearing (those who can hear loud sounds and are not deaf) and attributed deafness to "some lack" in the development of the fetus. He claims to have discovered the cochlea.

alerting devices   A compensatory device that alerts deaf and hard-of-hearing persons to a sound (doorbell, crying baby, telephone, timer) by activating a light signal.

These visual alarms often feature one or more flashing lights (one lamp or all the lights in the house). The lights are turned on either through direct wiring or by using a signal transmitted through the building's wiring system. Some systems can even alert to different sounds by using different light patterns for each sound. See also WAKE-UP ALARMS; Appendix III.

Alexander Graham Bell Association for the Deaf
A private, nonprofit organization serving as an information center, publisher and advocate of effective ways of teaching deaf and hard-of-hearing persons to improve their abilities to speak, speechread, use residual hearing and process spoken and written language. It also aims to empower those with hearing problems to function independently.

Since its inception in 1890 as the American Association to Promote the Teaching of Speech to the Deaf, the association has had one primary purpose: to promote the use of speech, SPEECH-READING and residual hearing by hard-of-hearing people.

Most of the first members of the group were articulation teachers who used the VISIBLE SPEECH method, a system of written symbols representing the anatomical formation of speech sounds, invented by Alexander Melville Bell (Alexander Graham's father). Since then, the association has grown into an international organization whose members fall into four categories: professionals in the deafness field, parents of hard-of-hearing children, deaf adults who can speak and speechread and others who believe in the importance of oral communication.

Although it began as an active proponent of speech for deaf people, the organization has gradually expanded its interests to include research, family support and financial assistance to help deaf students attend classes with hearing peers. It also sponsors workshops and biennial conventions and publishes the *Volta Review,* a professional journal published six times a year; *Newsounds,* a newsletter published 10 times a year; and *Our Kids Magazine.* In addition, the association sells books of interest to members through mail-order catalogs and presents books on various oral topics for teachers, parents and deaf and hard-of-hearing adults.

Three distinct sections within the organization focus on the needs of three specific groups: deaf adults (Oral Deaf Adults Section), parents (International Parents Organization) and teachers (International Organization for the Education of the Hearing Impaired).

Oral Deaf Adults Section
This voluntary, nonprofit service section was formed in 1964 to help improve the education, employment and social opportunities of deaf people. Members receive a newsletter, a membership directory and scholarship support and have access to programs designed to help parents of children with hearing problems.

International Parents Organization
This section provides special help to families of children with hearing problems who are interested in promoting aural/oral education. Membership is open to any member of the association and includes a magazine, *Our Kids Magazine,* family workshops, educational scholarships and a family support network throughout the United States and Canada.

International Organization for the Education of the Hearing Impaired
This special section, formed in 1967, promotes excellence in aural/oral education for deaf children and adults. The aims of this group include the development of effective oral education and communication programs, research into oral communication and an information exchange among educators. See also BELL, ALEXANDER GRAHAM; VOLTA BUREAU.

Alport's disease   A genetic disease that causes kidney inflammation in childhood, followed by a sensorineural hearing impairment in young adulthood and eye problems later in life. It is more common among men than women. There is no clear relationship between the extent of kidney disease and onset of deafness.

Treatment is supportive. The disease is not known to recur following transplantation.

alternate binaural loudness balance test The ABLB test measures RECRUITMENT (the abnormal rapid increase in loudness above the THRESHOLD level) with a device that allows the client to set controls so that the loudness of a tone heard by the defective ear matches the tone heard in the normal ear.

By repeating this comparison at several intensity levels, the presence or absence of recruitment can be identified. This test is used to diagnose a SENSORINEURAL HEARING LOSS affecting primarily one ear.

alternative listening systems See ASSISTIVE LISTENING SYSTEM.

Ambrosi, Gustinus (1893–1975) Born in Eisenstadt, Austria, this talented musician and sculptor was best known for his classic sculptures in bronze and marble.

A child prodigy on the violin, he lost his hearing at the age of six after a bout of meningitis and smashed his treasured instrument when he realized he could no longer hear. However, as Ambrosi grew to adulthood he began to consider his deafness a blessing in disguise.

Finding he was no longer able to continue in music, Ambrosi studied woodcarving at the age of eight and became an apprentice at 14 with a sculpting firm in Prague. Within five years he had won two major art prizes, and in 1908 Emperor Fran Joseph gave him lifetime use of an atelier.

Considered a Renaissance man, Ambrosi was a gifted poet, graphic artist and philosopher, although he was known primarily for his lifelike busts.

When old age began to interfere with his ability to sculpt, Ambrosi committed suicide on July 1, 1975, in Vienna.

American Academy of Audiology A professional membership organization of AUDIOLOGISTS that provides an annual national meeting to exchange research and information about hearing science and hearing aids. The group does not provide consumer outreach. See also Appendix II.

American Academy of Otolaryngology–Head and Neck Surgery The largest professional organization in this field, representing physicians who specialize in the treatment and surgery of the ear, nose and throat and related structures of the head and neck. It provides continuing medical education and various professional publications and also presents the interests of otolaryngologists to legislators. Its annual convention includes an intensive continuing education program offering a wide range of courses in the latest research and advanced techniques in cosmetic facial reconstruction, cancer surgery, patient management and treatment of allergic, sinus, laryngeal, thyroid and esophageal disorders.

The association publishes leaflets related to ear problems and a monthly journal, *Otolaryngology-Head and Neck Surgery* and also provides physician referrals. See also OTOLARYNGOLOGIST; Appendix II.

American Annals of the Deaf The oldest professional educational journal in the United States, *American Annals of the Deaf* is published jointly five times a year by the CONVENTION OF AMERICAN INSTRUCTORS OF THE DEAF (CAID) and the CONFERENCE OF EDUCATIONAL ADMINISTRATORS SERVING THE DEAF (CEASD).

The journal, which was first published in 1847 by the faculty of the AMERICAN SCHOOL FOR THE DEAF in Hartford, Connecticut, has passed through many different editorial hands. Its primary focus is to publish information of broad interest to those concerned with the education of deaf people. This information includes statistics on deafness, research into the psychology and sociology of deafness, conference reports and philosophical discussions. In addition, the publication includes an annual directory of services for the deaf. See also Appendix II.

American Association of the Deaf-Blind An organization that promotes better opportunities and services for deaf-blind people and assures that a comprehensive, coordinated system of services is accessible to all deaf-blind people, enabling them to achieve their maximum potential through increased independence, productivity, and integration into the community. The biannual conventions provide a week of workshops, meetings, tours and recreational activities. The group also publishes *The Deaf-Blind American.* See also Appendix II.

American Association to Promote the Teaching of Speech to the Deaf

The original name of the ALEXANDER GRAHAM BELL ASSOCIATION FOR THE DEAF, this group—founded in 1890—first changed its name to the Volta Speech Association for the Deaf in 1948 and then changed to its present name in 1953. See also Appendix II.

American Athletic Association of the Deaf (AAAD)

Founded in 1945, this group was established to encourage athletic graduates of deaf schools to continue in sports competition. It promotes intramural competition among deaf athletic clubs, supervises regional tournaments and, since 1957, gives financial support to deaf athletes wishing to participate in the WORLD GAMES FOR THE DEAF.

From the early 1900s, deaf athletes discussed the possibility of having a national basketball tournament for deaf people. In 1945 the first competition for the National Basketball Champion of the Deaf was held in Akron, Ohio, pitting top players from teams in Akron, Buffalo, Philadelphia, Kansas City and Los Angeles. (Buffalo won the tournament.) At the same time, members from the deaf clubs all over the country voted to make the tournament an annual event and formed the American Athletic Union of the Deaf to oversee its organization. The AAUD later changed its name to the American Athletic Association of the Deaf to avoid its being confused with the Amateur Athletic Union of the United States.

After the AAAD became affiliated with the Comité International des Sports des Sourds, sponsor of the World Games of the Deaf, the AAAD was able to hold three World Games for the Deaf in the United States: summer games in Washington, D.C. (1965) and in Los Angeles (1985) and winter games in Lake Placid, New York (1975).

The AAAD sponsors annual basketball and softball tournaments, names an annual Athlete of the Year and hosts an AAAD Hall of Fame to honor outstanding deaf athletes, coaches and sports figures. In addition, AAAD is affiliated with four national athletic organizations (skating, ice hockey, tennis and volleyball), the U.S. Olympic Committee's Handicap in Sports Committee and the Amateur Softball Association. See also Appendix II.

American Coalition of Citizens with Disabilities

This national nonprofit group, founded in 1974 by the directors of about 150 disabilities groups, was the only one of its kind directed by disabled people. Although no longer in existence, at one time it promoted the human and civil rights of America's 30 million disabled people on local, state and national levels, encouraged research and training and provided information and referral programs.

The coalition also published the *ACCD NewsNet,* which covered disability-related issues and books related to disabilities. See also Appendix II.

American Deafness and Rehabilitation Association (ADARA)

A nonprofit, interdisciplinary group that promotes efforts to improve and expand rehabilitation services for deaf people, encourage research in deafness and promote the recruitment and training of professionals to work and communicate with deaf individuals.

Formerly called the Professional Rehabilitation Workers with the Adult Deaf (PRWAD), the organization was founded at a national conference of the Rehabilitation Services Administration in 1966. At that time, there was no national group serving those who worked with deaf people (the Convention of American Instructors of the Deaf was only interested in education and teachers, and the National Rehabilitation Association had no section for those who worked with deaf clients). The PRWAD welcomed rehabilitation counselors, psychologists, social workers and other professionals whose clientele were mostly deaf people.

After several years of debate, the name was changed to its present form during the group's 1978 convention, placing "deafness" before "rehabilitation."

Today, ADARA works closely with other organizations to develop legislation serving the needs of deaf people and publishes the quarterly *Journal of the American Deafness and Rehabilitation Association* as well as various monographs sold as separate publications. The association also organizes national and regional conferences, workshops, training seminars and continuing education programs.

Although ADARA does not conduct research itself, its conferences and publications provide scientists with information and bibliographical support. The biennial conference provides a forum for professionals to learn about developments in the field, special problem areas and new treatments and advances. Several states have chapters that continue the work of the national group at the local level.

ADARA has grown from a group of about 300 in 1967 to more than 2,000 members in 1991. Separate sections within the organization address DEAF-BLINDNESS, mental health counseling, social work, and vocational and psychological assessment. See also JOURNALS IN THE FIELD OF DEAFNESS; Appendix II.

American Hearing Research Foundation   A nonprofit agency that promotes and finances medical research into the causes and treatments of deafness, hearing problems and balance disorders, encourages collaboration between clinical and laboratory research and works to broaden teaching and professional aims. The association funds eight to 10 projects a year, with an average grant of $20,000. The projects cover how hearing and balance functions are lost and regained and how to preserve the function patients still have. See also Appendix II.

American Humane Association   A national federation of local, state and regional animal care and control agencies that started the first formal hearing ear dog training program in 1976 and helped create other training programs across the country.

Today, American Humane's Center for Hearing Dog Information assists local hearing dog training programs through publications and training aids and helps deaf individuals obtain dogs of their own. See also CENTER FOR HEARING EAR DOGS; HEARING EAR DOGS; Appendix II.

American Laryngological, Rhinological and Otological Society   A national society of OTOLARYNGOLOGISTS and head and neck surgeons that provides continuing educational opportunities for its members through its meetings. Four section meetings and an annual meeting are held each year. See also Appendix II.

American manual alphabet   See FINGERSPELLING.

American Ministries to the Deaf   An evangelical organization whose aim is to proclaim the gospel of Jesus Christ among deaf people around the world. See also Appendix II.

American Otological Society   A professional organization whose mission is to advance and promote medical and surgical OTOLOGY, including the rehabilitation of hearing impairment, and to encourage and promote research in otology and related disciplines. See also Appendix II.

American School for the Deaf   The oldest school for deaf students in the United States. It offers a wide range of programs guided by the TOTAL COMMUNICATION philosophy—a philosophy implying acceptance of all methods of communication (speech, speechreading, aural, oral, American Sign Language and other manual communication systems).

The school began as a joint collaboration between THOMAS HOPKINS GALLAUDET, a young Andover, Massachusetts divinity student, and Dr. MASON FITCH COGSWELL, a surgeon and professor at Yale Medical School. When Dr. Cogswell saw Gallaudet's success at teaching Cogswell's young deaf daughter, he was inspired with the idea of reaching other hard-of-hearing students around the country. Gallaudet was sent to Europe by Cogswell and the Hartford, Connecticut city fathers to study both the French and English methods of teaching deaf students.

However, when Gallaudet arrived in England, he discovered that the founder of the English method demanded payment in turn for sharing his knowledge of deaf education. Unable to pay, Gallaudet continued on to France.

In Paris, Gallaudet worked closely with ABBÉ ROCH-AMBROISE CUCURRON SICARD, director of the French Institute for the Deaf (now the Institut National des Jeunes Sourds) and his two assistants, JEAN MASSIEU and LAURENT CLERC. Eventually, Gallaudet returned to the United States with Clerc to set up a school for deaf students in Hartford.

The American School for the Deaf (originally known as the American Asylum for the Education and Instruction of Deaf and Dumb Persons) opened its doors April 15, 1817, with a class of seven students.

Immediately successful, it became the first recipient of state aid to elementary and secondary education in the United States when the state government awarded the school a legislative grant in 1819.

Since then, almost 5,000 students have graduated from this school, which has evolved from a small educational institution for deaf children to a multifaceted organization offering more than 75 different programs and services to the deaf community and the general public, including:

- Parent-Child Counseling Program—a home-based early intervention program serving families of hard-of-hearing infants and children through school age.
- PACES program—comprehensive and highly structured psychoeducational and dormitory life for emotionally and behaviorally disordered hard-of-hearing children and adolescents.
- Adult Vocational Services—New England's center for vocational rehabilitation services for hard-of-hearing individuals seeking job training and skills necessary for employment. The comprehensive resource center serves deaf people who need help preparing for, finding and keeping jobs.
- Community Audiological Services—a comprehensive hearing health care service including hearing tests; hearing aid evaluations, dispensing, fitting and repair; earmold impressions; and electroacoustical analysis of hearing aids and amplifications equipment.
- Camp Isola Bella—a recreational residential summer camp for deaf children between ages six and 18, located in the southern Berkshire hills of Salisbury, Connecticut.

Other services at the American School for the Deaf include preschool and kindergarten programs; academic and vocational instruction; residential opportunities; extracurricular, cultural and social activities (scouting, athletics, Junior Achievement, student body government); professional consultation and training; and summer recreation and education programs. See also Appendix II.

American Sign Language (ASL)   A visual-gestural language used as a primary means of communication by a very large portion of the deaf population in the United States (estimates suggest between 100,000 to 500,000 people). Often called the language of deaf people, ASL has a unique grammar and syntax and is unrelated to English, although it reflects English influences. It also features FINGERSPELLING (the manual alphabet) to spell out words, including proper names and technical phrases. Some deaf individuals use sign exclusively, others use ASL in combination with SIGNED ENGLISH.

For many years, ASL was not considered a language at all. Critics claimed it lacked grammatical structure and warned that it relegated deaf people to an isolated subculture. Because ASL was considered "grammatically incorrect" by many educators, its usage was forbidden in schools and educational programs for deaf children. Thus, for years ASL was considered a suppressed language, despite its wide use by deaf children and adults from one generation to the next.

However, on the basis of new research, linguists today believe ASL is indeed a language—a visual language that includes many nonmanual features, including facial expressions and body language. It is passed on from parents to children; children whose parents are deaf and fluent signers learn ASL as a first language.

Many linguists believe that it is only when sign language differs completely from English that it may properly be called AMERICAN SIGN LANGUAGE, although some use ASL as a catch-all term to describe a whole range of manual communication.

At one extreme of the sign language continuum is FINGERSPELLING, in which handshapes are used to spell out each word of the English language while speaking or moving lips. This method (also called the Rochester method or visible English) is occasionally used in a few schools, but it is an unpopular method of communication and can be tiring to use and interpret.

Farther along on the continuum are MANUALLY CODED ENGLISH systems, which use fingerspelling but also include signs and markers. The most common forms of this system are SIGNED ENGLISH and SIGNING EXACT ENGLISH, which base their signs on ASL but include other aspects of the English language.

They often use the first letter of the word (also called initialization) with the basic movement of the sign to give hints to the intended word. These systems also include markers for prefixes, suffixes, plural endings and tenses, together with signs for articles, infinitives and all forms of the verb "to be." Although this system is often used in schools, it is not used by deaf adults except for some initial signs and endings that have found their way into popular usage.

In the middle of the sign language continuum is a system called PIDGIN SIGN ENGLISH (PSE), the system used most often by hearing people learning to communicate with deaf people.

PSE combines the English language with the vocabulary and nonmanual features of ASL and is the preferred method of communication by many deaf people. Signs for definite and indefinite articles are omitted, and only one sign is used for the verb "to be" unlike the manually coded English systems.

Finally, American Sign Language, when used in its true sense to mean the patterns used by deaf persons when they communicate in sign in a non-English style, is at the other end of the sign language continuum.

Studies have shown that signs used this way are indeed a recognizable language with its own grammatical pattern, and nonmanual behaviors are an important part of this system. Neither articles nor speech are used, although fingerspelling is used for proper names.

In the United States, variations in ASL can often be traced to different residential schools and educational programs for different deaf communities. For example, the segregation of black deaf students in the South resulted in a variation of ASL used by the majority of the white population. It featured different words and even some different grammatical structures.

The acceptance and resultant surge in the use of ASL by both deaf and hearing people is reflected in the increase of ASL classes, videos and instructional books. Today, ASL has been incorporated with Signed English, speech, speechreading and other modes of communication in many educational programs for deaf students from elementary to postsecondary levels.

Still, there is some resistance to the use of ASL, especially in education where many school officials acknowledge the language but do not officially recognize it as a teaching tool. Despite research to the contrary, these school administrators believe teaching is ASL will interfere with the development of English skills.

In fact, there is still disagreement among deaf people themselves about ASL. Many find a source of pride and an example of cultural identity in the language, but others feel more ambivalent about its use in the wider hearing society. See also SIGN LANGUAGE; SIGN LANGUAGE INTERPRETERS; SIMULTANEOUS COMMUNICATION; TOTAL COMMUNICATION, Appendix XII.

American Sign Language Teachers Association

A national professional organization of AMERICAN SIGN LANGUAGE and deaf studies teachers (formerly known as the Sign Instructors Guidance Network, or SIGN). SIGN was originally formed in 1975 by the NATIONAL ASSOCIATION OF THE DEAF Communicative Skills Program (CSP) to meet the increasing demand for qualified ASL teachers. To promote high quality instruction, teacher evaluations were held in conjunction with biennial NAD conventions and other ASL-related conferences since 1976. Local SIGN chapters were established in 1985, and by 1992 members of SIGN overwhelmingly endorsed a proposal to rename the organization to the American Sign Language Teachers Association (ASLTA).

By 1999, ASLTA had expanded to 25 local chapters. It publishes a newsletter, advocates for legislation recognizing ASL as a language and promotes the hiring of certified teachers of ASL. ASLTA has more than 800 members, including more than 200 certified teachers of ASL. The organization aims to provide an effective avenue for ASL and deaf studies teachers to exchange information on language and culture, instructional methods, materials and evaluation techniques. See also Appendix II.

American Society for Deaf Children (ASDC)

An organization providing advocacy, information and support to more than 20,000 parents, professionals and families with deaf or hard-of-hearing children. The organization was founded in 1967 by members of the CONVENTION OF AMERICAN INSTRUCTORS OF THE DEAF and promotes TOTAL COMMUNICATION as a way of life for deaf children and their families.

ASDC is the only national, independent, non-profit organization whose sole purpose is to provide support, encouragement and information about deafness to families of deaf and hard-of-hearing children. The fundamental goal of ASDC is to improve education for deaf and hard-of-hearing students and to involve parents in the decision-making process.

Its "Two Years of Love" program includes a range of personalized services presented to a family with a deaf child—ASDC membership and a monthly shipment of books, toys, letters and journals.

In addition, the group provides a speakers' bureau, sponsors task forces, holds regional meetings and a biennial convention, and publishes various brochures, position papers and a quarterly newsletter, *The Endeavor.*

Parent groups can become affiliate members of ASDC, and organizations, agencies and educational institutions can become organization-affiliate members. See also Appendix II.

American Speech-Language-Hearing Association (ASHA)

The national professional and scientific organization founded in 1925 for speech language pathologists and audiologists concerned with communication disorders. The group provides information and a toll-free helpline number for individuals with questions about speech, language or hearing problems.

ASHA maintains high standards of professional competence, develops good clinical service programs, stimulates research and offers continuing communication about speech and hearing.

New members must hold a graduate degree (or equivalent) in speech-language pathology, speech and hearing science, audiology or allied disciplines. Members in independent clinical practice must meet specific requirements in order to receive the Certificate of Clinical Competence.

Publications include three quarterly publications, *Journal of Speech and Hearing Disorders, Journal of Speech and Hearing Research* and *Language, Speech and Hearing Services in Schools* in addition to monographs, reports and directories. See also JOURNALS IN THE FIELD OF DEAFNESS; Appendix II.

Americans with Disabilities Act   This law signed in 1990 guarantees a number of rights to all handicapped Americans in four important areas: employment, transportation, public services and telecommunications.

Specifically, the law applies to deaf people as follows:

- A deaf person cannot be denied a job if that person is qualified for the job. Businesses must make "reasonable accommodation" for deaf employees—including TDD (TELECOMMUNICATIONS DEVICE FOR THE DEAF) availability and interpreters.

- Medium- and large-sized hospitals, libraries, museums, hotels, restaurants, stores, parks and zoos must make interpreters and TDDs accessible for deaf patrons.

- By 1993, the United States must have developed a TDD relay system for all its deaf citizens, which will allow deaf people to call anyone anywhere at anytime.

- All public service announcements produced or funded by the federal government must be closed captioned. In hotels and hospitals, closed captioning must be made available on request in hotels with TVs in at least five rooms; all hospitals that provide TVs must provide access to closed captions.

A TDD relay system takes telephone calls in voice and transfers them to a TDD and vice versa. This new national relay system will give deaf people equal access via telephone to libraries, doctor's offices and so forth. In addition, the law provides that all emergency services must have TDD access. See also TELEVISION DECODER CIRCUITRY ACT OF 1990.

American Tinnitus Association This nonprofit group founded in 1971 provides education and information about TINNITUS to patients and professionals in addition to raising money for research.

Founded by Dr. Charles Unice, the organization offers a wide range of services, including information and a resource center, referral to a worldwide network of tinnitus clinics, local self-help groups and activities, professional workshops and seminars, counseling and guidelines for organizing tinnitus self-help groups and publishes a newsletter about tinnitus. See also Appendix II.

Ameslan See AMERICAN SIGN LANGUAGE.

amoxicillin This broad-spectrum penicillin is one of a group developed to treat bacteria and is frequently prescribed for the treatment of ear infections (OTITIS MEDIA.) Amoxicillin is also useful in treating infections caused by certain types of bacteria leading to cystitis, bronchitis, etc., and is sensitive to penicillinase, an enzyme that makes penicillin ineffective.

amplification See HEARING AIDS.

amplified hearing aid See HEARING AIDS.

amplified telephone See ASSISTIVE LISTENING DEVICES.

amplitude One of three measurements detecting the vibration of a sound wave (the other two are wavelength and frequency). Amplitude is the vertical vibration that reflects the intensity of sound.

ampulla The expanded end of the semicircular duct contained in each SEMICIRCULAR CANAL of the inner ear.

anacusia Term meaning total deafness. Also spelled *anakusis* or *anacusis*.

anacusis See ANACUSIA.

anoxia The complete loss of oxygen within a body tissue that can kill cells unless corrected very quickly. Anoxia is very rare, as opposed to hypoxia (reduced oxygen supply).

Anoxia and hypoxia are the most frequent causes of damage to the ORGAN OF CORTI (the body's hearing organ) during birth, since any disturbance of the infant's breathing or circulation can cause loss of oxygen in the blood.

Anoxia can result from long labor, heavy sedation of the mother, obstruction of the baby's respiratory passages with mucus, poor lung development or congenital circulatory or heart defects. The only treatment for anoxia is prevention of these conditions.

antibiotics and deafness Studies have shown that aminoglycoside antibiotics can harm hearing when treatment is continued for more than 10 days.

These antibiotics include amikacin, gentamicin, kanamycin, ribostamycin, tobramycin, netilmicin, dihydrostreptomycin, neomycin and streptomycin. Neomycin is considered the most toxic of all drugs to the cochlea, and damage may result in hearing loss that continues irreversibly after treatment is stopped. Warning signs may include tinnitus or impaired balance, but these symptoms do not always occur.

Other types of antibiotics, including erythromycin and viomycin, can also cause hearing loss. However, cases of erythromycin ototoxicity (hearing loss and tinnitus) can be reversed once the drug is discontinued. Only large doses (more than four grams per day) have been associated with erythromycin toxicity. Viomycin, on the other hand, can cause permanent hearing loss. See also OTOTOXIC DRUGS.

antitragus   A bump on the outer ear opposite the tragus (located in front of the ear canal). The antitragus projects cartilage in the outer ear near the opening of the ear canal.

anvil   The middle of the three bones in the MIDDLE EAR that transmit sound vibrations, also known as the incus. The body of the incus is tightly bound to the head of the malleus (hammer); as the eardrum membrane moves, these two OSSICLES move in and out as a unit. With moderate sound, the third bone of the ossicles (the stapes or stirrup) moves with them, and all three then vibrate as a single mass, transmitting the vibration across the middle ear to the fluid-filled inner ear, the ORGAN OF CORTI, through the neural pathway and on to the central nervous system and the brain.

aphasia   A disturbance in the ability to speak, write and/or comprehend and read, aphasia is caused by damage to the brain rather than by a problem with hearing or sight. Most often, head injury or a stroke in the dominant cerebral hemisphere—especially the Wernicke's and Broca's areas important for language—causes the brain damage that results in aphasia.

Some recovery can be expected following head injury or stroke with speech therapy. In general, the more severe the aphasia, the less chance for recovery.

Architectural and Transportation Barriers Compliance Board   This independent federal agency is responsible for enforcing the ARCHITECTURAL BARRIERS ACT of 1968, which prohibits architectural barriers to the handicapped in federally-funded buildings and public transportation systems. (These buildings cannot have barriers to people in wheelchairs or using crutches or who are blind or deaf. Buildings and transportation systems covered by this act must meet the minimum standards for accessibility established by the American National Standards Institute.)

Any person who believes there has been a violation of the act in a building built with federal funds can file a written complaint with the board describing the problem and giving the name and address of the building.

The board, which investigates every complaint it receives, first seeks voluntary compliance in a friendly, informal way if a violation is found. If no informal resolution is possible, the board's executive director may begin legal action by filing a citation before an administrative law judge, who then calls a hearing. (The person bringing the complaint does not need to appear at the hearing and will remain anonymous unless specific permission to reveal the name is given in writing.)

After the hearing the judge makes the final decision. If the judge's decision supports the board's findings, the judge may issue an order requiring correction of the problem within a specific amount of time.

The board also has a range of other responsibilities, including the development of advisory standards and provision of technical assistance to groups covered in the civil rights section of the Rehabilitation Act of 1973. See also LEGAL RIGHTS.

Architectural Barriers Act   Also known as Public Law 90–480, this 1968 law requires federally-funded buildings and public transportation systems to be accessible to handicapped persons. This law applies to those with vision and hearing problems in addition to those in wheelchairs or with other physical handicaps.

The act also sets minimum standards for the design and construction of buildings under the supervision of the General Services Administration, the Department of Housing and Urban Development, the Defense Department and the U.S. Postal Service. These four agencies issued joint standards (the Uniform Federal Accessibility Standards) that include specifications for visual warning alarms, a permanently installed or portable listening system for hard-of-hearing people and at least one volume control on public telephones.

In order to enforce the act, Congress created the ARCHITECTURAL AND TRANSPORTATION BARRIERS COMPLIANCE BOARD in its Rehabilitation Act of 1973 (section 502), giving the board power to conduct investigations and issue orders of compliance. Those who don't comply can face withholding of federal funds. See also LEGAL RIGHTS.

Aristotle (384 B.C.–324 B.C.) Ancient Greek philosopher who coined the term *deaf and dumb*. "Men that are deaf are in all cases also dumb," he wrote, "that is, they can make vocal sounds, but they cannot speak." Although Aristotle's use of the term *dumb* meant speechless, it came to take on other, more negative connotations (such as stupid or unable to comprehend). The negative connotations of this word have deeply influenced the rights of deaf people from Aristotle's time up to this day.

ASCII The language of most personal computers in the United States, this data code standard (the American Standard Code for Information Interchange) was adopted in 1968 by the federal government in response to the rapid growth of computers.

The code is composed of 128 characters, including the upper and lower case alphabet, numerals and many special characters. It is used by more than 20 million personal computers in the United States and is the accepted language for most data communications.

Although it is not the language of the TDD (TELECOMMUNICATIONS DEVICE FOR THE DEAF), some more modern TDD machines offer a combination of ASCII and the traditional BAUDOT CODE, allowing TDD users to communicate with personal computers over the telephone lines.

ASL Access A nonprofit organization providing videos about AMERICAN SIGN LANGUAGE to public libraries. The video topics include information about ASL, ASL literature, deaf history and informational videos in ASL. ASL Access encourages people to learn or improve ASL skills, to appreciate ASL literature, to provide information in ASL, and to produce ASL video recordings. ASL Access also tries to help libraries acquire ASL resources as a service to communities. See also Appendix II.

aspirin and deafness High doses of aspirin can cause TINNITUS and a hearing loss of up to 40 decibels—both directly related to the amount of the drug in the blood.

Although many drugs can be toxic to the delicate sensory tissue of the ear and can cause permanent hearing loss, aspirin is unusual in that the inner ear hearing loss it causes is reversible. Both hearing loss and tinnitus will disappear within one to three days after drug treatment is stopped. Normally, more than 12 aspirin tablets per day must be taken before there is a danger of hearing loss, although each person's sensitivity to the drug varies.

Patients with nerve deafness may also notice that aspirin will have a greater effect on hearing at lower frequencies.

Drugs containing quinine may also cause a similar, reversible hearing loss.

assistive listening devices Personal devices that can be used by hard-of-hearing people to improve their hearing and comprehension under a wide variety of circumstances. Hearing loss may interfere with daily communication on many occasions. A hearing aid usually helps, but some situations may still present a problem—it might be hard to hear in a noisy restaurant or in a business meeting where the speaker is at a distance from the listener. The telephone can present a special problem where even a hearing aid is not of help.

There are many assistive communication devices for people with hearing loss. Information about these devices can be obtained from an OTOLARYNGOLOGIST, AUDIOLOGIST or hearing aid dispenser.

There are many types of these devices, including those that offer input to the ear, extension microphones and telephone and television devices.

Input to the Ear

There are several ways that listening devices can provide sound directly to the ear.

Induction A magnetic field capable of transmitting sound can be generated by a coil connected to the sound source, transmitting sound to a specifically-equipped hearing aid. This coil can be a loop of wire strung around a room, worn around the neck, embedded in a small, flat plastic device hooked over the ear or placed in the receiver of a compatible telephone. A second coil that picks up this magnetic signal is built into many HEARING AIDS. Called a TELECOIL, it is activated by use of the "T-switch" on hearing aids.

One advantage of the T-mode is that the microphone in the hearing aid is usually turned off, so background noise does not interfere with the sound from the induction system. For hearing aids without a T-switch, special receivers are available that have a telecoil that picks up and amplifies the induced sound.

Direct audio input Direct audio input (DAI) makes it possible to transfer sound directly to the hearing aid, taking advantage of the hearing aid's amplification and eliminating through-the-air noise. With some aids, the DAI signal can be heard while in the T-mode, turning off the microphone and further eliminating background noise. The hearing aid must be equipped to accept a DAI attachment.

Earphone Earphones are generally used by people not yet fitted with a hearing aid or whose aid has neither a T-switch nor DAI capability.

Speaker For people with a mild hearing loss, a loudspeaker close to the ear is enough to improve comprehension.

Extension Microphones

The purpose of extension microphones is to extend the microphone closer to the sound source rather than rely solely on the microphone built into the hearing aid. Because microphone sensitivity drops rapidly with distance, an extension makes the signal stronger and tends to minimize background noise.

There are several types of extension microphones, including hard-wired, amplified and wireless.

Hard-wired This type of extension microphone consists solely of an additional microphone connected via cable and coupled to the hearing aid either by earphones, induction (neck loop or ear hook) or DAI. Most devices need an amplifier worn in the pocket, on the belt or held in the hand, but there are palm-sized models combining microphone with amplifier. Recent "super-directional" models have become available that make it possible to accurately pick up a voice 6 to 10 feet away if there is not too much background noise.

Amplified For people who need less amplification and don't wear a hearing aid, there are amplified microphones attached to a battery powered pocket/belt amplifier. The amplifier can be connected to the ear by an earphone or a built-in speaker held close to the ear. As with the hard-wired microphone, the amplified microphone cable can be as long as needed.

Wireless (Personal FM system) Considered the ultimate in extension microphones, this transmitter can broadcast 150 to 300 feet without connecting cables and can provide for another microphone in addition to the one built in. Receivers can use earphones, induction couplers or DAI but have no built-in speaker. Each unit is about the size of a cigarette package and can be useful in public auditoriums if the receiver frequency matches the one being broadcast. The transmitter can be connected directly to the sound source, such as a TV or a microphone; the sound is carried on a specific FM radio frequency through the air until it reaches an FM receiver tuned to the same frequency. The receiver changes the signal, and the electrical energy is sent to the ear through a headset or a hearing aid. If a hearing aid with a telecoil is used, it can connect to a necklace loop attached to the receiver.

FM systems can be very helpful for people with a profound hearing loss.

Telephone Devices

The telephone is often one of the biggest obstacles in communication for a deaf person because the sound is frequently distorted and visual cues are impossible.

The hearing aid telecoil was developed in America to take advantage of a defect in telephone design—the fact that the magnetic signal leaks and that leak can be picked up by a hearing aid equipped with a T-switch. In the United States, all telephones sold must be labeled "Hearing Aid Compatible," and all public phones, by law, must meet these requirements.

Minimizing feedback There are telephone attachments that minimize the feedback that occurs when the telephone receiver is held against a hearing aid. For a less expensive approach, a plastic-foam filled cap designed for telephone comfort can be slipped over the receiver instead. Using a T-switch on the hearing aid with a compatible phone will also eliminate feedback.

Amplifying handset An amplifying handset is available that features an amplifier built into the receiver, with a wheel for adjusting volume. Some models have another push button that gives additional volume as well. There is also a modular portable amplified handset that may be substituted for unamplified handsets of similar modular units when away from home.

Attachable portable amplifier There are two types of attachable portable amplifiers. One increases the audio signal from either a model that slips over the handset receiver or a small box-shaped model that plugs into the modular fitting at the base of the phone and amplifies the signal there. The second type slips over the receiver and converts the audio signal into a strong magnetic signal that is picked up by the T-switch of a hearing aid. There is also an attachable amplifier that combines both types.

TDD A TELECOMMUNICATIONS DEVICE FOR THE DEAF (TDD) is a visual typewriter connected to the telephone line by a modular plug or acoustic modem with the conversation appearing on a moving screen above the keyboard.

Television Devices

There are several ways to improve sound for the hard-of-hearing TV watcher.

Hard-wired If a listening jack is provided in the TV set, a hard-of-hearing person can simply plug in earphones.

Amplified A cable can be connected from the listening jack of the TV to the microphone jack of a portable amplifier, or an extension microphone can be mounted near the TV speaker if there is no listening jack available on the TV.

TV band radio A small portable radio that receives both UHF and VHF audio broadcasts of the TV, with usually better sound quality, can be placed nearby, the radio's speaker or its earphone can be used.

Audio induction loop For people with a T-switch-equipped hearing aid, this method will eliminate background noise. An amplifier that converts the TV audio signal to an induction signal is needed, and either a neckloop or a loop system around the wall or under the viewer's chair can be used. Loop and/or wire can be permanently installed, avoiding a cable stretched across the room.

Infrared light This method picks up the TV sound with a microphone and then transmits it by invisible infrared light (the same technique used for TV remote control units). A viewer wears a stethoscope or a clip-on receiver; sound is transmitted to the ear via either earphone, neckloop or DAI. See also ASSISTIVE LISTENING SYSTEMS.

assistive listening systems In a large room, a person with a hearing problem may have trouble understanding speech even when using the most powerful hearing aid. Background noise and vibration can compound hearing problems and interfere with a hearing aid's ability to pick up specific sound.

Because of this, large public meeting rooms, concert halls, auditoriums and churches are sometimes equipped with one of a number of different alternative listening device systems that help hard-of-hearing people. These include AM systems, FM systems, infrared systems and AUDIO LOOP SYSTEMS.

Association of Late-Deafened Adults This group serves as a resource and information center for late-deafened people and works to increase public awareness of the special needs of ADVENTITIOUS DEAFNESS. It offers a publication, *ALDA NEWS*. See also Appendix II.

atresia The absence or closing of the ear, which usually occurs during development of the fetal external ear, external ear canal or middle ear, and usually affects only one ear. It is an uncommon birth defect, occurring in one out of every 30,000 live births. Atresia of the external ear can follow burns, tumors, accidents and infections.

Surgery can repair the ear's appearance and restore hearing by creating a passage for sound to reach the inner ear. Complete external and middle ear atresia in one ear only usually causes a 60 decibel (dB) hearing loss for speech. Hearing loss after surgery depends on the severity of the ear's malformation, but 50 percent of the time there is generally at least a 20 dB improvement.

audiogram A graph produced as part of certain hearing tests, and used to represent at what level of loudness an individual can hear sounds of different frequencies.

The audiogram form is arranged so that octave and half-octave frequencies range across the top with the frequency increasing from left to right. The hearing level scale on the left side of an audiogram shows the strength of the test sound in decibels. See also AUDIOMETER; AUDIOLOGIST; AUDIOMETRY.

audiologist A licensed and/or certified professional trained to identify and measure hearing loss and rehabilitate those with hearing and speech problems.

Audiologists are trained to determine where hearing loss occurs. They also assess the effect of the hearing loss on the ability to communicate and offer hearing aid evaluation and orientation, auditory training, training in speechreading techniques and speech conservation and counseling. Audiologists are not physicians and thus cannot treat infections or other ear diseases.

Services

Audiologists work in a wide variety of settings, including universities, hospitals, schools, medical offices and private practice.

When employed by a university, audiologists may teach, supervise clinical practice and direct clinical services.

At medical centers, hospitals and rehabilitation agencies, audiologists test hearing, including the pre- and post-operative evaluation of otologic surgical patients. Referrals come from a wide variety of professionals, including OTOLARYNGOLOGISTS, neurologists, neurosurgeons, pediatricians, geriatricians, family doctors and internists. In hospitals with acute care pediatric nurseries, audiologists direct hearing screening programs for infants at risk for hearing problems. In addition, hospital audiologists often dispense hearing aids and, in veterans' hospitals, test and rehabilitate veterans with hearing problems.

Since most school districts require some type of hearing screening tests for students, audiologists serve as directors of these programs and work with teachers to help with special educational needs of students with hearing problems. In schools with special classes for students with hearing problems, audiologists equip and maintain classroom amplification systems.

Audiologists are also employed by private practice physicians (especially otolaryngologists) to test hearing, evaluate vestibular function and dispense hearing aids.

Recently, audiologists have begun branching out into private practice themselves, primarily to dispense hearing aids directly to clients with hearing problems. What separates them from traditional hearing aid commercial dealers is the in-depth professional rehabilitation program they can offer their customers.

Audiologists in private practice also work with industry to protect the hearing of employees in noisy environments, as required by the Occupational Safety and Health Act and the Workman's Compensation program.

Finally, community hearing and speech centers employ audiologists to work with adults and children as rehabilitation specialists to test hearing, select hearing aids and help improve speech and reading skills.

Tests

Audiologists use both formal and informal tests to determine a person's ability to hear and understand. Although these tests usually measure hearing abilities, the audiologist may also test skills at interpreting gestures and facial expressions.

The audiologist routinely tests three aspects of hearing: the degree of hearing ability, the kind of hearing loss (if any) and the ability to understand speech under different conditions. See also AUDIOMETRY.

Training

An audiologist needs a bachelor's degree in speech-language pathology or a related field, a master's degree in audiology and a certificate of clinical competence in order to practice independently. Some states also require a license.

The certificate of clinical competence is widely acknowledged as evidence that the person is able to give independent audiologic services to children and adults with hearing problems. This standards program was set up by the American Speech-Language-Hearing Association (ASHA) in 1952, and certification standards are set by the Council on Professional Standards in Speech-Language Pathology and Audiology. Their certification is "CCC-A" (Certificate of Clinical Competence) from the American Speech-Language-Hearing Association.

In order to take the certification exam, audiologists must have completed a master's degree and a minimum number of credits covering both the normal and disordered processes of hearing, speech and language. In addition, an applicant must have completed at least 300 hours of supervised clinical experience within the academic program, at least half of which is at the graduate level, followed by nine months of full-time professional experience under the supervision of a certified audiologist.

In order to attain certification, the applicant must then pass the National Examination in Audiology, a written test covering basic auditory sciences and clinical issues. Audiologists are not required to be active members in ASHA in order to be certified. Dispensing audiologists are usually more trained than a "hearing aid dispenser," who is licensed by the state but who has no college degree.

audiology   The study of the entire field of hearing, including the nature and conservation of hearing, identification and assessment of hearing loss and the rehabilitation of all those with hearing impairments.

Within the field, there are specialities of diagnostic work, rehabilitation, research and teaching. See also AUDIOLOGIST; AUDIOMETRY.

audio loop   A loop of cable (also called an induction coil) through which electricity passes, creating an electromagnetic field that can be converted into audible sounds by someone wearing a hearing aid equipped with a special device called a TELECOIL or T-coil. The loop can be worn around the neck or—as in part of an AUDIO LOOP SYSTEM—placed around the room, under the carpet and so forth. See also ASSISTIVE LISTENING DEVICES; ALTERNATIVE LISTENING SYSTEMS.

audio loop system   In a large room, a person with a hearing problem may have trouble hearing even with the most powerful hearing aid. Back-ground noise can compound hearing problems and interfere with a hearing aid's ability to pick up sound. To alleviate this problem, large public meeting rooms can be equipped with an audio loop system that utilizes a loop of wire placed around an entire room, a microphone and an amplifier. The electric current flowing through the loop creates an electromagnetic field that can be picked up by anyone wearing a special hearing aid sitting near or within the loop. Portable receivers are available for people without the special hearing aids.

The system's microphone picks up sound and changes it into electrical energy that is then amplified and sent through the coil of a wire (known as an induction loop) strung around a room. The electrical energy flowing through the wire coil creates a magnetic field that can be picked up by a hearing aid containing a very small coil of wire called a TELECOIL, or T-coil.

The telecoil is activated by the T-switch and acts as an antenna that picks up the electromagnetic energy and delivers it to the hearing aid's receiver, where the energy is converted to sound.

An induction loop may be connected to a microphone or plugged directly into a TV or stereo jack. It can be coiled around a room, desk or chair or can be worn around the neck or in the ear (as a silhouette inductor). But a hearing aid cannot be used with a loop system unless it also contains an electromagnetic device (the telecoil). See also ASSISTIVE LISTENING DEVICES; ALTERNATIVE LISTENING SYSTEMS.

audiometer   An electronic device used to test hearing that produces simplified PURE TONES or speech of a defined intensity and frequency. The audiometer includes a signal generator, an amplifier, an attenuator (which controls and specifies the intensity of sounds) and an earphone.

The hearing in one ear is measured over the full range of normally audible sounds, usually ranging up to 100 DECIBELS (dB) in steps of five. The 0 dB level represents normal hearing for young adults in favorable laboratory conditions.

There are several types and classes of electric audiometers, divided into two main types: pure tone and speech. A single instrument may be designed to serve both functions.

Pure Tone Audiometers

These devices provide pure tones of selected frequencies and of calibrated sound-pressure levels, including wide range (which cover most of the human auditory range in frequency and sound pressure level) and must include the means for AIR CONDUCTION and BONE CONDUCTION tests and masking. A limited-range pure tone audiometer offers a more restricted range of frequency or sound pressure level, and may only allow air conduction tests. A narrow-range audiometer offers limited range of frequency and sound pressure levels. Audiometers vary in scope from limited to wide range.

Speech Audiometers

A speech audiometer provides spoken syllables, words or sentences at known sound-pressure levels. It can be a separate unit but more often is a function included on diagnostic audiometers.

Automatic Audiometers

These units provide both interrupted and continuous stimuli and may be operated by the client. The Békésy audiometer is a classic example of an automatic audiometer. They have largely been replaced by electrophysiologic testing.

Immitance Equipment

Tests with this device include tympanometry, static measurements, acoustic reflex threshold determination and acoustic reflex decay. See also AUDIOMETRY.

audiometric zero   The zero reference setting for the tone-intensity control at each selected frequency on a pure-tone audiometer. The tone intensity at zero is assumed to represent the average normal hearing threshold at each frequency used for testing. See also AUDIOGRAM; AUDIOMETER; AUDIOMETRY.

audiometrist   A person without a degree in AUDIOLOGY who has been given informal training in the administration of hearing tests. An audiometrist must work under the supervision of an audiologist or a physician, and can neither diagnose hearing disorders nor interpret AUDIOGRAMS. See also AUDIOMETRY.

audiometry   Measurement of a person's ability to hear through the use of hearing tests that provide accurate and quantitative results. Tests can determine if a HEARING LOSS exists, the amount and nature of the hearing loss and can yield some indication of the benefits that are possible through available treatment.

Basically, hearing tests measure sensitivity (the level at which a person can first detect sound) and DISCRIMINATION. A person's hearing loss is measured in DECIBELS (dB); however, two people with the same decibel loss may actually perceive speech quite differently, depending on the amount of structural damage to the ear and the age at onset of hearing loss.

Many methods have been used in the past to measure hearing, including monochords, whispered voice, watch ticks and whistles. Today, there are five basic types of hearing tests: screening or identification audiometry, routine diagnostic audiometry, acoustic-immitance audiometry, special audiometric tests and electrophysiologic tests.

Screening or Identification Audiometry

Used to measure hearing of large groups, such as schools or industry, the audiologist can use a screening test to rapidly sift through the majority of hearing clients to identify the few with hearing loss. These tests are for detection of loss, not for description nor quantification. The most common is the pure tone sweep check tests.

Every child should have a hearing test as part of a school screening during the first two years of school and routinely throughout the school years, according to the Better Hearing Institute. The institute also recommends that every adult who is regularly exposed to high noise levels should have a hearing test at least once a year.

Routine diagnostic audiometry includes both air and bone conduction tests.

Pure Tone Air Conduction

Air conduction refers to the process by which stimuli travels through air to the ear's conductive mechanism, which stimulates sensory endings of the eighth cranial nerve. This test evaluates how softly a client can hear across the spectrum of frequencies and measures the threshold of sound detection—the lowest hearing level at which the client responds correctly to pure tones 50 percent of the time.

Pure Tone Bone Conduction

Bone conduction is the process by which sound vibrates the skull and thus the cochlear mechanism, bypassing the conductive apparatus of the ear. This test is designed to bypass the air conduction pathway and stimulate the cochlea. It also provides data on sensorineural mechanisms and the cochlear system.

The air bone gap (the difference between the thresholds measured by air and bone conduction) are attributed to pathological states in the outer or middle ears. Patients whose bone conduction results are normal or near normal and who have significant hearing loss by air conduction tests may be candidates for surgical or medical treatment.

Pure tone bone and air conduction tests measure hearing through the use of pure tones (a single frequency) by sending a tone through earphones to one ear at a time. The decibel loudness when these sounds can first be heard is the pure tone hearing threshold (or hearing level) for that frequency. People with normal hearing will usually hear each pure tone frequency at the zero point or close to it; people with a hearing loss will only hear pure tones much louder than zero.

Pure tones are usually in octave or half-octave steps, and cover the frequencies between 250 and 8,000 hertz (Hz). Because speech falls within this range, it is possible (in a limited fashion) to measure a person's ability to hear a conversation by testing with pure tones. The disadvantage of testing hearing with pure tones is that the sounds heard every day are not pure tones, but complex ones.

With the electronic AUDIOMETER, it is possible to measure a person's threshold of hearing for a series of pure tones at 11 different frequency points, starting at 125 cycles per second and ending at 8,000. This includes the three octaves between 500 and 4,000 Hz that are most important for speech. Audiograms test hearing at most of these 11 points.

When there is a large difference between the hearing thresholds of two ears, the AUDIOLOGIST will mask the better ear to prevent it from responding and giving a false reading while the poorer ear is tested. The better ear is masked by presenting a band of noise through the earphone at about the same frequency as the one being tested.

In addition to air and bone conduction tests, there are a number of special audiometric measures.

Speech Audiometry

Pure tone thresholds tell the nature and extent of the hearing loss, but don't reveal the extent of communication problems. In addition to pure tone tests, a hearing evaluation often includes some measurement of a person's sensitivity to speech (or the lowest level at which speech is heard). In speech audiometry, the clinician gives verbal messages (live or taped) through earphones or loudspeakers to determine the lowest level the client can hear two-syllable words (spondees) well enough to repeat them (the speech reception threshold) and how clearly the client can discriminate one-syllable words while listening at a comfortable level (speech discrimination, or word recognition). The speech discrimination test determines the person's ability to understand important sounds (primarily consonants) and measures how well a person can discriminate speech at intensities 30 to 40 decibels (dB) above the speech reception threshold. (See chart on interpretation of discrimination scores, page 24.)

Speech audiometry results are important because patients with hearing loss in one ear with poor discrimination at high loudness levels may require additional audiometric or X-ray studies to rule out possibility of a tumor on the hearing nerve. Secondly, speech discrimination results may be beneficial in predicting the extent to which a person with sensorineural hearing loss will benefit from a hearing aid.

Acoustic-Immitance Tests

Immitance tests measure the response of the eardrum, ossicles and small muscles attached to the ossicles. Immitance is a measure of how easy it is to transfer sound energy from the external ear through the middle ear to the COCHLEA.

The measure of ACOUSTIC IMMITANCE can be defined as either acoustic admittance or acoustic impedance. "Admittance" refers to how easily energy flows through a system, while "impedance" represents the opposition to the flow of energy. A system with high acoustic impedance to the flow of sound will have low acoustic admittance, and vice versa. The most common acoustic-immitance test is the tympanogram, a measure of eardrum stiffness as a function of air pressure change. It can determine with a good degree of accuracy whether there is fluid behind the eardrum or whether air pressure condition in the middle ear is abnormal.

Another acoustic-immitance test is the acoustic reflex test, which is helpful in testing young children. This tests measures the reflex contraction of muscle in the middle ear.

Acoustic immitance tests are used as an adjunct to hearing tests, since a patient may have a significant ear disease with little hearing loss. While most hearing tests can uncover type and degree of hearing loss, they may not reveal specific ear diseases. Unlike most hearing tests, acoustic-immitance can reveal middle ear disorders without requiring any active participation by the patient. This is particularly helpful in the testing of young children.

Special Audiometric Tests

These determine whether a sensorineural loss is located in nerve endings in the inner ear or hearing nerve. They include tone decay tests, the short increment sensitivity index (SISI), loudness balance tests and Békésy audiometry. These have largely been replaced by electrophysiologic tests.

Electrophysical Tests

Other tests that do not require the client to give a conscious response include electrophysical tests: electroencephalic (EEG) audiometry and evoked response audiometry. For the very young, hearing thresholds for pure tones can be deciphered from these electrophysical methods.

The electroencephalogram is a graphed representation of the electrical activity of the brain but is not widely used. With this method, a click causes a small variation in the electrical potentials recorded by the EEG. Through the aid of a computer and repeated presentation of clicks, the child's auditory threshold can be determined. Although very closely matching findings from conventional audiometry,

INTERPRETATION OF DISCRIMINATION SCORES

Discrimination Score	Interpretation
90–100 percent	Excellent understanding of speech
80–88 percent	Good understanding of speech
70–78 percent	Fair understanding of speech
60–68 percent	Poor understanding of speech
0–58 percent	Marked reduced understanding of speech

the EEG readings cannot pinpoint the site of any hearing problem.

As nerve impulses pass through the lower levels of the brain from the auditory nerve on their way to higher brain centers, they make connections in the brainstem near the base of the skull. The most widely used electrophysiologic test is the AUDITORY BRAINSTEM RESPONSE TEST (ABR), which measures this electrical activity in the brainstem to see how well certain portions of the auditory system in the brain respond to a presented stimulus.

This noninvasive test is useful for the detection of hearing loss in newborns and infants, for the medical diagnosis of auditory disorders (including tumors) and for confirming nonorganic hearing loss. The ABR can be performed on individuals of any age—even the youngest infant.

In the test, clicks or tone pips are fed into the ear and a computer analyzes the results to see if the brain activity changes. Rather than a true test of the entire process of hearing, the ABR determines whether auditory signals are reaching the brain. Development of new stimulus delivery systems and recording electrodes now permit the use of ABR for intraoperative monitoring and monitoring patients with head injuries.

Another type of electrophysical test is the ELECTROCOCHLEOGRAM, which measures impulses in the cochlear nerve by inserting a thin electrode through the eardrum into the promontory of the basal turn. This indicates how well the cochlea is functioning.

Who Tests Hearing?

Although general practitioners or pediatricians may test hearing in the office, these simple tests can give only crude, unreliable results. Much better results can be expected from two kinds of experts on hearing who cooperate on diagnoses and treatment: the AUDIOLOGIST and the OTOLOGIST.

The audiologist is a nonmedical professional with a master's or doctorate in audiology who is trained to evaluate hearing and knowledgeable about types of hearing loss and their management.

The otologist is a surgeon specializing in the diagnosis and treatment of diseases of the ear. Otologists may make their own audiograms or rely on an audiologist's findings. While speech pathologists may also have qualifications in audiology and may be very helpful with deaf children's speech, not all are experts in deafness.

In addition, a nonaudiometric test is sometimes used as a very basic way to test hearing. The most common of these are the tuning fork tests (WEBER, SCHWABACH and RINNE).

auditory adaptation   A perceived decline in loudness of a sustained acoustic signal commonly found in people with lesions of the cochlea or auditory (eighth cranial) nerve. People with normal hearing, when presented with the same sustained signal, experience no "tone decay" or decrease in loudness over time.

It is also possible to differentiate between lesions of the cochlea and the auditory nerve, since auditory nerve lesions cause a more rapid and extensive tone decay.

Auditory adaptation is measured by Békésy AUDIOMETRY or conventional tone-decay tests.

auditory agnosia   A defect, loss or failure in development of the ability to comprehend spoken words caused by disease, injury or malformation of the hearing centers of the brain. A person with auditory agnosia may or may not respond to an audiometric test or may give very different results at different times.

auditory analgesia   The control of pain by listening to music or WHITE NOISE through earphones, with the volume under control by the patient.

Because most subjects become less sensitive or insensitive to certain kinds of pain when listening to very loud noise or music, auditory analgesia is sometimes used in dental and obstetrical situations.

auditory aphasia   See AUDITORY AGNOSIA.

auditory brainstem response test (ABR)   As nerve impulses pass through the lower levels of the brain from the auditory nerve on their way to higher brain centers, they make connections in the brainstem near the base of the skull. The ABR measures this electrical activity in the brainstem and can determine how well certain portions of the auditory system in the brain respond to a presented stimulus.

This noninvasive test is useful for the detection of hearing loss in newborns and infants, for the medical diagnosis of auditory disorders and for confirming nonorganic hearing loss. The ABR can be performed on individuals of any age, even the youngest infant.

In the test, a brief tone causes a small variation in the electrical potentials that can be recorded from the scalp. Clicks or tone pips are fed into the ear, and a computer analyzes the results to see if the brain activity changes. Rather than a true test of the entire process of hearing, the ABR determines whether auditory signals are reaching the brain.

By repeating the stimulus up to 100 times and averaging the response by computer, the responses can be enhanced while eliminating random background electrical activity. This way, auditory thresholds can be established that are quite close to those that can be obtained in conventional AUDIOMETRY.

Development of new stimulus delivery systems and recording electrodes now permit the use of ABR for intraoperative monitoring and monitoring patients with head injuries.

auditory discrimination   The ability to discriminate one speech sound from another.

auditory evoked potentials   Slight electrical signals in the brain that have a characteristic pattern and occur in response to repetitions of identical sounds. The characteristic pattern, or wave form, indicates that the brain has responded to the test sound and, therefore, the sound must have been heard by the client. Tests of auditory evoked potentials are useful in those who cannot participate in hearing tests, such as the very young or the retarded. See also AUDIOMETRY; AUDITORY BRAINSTEM RESPONSE TEST.

auditory feedback   The ability to hear one's own speech, in which the output is fed back to the ear, producing a self-monitoring regulation of speech.

auditory-global method   See AUDITORY-ORAL METHOD.

auditory nerve   The part of the vestibulocochlear nerve (the eighth cranial nerve) concerned with the sense of hearing; also called the acoustic nerve or hearing nerve.

auditory nerve tumor   This type of tumor, located along the eighth cranial nerve, can cause hearing loss on the affected side and is usually slow-growing and benign. Although several types of tumors can grow on the auditory nerve, the most common is an acoustic neuroma (also called a neurinoma or Schwannoma). The cause of these tumors is unknown, except for the few that are associated with neurofibromatosis, a hereditary neurologic disorder.

Untreated, the acoustic nerve tumor first distorts the eighth cranial nerve and then, as it grows larger, presses on the seventh cranial nerve next to it. Eventually it can grow so large it protrudes from the canal into the brain behind the mastoid bone and, if untreated, can eventually cause death.

There are no typical symptoms, but people who have inner ear problems should be evaluated to eliminate the possibility of an acoustic neuroma. Most people with these tumors have hearing problems in one ear together with ear noise or tinnitus and sometimes have balance problems as well. Auditory, balance and hearing tests (including a brainstem auditory evoked response test and a CAT [computerized axial tomography] scan) can be used to diagnose the acoustic tumor.

Although the surgical removal of these tumors is complex and delicate, few patients die from the surgery because of modern technology and early detection. Still, long-term eye problems affect at least half of those who have had an acoustic neuroma removed, in addition to possible taste distur-

bances, problems with voice or swallowing and—if the facial nerve has been injured or removed during surgery—some degree of facial paralysis.

With small tumors, it may be possible to save what is left of the patient's hearing, but medium or large tumors have usually destroyed hearing, and this cannot be restored through surgery. The particular hearing problems common to people who have had acoustic neuromas include locating the direction of sound, hearing a person speaking softly and understanding speech in a noisy environment.

auditory neuritis   Inflammation of the auditory nerve that can follow scarlet fever or typhoid fever or other infections with high fevers. Hearing loss may be noted immediately, although deafness usually progresses over several days or weeks.

The insidious development of neuritis can cause sensorineural deafness very similar to PRESBYCUSIS but it occurs much earlier in life and is usually attributed to lack of oxygen, anemia, nonspecific viruses and LABYRINTHITIS (inflammation of the fluid-filled chambers of the inner ear).

auditory-oral method   A method of teaching speech to deaf and hard-of-hearing children. Proponents believe that using residual hearing is the most efficient way to develop speech. Therefore, children are encouraged to perceive speech of others through audition alone. This method is also referred to as acoupedic, aural-oral, auditory approach, unisensory-auditory and auditory-global. See also MULTISENSORY TEACHING APPROACH; SPEECH TRAINING.

auditory perception   The mental awareness of sound.

auditory rehabilitation   A variety of modern techniques are available to help people with HEARING LOSS. These include specialized programs for deaf children; customized personal HEARING AIDS; help for specific situations through the use of ASSISTIVE LISTENING DEVICES for telephone communication, television and group listening; COCHLEAR IMPLANTS; tinnitus maskers; tactile aids and alerting devices, and counseling (when necessary). See also AUDITORY TRAINING.

auditory training The process of teaching a person with a hearing loss to take full advantage of any sound cues that can still be heard. Like SPEECHREADING, auditory training can help people with hearing losses become aware of cues they might not notice otherwise. The form of auditory training used depends on when the person lost hearing and the type of hearing loss.

Auditory training helps children born deaf learn how to understand the weak or distorted sounds they can still hear; it can also help people with acquired hearing loss learn to pay attention to the act of listening and to separate background noise from speech. It also helps those with HEARING AIDS adjust to the task of using the device.

A person's need for auditory training depends on the ability to understand speech with or without a hearing aid. Often, auditory training is combined with speechreading training in a total AUDITORY REHABILITATION program.

aural Pertaining to the sensation of hearing or to the ear itself.

aural-oral method See AUDITORY-ORAL METHOD.

auricle See OUTER EAR.

Australia As many as as 1.7 million Australians have some degree of hearing loss. About 0.1 percent of the population is profoundly deaf. Most of these deaf or hard-of-hearing Australians are elderly and began to lose their hearing after finishing school. Only about 40,000 were born with hearing problems or lost hearing early in life. In addition, conductive hearing loss is particularly high among the aborigines, since most native Australian children have chronic suppurative OTITIS MEDIA. Australia has the lowest prevalence rate of deafness among those developed countries for which statistics were available.

Education

Because the educational system in Australia is administered at the state level, most families with children who cannot hear have access to some guidance and counseling during the child's early years. All states have a kindergarten/preschool service for children with hearing problems, generally with large centers in cities and satellite programs in rural areas. The preschools are usually special schools for deaf students, but children may also attend regular preschools if they wish.

As deaf children enter elementary school, services become more fragmented from state to state, although most states do have elementary day schools for deaf students. (When deaf education began in Australia at the end of the 19th century, there were large state residential schools, but by the end of World War II their enrollment dropped; today most deaf students commute to special schools.)

At the high school level, deaf students are generally taught academic subjects by elementary teachers; secondary teachers trained in deafness generally teach vocational studies. Because of the differing pattern of services among states, the educational level of deaf students in Australia ranges from superior to below normal.

There are no specialist higher-education services for Australians. Although deaf high school graduates have the ability to go on to universities, very few do so.

Communication

Because most deaf people in Australia lose their hearing late in life, they rely on HEARING AIDS and SPEECHREADING to communicate. Most schools and services supplement their oral-aural curriculum with a manual system, which is usually a mixture of signs, FINGERSPELLING and SIGNED ENGLISH. Occasionally, cued speech is used.

AUSTRALIAN SIGN LANGUAGE is a direct descendant of BRITISH SIGN LANGUAGE, introduced by the founders of two large state schools for deaf students. Although Catholic schools for deaf students at first used Irish Sign Language, today these Catholic schools rely on the oral method and use cued speech. There are few people left in Australia who use Irish-Australian Sign Language.

Because Australian Sign Language, like all sign languages, has a grammar alien to English, Australian educators believed it was less useful in schools and have tried to employ Signed English by adding various fingerspelled markers for grammar (tense, plurals and so forth) to Australian Sign Language. Australian aborigines developed an extended communication sign system of their own, and this is now used with deaf aboriginal children.

The National Acoustic Laboratories provide free hearing aids to all military personnel, senior citizens and Australians under age 21 (which allows most school-age children with hearing problems to be properly fitted with hearing aids). The labs are the second-largest provider of hearing aids in the world, and were founded in 1948 to produce hearing aids for the deafened veterans of World War II and children deafened by the rubella outbreaks in the early 1940s.

Organizations for the deaf include the Australian Association of Teachers of the Deaf, the Association of Welfare Workers with the Deaf and the Federation of Australian Deaf Societies.

Australian Sign Language   The sign language used by most deaf Australians incorporates the British two-handed system together with some use of the Irish and American one-handed alphabets.

The British two-handed system was brought to Australia in 1860 when the first two schools for deaf students were established; subsequent Irish Catholic schools introduced IRISH SIGN LANGUAGE.

A *Dictionary of Australasian Signs* was published in 1982 and includes the signs used in Australian schools in English word order.

autocuer   This assistive device is a speech processor that breaks units of speech down into cues. These cues are activated by tiny light-emitting diodes, which show up in digital form on special eyeglasses worn by the deaf person. As with CUED SPEECH, that person will have to read the lips of the speaker as well as the cues on the eyeglasses in order to get the whole message. Cues and lips can be lined up and read at the same time by moving the head. The equipment consists of the eyeglasses and a small boxlike speech processing microcomputer.

The autocuer was invented by Dr. ORIN CORNETT (the inventor of cued speech) and was developed by Dr. Cornett, Dr. Robert Beadles and a team of researchers in the North Carolina Research Triangle Institute's Center for Biomedical Engineering.

autoimmune inner ear disease (AIED)   This syndrome causes progressive hearing loss and/or dizziness triggered by immune cells that attack the inner ear. Usual symptoms include a relatively rapid reduction of hearing accompanied by TINNITUS (ringing in the ears), which occurs over a few months. Alternatively, there may be attacks of hearing loss and tinnitus that resemble MÉNIÈRE'S DISEASE and attacks of dizziness accompanied by abnormal blood tests for antibodies. About half of the patients with AIED also have balance symptoms.

Causes

The immune system is complex, and there are several ways that it can damage the inner ear. Several well-known autoimmune diseases such as systemic lupus erythematosis (SLE), Sjögren's syndrome (dry eye syndrome), COGAN'S DISEASE, ulcerative colitis, Wegener's granulomatosis, rheumatoid arthritis and scleroderma can cause or be associated with AIED. Still, AIED is rare and probably accounts for less than 1 percent of all cases of hearing impairment or dizziness. About 16 percent of patients with bilateral Ménière's disease and 6 percent of persons with Ménière's disease of any variety may be affected by immune dysfunction.

There are several ways that a person's immune system could begin to attack the cells of the inner ear. In one theory, damage to the inner ear triggers substances that provoke additional immune reactions. (This theory might explain the attack/remission cycle of disorders such as Ménière's disease). In the most commonly believed theory, antibodies or rogue T-cells could cause accidental inner ear damage because the ear shares common antigens with a potentially harmful substance, virus or bacteria that the body is fighting against. This is the favored theory of AIED.

There is increasing evidence that genetically controlled aspects of the immune system may boost susceptibility to common hearing disorders such as Ménière's disease. There is also evidence for a genetic vulnerability to ototoxic drugs such as gentamicin.

Diagnosis

The diagnosis of AIED is based on careful review of the patient's family history, findings on physical exam, blood tests and the results of hearing and vestibular tests.

Treatment

Treatment for patients with a classic rapidly progressive bilateral hearing impairment may include steroids (such as prednisone) for four weeks. In most patients who respond to steroids, a chemotherapy drug such as cytoxan or methotrexate can be used over the long term.

automatic audiometry   Hearing tests in which the audiometers are operated by the patient. See also BÉKÉSY AUDIOMETER.

bacterial labyrinthitis   See LABYRINTHITIS.

bacterial meningitis   See MENINGITIS; POSTNATAL CAUSES OF HEARING LOSS.

barotitis   See AERO-OTITIS MEDIA.

barotrauma   See AERO-OTITIS MEDIA.

Barry five slate system   A printed system to help deaf children learn to speak, read and write syntactically correct sentences.

Devised in 1899 by Katherine Barry, this system is similar to the five sentence parts system of Abbé Roch-Ambroise Cucurron Sicard. Barry's method utilized five large slates, each with one column, to help children categorize the parts of speech in sentences. Each slate contained one part of speech: subject, verb, object of the verb, preposition and object of the preposition.

basilar membrane   A flexible membrane that is attached to the bony shelf and divides the coil of the COCHLEA lengthwise into two compartments. On one side of the membrane is the PERILYMPH fluid of the SCALA TYMPANI; on the other side is the ORGAN OF CORTI. As sound vibrations disturb the perilymph fluid, they are transferred through the basilar membrane to the organ of Corti and on to the hair cells inside.

battery hearing aid   See HEARING AIDS.

Baudot code   A code invented by Emile Baudot in 1874 that recognizes 32 characters—the capital letters of the alphabet and six other characters. The Baudot code was chosen in the early 1900s as the language of the teletype (TTY) machines by inventor ROBERT H. WEITBRECHT, and the TDD (TELECOMMUNICATIONS DEVICE FOR THE DEAF) network is based on the language of the Baudot code.

A person with a TDD that uses Baudot code cannot communicate over the phone lines with a personal computer (which uses ASCII) since the TDD and the computer "speak" different languages.

However, it is now possible to buy a TDD with both Baudot and ASCII capability. A TDD user transmitting or sending over the ASCII code can process information about five times faster than when using the Baudot code; this speedier ASCII rate is called 300 Baud.

The ASCII capability feature on a TDD also allows the user to have access to many personal computer bulletin boards. While the number of these bulletin boards are constantly changing, estimates range from 1,500 to 5,000. See also ELECTRONIC MAIL.

Beethoven, Ludwig van (1770–1827)   A German musical genius widely regarded as one of the greatest composers who ever lived, Beethoven's life was marked by a heroic struggle against encroaching deafness. Some of his most important works were composed during the last 10 years of his life, when he was completely unable to hear.

During the first part of his life, his art stayed within the bounds of 18th-century technique. However, he experienced a change in direction as he gradually realized he was becoming deaf. The first symptoms appeared in 1800 before he was 30, and by 1802, when he could no longer deny that his hearing disorder was both permanent and progressive, he considered suicide. "But only Art held back," he wrote, "for it seemed unthinkable for me to leave the world forever before I had produced all that I felt called upon to produce."

As his hearing became worse, his piano playing degenerated, although he continued to appear in public from time to time. By 1819 he was totally deaf, and friends communicated to him using "conversation books" in which they wrote down questions and he replied orally.

By 1824, Beethoven finished his last large-scale work—the Ninth Symphony—with the aid of a type of audiophone. Holding a "sound stick" in his teeth with one end touching the piano, Beethoven would feel sound vibrations traveling through the stick to his teeth, the bones of his skull and into his inner ear.

At the end of the premiere of the Ninth Symphony, Beethoven, as conductor, stood alone in front of his orchestra. Totally deafened, he was unable to hear the thunderous applause and stood unaware until one of the soloists made him turn to face the audience.

Beginnings for Parents of Children Who Are Deaf or Hard-of-Hearing   A nonprofit agency established to provide emotional support and objective information to parents of deaf and hard-of-hearing children. The mission of the organization is to help parents be informed so that they can be knowledgeable decision makers. Beginnings can help parents work with schools to get appropriate services for a child, give information on assistive listening devices and provide referrals to other organizations. See also Appendix II.

behind-the-ear hearing aids   These devices include a microphone, amplifier and receiver inside a small curved case worn behind the ear and connected to the EARMOLD by a short plastic tube. It can help all but the most severe hearing loss. Batteries are located in the base of the aid.

Some models have a tone control, volume control and telephone pickup device (T-switch), although all types of aids will amplify speech from the phone if the phone receiver is brought close enough to the hearing aid's microphone. See also HEARING AIDS; TELECOIL.

Békésy, Georg von (1899–1972)   The inventor of the modern theory of BASILAR MEMBRANE resonance,

this Hungarian-born communications engineer wanted to understand the difference between the quality of the human ear and the telephone system. While director of the Hungarian Telephone System Research Laboratory, he studied long-distance communication problems and became interested in the human hearing mechanism.

He studied the inner ear by building mechanical models of the COCHLEA. From this work, he developed his traveling-wave theory, which describes how a sound impulse sends a wave sweeping along the basilar membrane, increasing its amplitude until it reaches a maximum when it falls off sharply until the wave dies out. The point of greatest amplitude is the point at which the frequency of the sound is detected by the ear. He developed highly sensitive instruments that made it possible to understand the hearing process, differentiate between types of deafness and choose proper treatment.

Von Békésy also found that high-frequency tones were perceived near the base (or entrance) of the cochlea and lower frequencies toward its end. He also discovered that location of nerve receptors are most important in determining pitch and loudness. For this theory, Békésy received the Nobel Prize in physiology and medicine in 1961. See also BÉKÉSY AUDIOMETER.

Békésy audiometer   An instrument developed by GEORG VON BÉKÉSY in 1947 to provide automatic AUDIOMETRY. This device automatically tracks auditory thresholds for tones on a moving chart.

With the Békésy audiometer, the client makes his own audiogram tracing by pressing a button as long as he can hear a pure tone given during a hearing test. As the button is pushed (threshold response), the tone automatically decreases in intensity. When the button is released, the sound gradually increases again until the patient taps the button to indicate that he can again hear it. As the frequency is slowly increased, a graphic recording is made that produces a complete AUDIOGRAM in less than 10 minutes.

Auditory thresholds for pulsed and sustained tones are recorded, and the audiograms are evaluated on the basis of the separation between threshold tracings for pulsed and sustained tones. This procedure is basically a test for auditory adaptation for the sustained tone since most people, both deaf and with normal hearing, show adaptation for pulsed tones.

In a sweep-frequency Békésy audiometer, thresholds can be charted as a function of frequency; a fixed-frequency Békésy audiometer charts thresholds as a function time at a given frequency. See also BÉKÉSY AUDIOMETRIC TEST.

Békésy audiometric test   A special hearing test that is given to older children and that can sometimes detect certain types of hearing problems of the inner ear and of the hearing nerve beyond the inner ear.

With the Békésy automatic recording audiometer, the patient controls the level of the tone by pressing a button as long as he can hear the tone. As the button is pushed, the tone automatically decreases in intensity. When the button is released, the sound gradually increases again until the patient taps the button to indicate that he can again hear it.

As the frequency is slowly increased, a graphic recording is made that provides a complete AUDIOGRAM in less than 10 minutes. See also AUDIOMETRY; BÉKÉSY, GEORG VON; BÉKÉSY AUDIOMETER.

Belgian Sign Language (BSL)   The sign language of BELGIUM includes many regional dialects. Although the country has two official languages (Dutch in the north and French in the south), sign languages in these two areas are quite similar, possibly because the deaf schools in Brussels have included students from both sections of the country.

Belgian Sign Language began in schools for deaf students and was based on signs from the old FRENCH SIGN LANGUAGE. Although this country has been traditionally oralist, support for BSL and both the manual codes of Signed Dutch/Signed French (used in communicating between deaf and hearing people) has been growing.

Belgium   The deaf population in Belgium reflects the deep communication divisions between the Flemish and French-speaking natives. The provision of services for deaf Belgians, therefore, depends on the difference between the two groups.

The total number of deaf students in the country is about 610,000. Because early diagnosis is stressed in Belgium, most deaf children are diagnosed by the age of one. It is one of the few countries in which deafness rates are declining.

Education/Communication

For many years, as in most of Europe, Belgian teachers stressed the oral method of education. Manual communication, although not repressed, was not encouraged. Gradually, Belgian educators have decided that an exclusively oral education does not benefit all students; now many promote a combination of oral and manual communication in order to acquire a command of spoken language.

Cued speech is very popular, as is a Belgian invention called AKA (alphabet of assisted kinemes, or lip movements), which is used to complement spoken language in order to make speechreading easier. In addition, the total communication method using Signed French together with speech is used as an alternative to cued speech or in combination with it. Signed French is based on signs of BELGIAN SIGN LANGUAGE.

Mainstreamed students must learn through speechreading, hearing aids or written material, since there are no sign language, cued speech-interpreters or deaf teachers to help deaf students in schools for hearing students.

Services

Special education is free in Belgium, and the national health service helps pay for hearing aids. All Belgian families receive allowances for children, which are doubled for deaf children.

Little has been done to make television or telephone accessible to deaf consumers, although the national French-speaking television network provides sign interpretation five days a week. There is no systematic captioning system.

Bell, Alexander Graham (1847–1922)   This Scottish-born American inventor dedicated his life to improving methods of communication for deaf students, and was instrumental in instituting the oral method of deaf instruction at almost every school in the United States.

Born in Edinburgh, the son of Melville and Eliza Bell, Alec (as he was then known) was a brilliant child whose interest in inventions would preoccupy him for the rest of his life. With his father, he was also interested in speech disorders and elocution, in part because his mother had severe hearing problems since her childhood. However, she could speak well, used an EAR TRUMPET (a mechanical device to improve hearing), and played the piano.

Bell's father was a pioneer of the "VISIBLE SPEECH" system, in which he tried to develop a universal language for mankind. This system described oral sounds through written symbols and was created in order to improve elocution. Although the system was not originally designed to be used in teaching deaf students, a British teacher recognized its potential and began working with young Alec Bell. With the success of his first experience in teaching deaf students with visible speech, Bell accepted an invitation to teach the method at the Boston School for Deaf Mutes in 1870.

Three years later, Bell was hired as a private teacher for 15-year-old Mabel Hubbard; in 1877 the two were married, forming a union that lasted for 45 years. This remarkable woman was one of the strongest influences on Bell and helped shape his theories of education for deaf children.

In New England, Bell taught instructors at leading schools of deaf students the visible speech system but discovered that, in the long run, the symbols were too abstract for the teacher to apply, and the system fell into disuse.

During this time in New England, Bell began to promote his belief in day schools, instead of the residential facilities then common for deaf students. His first day school was started in 1878 in Scotland with three pupils. Back in the United States, Bell opened a day school in Washington, D.C. in the same building as a kindergarten class for hearing students; his hope was that the two groups would mix.

Bell was an ardent supporter of the ORAL APPROACH, and as he grew older, he focused his efforts on promoting oralism and founding schools to teach deaf students to speak. He was considered the champion of oral education in America and believed it was an educator's job to help deaf students speak English and read lips. He objected strongly to SIGN LANGUAGE because he believed it would prevent students from achieving integration into the hearing world.

Although some proponents of the MANUAL APPROACH argued that sign was the natural language of deaf people, Bell disagreed. He agreed that sign language was of great benefit in developing the intellect, but integration into society was far more important to him than developing the mind. Bell strongly believed that all deaf children could be taught to speak and read lips.

Because of his strong opinions against sign language—he considered a signing deaf adult a "failure"—many deaf adults hated him. They saw his attempts to eliminate sign language as an attack on their culture and identity.

Bell was also a supporter of eugenics, the science of improving hereditary characteristics through controlled mating, and opposed marriages between deaf people because he believed it would eventually create a race of deaf people. After studying statistics of deaf families, he concluded that deafness was often inherited and that those who inherited deafness should only marry hearing people. He wanted to have marriages between people with inherited deafness outlawed but gave up this idea when he decided that such legislation was unrealistic. He advocated that deaf students should not be segregated in schools, that deaf teachers should no longer be hired to teach deaf students and, of course, that sign language should be abolished.

It is not surprising that most of these ideas made him even more unpopular among the deaf population, at least among those who had adjusted to their inability to hear and considered themselves normal. But Bell, dreaming of a utopian society and brought up in a family that prized oral communication, saw deafness as a problem for society, not as an individual condition.

Bell also gave financial support to the cause of oral education. On May 8, 1893, young HELEN KELLER attended groundbreaking ceremonies for Bell's VOLTA BUREAU, an international information center promoting the oral education of deaf people. In 1890 he used his share of royalties from the invention of the Graphophone (a type of tape recorder) to finance the American Association to Promote the Teaching of Speech to the Deaf (AAPTSD) (now called the ALEXANDER GRAHAM BELL ASSOCIATION FOR THE DEAF). Today this association is a leader in the support of oral education, organizing meetings and conventions, lobbying and publishing a journal, the *Volta Review,* in its efforts.

Bell had an extraordinary impact on the educational methods used to teach deaf students in this country. When Bell formed the AAPTSD, only about 40 percent of deaf students were taught to speak. At the time of his death 30 years later, that number had risen to more than 80 percent.

Berthier, Jean-Ferdinand (1803–1886)   A political leader of the French deaf nation, Berthier was born in Louhans, France, and became the most outstanding advocate for deaf people in 19th-century France.

A firm believer in promoting public understanding of deafness, he also supported "natural sign language" and thought it helped students learn written French.

Berthier attended the famous Institut National de Jeunes Sourds in Paris and was the first deaf man to receive the Legion of Honor medal. He spent his life fighting negative attitudes toward deaf people, testifying before parliament to revamp laws dealing with (or ignoring) deaf people, and researching the history and heritage of deaf people. See also INSTITUT NATIONAL DES JEUNES SOURDS.

Better Hearing Institute   A nonprofit educational organization that offers general information about hearing loss and help available through medicine, surgery, amplification and rehabilitation. It also distributes films, technical information, news and human-interest features, and maintains a Hearing Help-on-Line website at http://www.betterhearing.org. Founded in 1973, the organization is supported entirely by private donations. See also Appendix II.

BI-CROS hearing aid   BI-CROS (bilateral contralateral routing of signal), aids, usually of the eyeglass type, used for those with an unequal hearing loss in both ears, one of which cannot be helped by amplification.

Unlike the CROS HEARING AID, which utilizes only one microphone, the BI-CROS system uses two microphones (one above each ear) sending signals to a single amplifier. Sound is picked up by microphones in both ears, transmitted to a single receiver and transferred to the better ear via a conventional earmold. See also HEARING AIDS.

Bilingual, Hearing- and Speech-Impaired Court Interpreter Act   This law, enacted by Congress in 1979, amends the 1978 Court Interpreters Act and requires the court to appoint a qualified interpreter for deaf, speech-impaired or non-English speakers in any criminal or civil action initiated by the federal government.

The director of the administrative office of the U.S. Courts determines the qualifications required of court-appointed interpreters. Each district court must maintain a list of certified oral and manual interpreters for deaf people, obtained in consultation with the NATIONAL ASSOCIATION OF THE DEAF and the REGISTRY OF INTERPRETERS FOR THE DEAF. The interpreter's services are paid for by the federal government.

However, an interpreter is *not* provided for a deaf person who initiates a lawsuit. Although many states will provide an interpreter for a deaf defendant in a criminal trial, few offer one at the time of arrest or in a civil case. See also LEGAL RIGHTS.

binaural   Pertaining to both ears.

binaural hearing aids   Two complete HEARING AIDS, one in each ear. Any type of hearing aid may be worn in both ears, if the listener can tolerate two aids and can benefit from amplifying residual hearing in both ears.

Some wearers find that the binaural system increases directional sense and helps separate desired sound from unwanted background noise. Although it is sometimes assumed that using an aid in each ear should improve hearing, tests of people wearing these aids do not always support this theory.

bionic ear   A popularized misnomer for the COCHLEAR IMPLANT.

body hearing aid   Also known as "on-the-body" aids, these devices feature a microphone and amplifier that are larger than in other HEARING AIDS and are carried inside a pocket or attached to clothing in a case about the size of a cigarette case. The external receiver attaches directly to the EARMOLD, and its power comes through a flexible wire from the amplifier.

The devices always include a volume control and on/off switch and may also offer tone control and a microphone/telephone selection switch (T-switch) that disconnects the microphone and allows the electromagnetic pickup of telephone conversations without background noise.

On-the-body hearing aids are more powerful and easier to adjust than smaller devices. However, their size and body location and the problem of noise from clothing make this aid an unpopular choice. These aids are still in use by people who need larger controls and for infants who are not old enough to wear ear-level hearing aids. See also TELECOIL.

bone conduction   Sound transmitted from the source through the skull bones directly to the COCHLEA, which is partly how we hear our own voice. The resulting sound is indistinguishable from air conduction signals. Bone conduction sounds reach the cochlea by several routes, unlike air conduction. Vibrations are sent through the skull wherever contact is made, reaching both ears almost at the same time.

With higher frequencies, the skull vibrates in segments, and these vibrations are transferred to the cochlear fluids by directly compressing the otic capsule (the body enclosure surrounding the inner ear). The resulting movements of the basilar membrane can stimulate the ORGAN OF CORTI. This form of conduction is known as compression bone conduction.

With frequencies below 1500 hertz, the skull moves as one rigid piece. Because the OSSICLES are only loosely attached to the skull, they are less affected than the cochlea and the OVAL WINDOW and move less freely. As a result, the oval window moves with the footplate of the stapes in a type of bone conduction known as inertial.

Because the ear disease OTOSCLEROSIS hardens the stapes, this interferes with inertial bone conduction but does not affect compressional bone conduction.

bone conduction test   See AUDIOMETRY.

bone conduction vibrator   An instrument placed on the mastoid bone behind the external ear as a way to present pure tones as part of bone conduction audiometry.

bone conductor hearing aids   Bone conduction aids are mostly for people with conductive hearing loss that has not been effectively treated by surgery. This type of HEARING AID, which allows sound to be heard through the bone behind the ear, is used when the ear canal is closed or drainage from the ear is poor.

bone hearing level   A measurement, determined through part of a hearing test, that indicates how well pure tones are heard through the bone behind the ear. See also AUDIOMETRY.

Bonet, Juan Pablo (1579–1623)   The author of the first published book of oral teaching methods for deaf people. Bonet was born on July 1, 1579, in a little town in Spain, Torres de Berrellén. After serving in the army and learning Italian and French, he was hired as secretary by the duke of Frias. The duke's second son, Luis, was deaf, and Manuel Ramírez de Carrión was employed to teach Luis, using the methods developed by PEDRO PONCE DE LEÓN. Bonet spent some time watching Ramírez and took over the education of Luis when Ramírez left.

After about three years, Bonet published *Simplification of the Alphabet and the Art of Teaching Mutes to Speak,* in which he explained the Ramírez de León technique. The text was not his own method, but by writing down the system, Bonet was able to interest a wide variety of European teachers in the possibility of oral education for deaf children.

Bonet believed in teaching reading and spelling, speech instruction and fingerspelling. However, he did not support the teaching of speechreading.

bony labyrinth   See LABYRINTH, INNER EAR.

Bove, Linda (b. 1945)   One of the most influential deaf women in the performing arts, this totally deaf actress may be best known for the character she played in public television's *Sesame Street.*

In addition, Bove is a founding member of both the NATIONAL THEATRE OF THE DEAF and the Little Theatre of the Deaf, and remains the National Theatre's ambassador-at-large.

Bove was born congenitally deaf in Garfield, New Jersey, to deaf parents and graduated from GALLAUDET UNIVERSITY, where she had been active in drama. She toured internationally with the National Theatre of the Deaf, and in 1973 she played "Melissa Hayley," a deaf character on the television soap opera *Search for Tomorrow;* other TV appearances include *The Dick Cavett Show, Happy Days* and *A Child's Christmas in Wales.* She first appeared on public television's *Sesame Street* in 1971; by 1976 she was a permanent member of the cast, portraying a deaf member of the neighborhood.

Boys Town Research Registry for Hereditary Hearing Loss   The registry matches families and individuals with hearing loss with collaborating research projects involving hereditary deafness. Participants provide demographic, genetic, audiologic and medical information to assist making that match. Information is kept confidential. The registry's publication, *Hereditary Deafness Newsletter of America,* is written for families and nongenetic clinical and research professionals.

Bragg, Bernard (b. 1928)   A cofounder of the NATIONAL THEATRE OF THE DEAF, Bernard Bragg is an actor, mime, director and lecturer known for his development of "sign-mime," a variation of sign language that features graceful, poetic body movement and motion to highlight dialogue.

Born deaf to deaf parents in Brooklyn, Bragg graduated as class valedictorian from the New York School for the Deaf and went on to GALLAUDET UNIVERSITY where he excelled in dramatics as an actor and director, and received the Teegarden Award for poetry upon graduation. His father, Wolf Bragg, was a talented actor who had performed in a deaf amateur theatrical group. At that time, there was no deaf professional theater.

Armed with a master's degree in education, Bragg taught for 15 years at a California school for deaf students, where he also performed for Marcel Marceau. The celebrated French mime then invited Bragg to study with him in Paris; after Bragg's return to California, he began performing in small clubs in San Francisco and was named one of the best small club performers by *Life* magazine.

Internationally, Bragg has served as artist-in-residence with the Moscow Theatre of Sign Language and mime and served on the U.S. Intelligence Agency's Overseas Speaker's Program in 1977, traveling all over the world conducting workshops in sign for both deaf and hearing audiences.

He currently serves as artist-in-residence at Gallaudet University.

Braidwood, Thomas (1715–1806)   A pioneer Scottish educator of deaf people best known for his refusal to pass on his methods in oral instruction to anyone outside his own family. This reticence was responsible for the early emphasis on manual education of deaf students in the United States.

Thomas Braidwood taught his first deaf pupil in 1760 and was so pleased with his success in helping the boy speak and understand language that he decided to concentrate on teaching deaf students.

His first school, the Academy for the Deaf and Dumb, opened in Edinburgh in the early 1760s. By 1779, the academy had 20 pupils who were taught to speak, read and write. Although his exact methods were not divulged, it was known that he based his method on the articulation theories of educator Thomas Wallis. This was an oral method, but the use of natural signs and the manual alphabet was not forbidden.

In response to an offer from King George III to set up a school for deaf students in London, Braidwood opened Grove House in 1792 and then a separate school for needy deaf children, where Braidwood's nephew Joseph Watson was headmaster.

Braidwood's schools were successful, but the oath of secrecy kept by the Braidwood family had important consequences for the future of deaf education in the United States. THOMAS HOPKINS

GALLAUDET, who had studied the manual communication system in France developed by ABBÉ ROCH-AMBROISE CUCURRON SICARD, came to Britain to learn the oral method from Braidwood.

When he got to London, he found that the three English schools for deaf students were all controlled by the Braidwood family, who were unwilling to share their methods freely, as was the custom at the time.

Consequently, Gallaudet returned to Paris to study the French manual system, which he subsequently introduced into the United States. This method became the basis of deaf education and communication in U.S. schools for deaf children.

brainstem audiometry See AUDITORY BRAINSTEM RESPONSE TEST.

brainstem auditory evoked potential See AUDITORY BRAINSTEM RESPONSE TEST.

brainstem evoked potential See AUDITORY BRAINSTEM RESPONSE TEST.

brainstem testing See AUDITORY BRAINSTEM RESPONSE TEST.

Brazil Deaf citizens in Brazil receive limited funds from the state and federal government for diagnosis, treatment, education and rehabilitation. Free diagnosis of simple cases of deafness and routine prescription of hearing aids are provided by the government through its own otolaryngologists and through agreements with private clinics. The state mandates minimal educational and treatment provisions and helps finance the training of teachers for deaf students. Numerous private charitable groups also serve deaf Brazilians. Many large cities maintain good private clinics and professionals, but the treatment cost is often beyond the reach of many Brazilians.

Although there are no exact figures, estimates suggest that there are up to 9.6 million deaf and hard-of-hearing Brazilians. More than half of the deaf students who receive assistance attend school in special classes, one-fourth are in integrated classes, and one-fifth attend special schools.

The predominant philosophy in the schools and programs for deaf citizens throughout the country is to integrate deaf people into the hearing world by developing speech and speechreading skills and utilizing residual hearing. The use of sign language was discouraged between 1950 and 1970, but today its use is spreading slowly across the country.

Brazilian Sign Language A number of dialects make up Brazilian Sign Language, but communication among people is surprisingly easy for so large a country.

Although Brazilian schools for deaf students became completely oral after the Milan Congress in 1880, there has been more interest in Brazilian Sign Language since the 1970s, and at least one school has adopted the educational philosophy of TOTAL COMMUNICATION.

Brazilian Sign Language is similar to both American and European sign languages, and its one-handed manual alphabet is quite similar to the French system. In Brazilian Sign Language, fingerspelling is used for proper names, fingerspelled signs, technical terms and negative emphasis. The system utilizes hand and body movements, facial expressions, eye gaze, pauses and changes in the rhythm of signing to indicate grammatical and structural meanings, and the space around the body provides an important frame of reference, indicating spatial agreement between verbs and subjects/objects, reference for directional verbs and so forth.

Breunig, H. Latham (b. 1910) A chemist, statistician and leading proponent of oral education, Breunig founded the Oral Deaf Adults Section of the ALEXANDER GRAHAM BELL ASSOCIATION FOR THE DEAF. Along with two others, he set up Teletypewriters for the Deaf, Inc., to acquire and recondition surplus teletypewriters donated by American Telephone and Telegraph.

Born in Indianapolis, he lost part of his hearing when he was three years old, a condition exacerbated by an attack of scarlet fever at age five. Two years after that, a skull fracture left him with a 115 dB loss. He attended the Clarke School for the Deaf in Northampton, Massachusetts, where he met his future wife, and then attended a public school, where he worked on the school newspaper, became an Eagle Scout and was accepted into the National Honor Society.

He received a degree in chemistry from Wabash College in Indiana and completed his Ph.D. at Johns Hopkins University. While a full-time researcher with the pharmaceutical firm of Eli Lilly, Breunig was active in national organizations for deaf people and was director of the Indianapolis Speech and Hearing Center for 21 years. Committed to the idea that deaf people need to be able to communicate with the hearing world in order to take advantage of opportunities, he attributed his own success in business and as a professional chemist to his ability to speak and speechread.

Brewster, John, Jr. (1766–1854)   Considered one of New England's most accomplished folk artists, he was also one of the most successful traveling artists of his day.

Brewster was born deaf to hearing parents, Dr. John and Mary Brewster, in Hampton, Connecticut. Able to communicate in sign language and adept at an early age in art, he obtained several commissions for portraits of family and friends despite a lack of formal training.

Brewster faced great difficulties as an independent artist forced to communicate constantly with strangers in inns or homes. He traveled by horseback in Massachusetts and Maine and was gifted at capturing a model's personality in his portraits.

When the Connecticut Asylum for the Education and Instruction of Deaf and Dumb Persons opened in Hartford (now the American School for the Deaf), Brewster, at the age of 54, was one of its first six pupils. During the three years he lived at the school, he was able to support himself through painting. He left the school in 1820 to continue painting. His paintings hang today in museums in Maine, Massachusetts and New York.

Bridgman, Laura Dewey (1829–1889)   The first deaf and blind person to be educated in the United States, Laura Bridgman was born in Hanover, New Hampshire, to a successful farm family. Always a delicate child, at age two she contracted scarlet fever, which destroyed her sight and hearing and left her ill for two years. During this time, she for-got the few words she had learned to speak before her illness, and she retreated into silence.

Bridgman was introduced in 1837 to Samuel Gridley Howe, the founder of the Perkins Institution for the Blind in Boston. Although Laura could barely communicate with her family (she understood shoves and pats on the head), Howe was convinced she was extremely bright and would benefit from instruction.

Her parents brought her to Perkins in 1837, where Howe constantly worked with her to establish a form of communication using labels with raised letters pasted on common objects. When she finally learned that the labels actually represented objects, the greatest obstacle to meaningful communication had been crossed. At Perkins, she studied a variety of subjects, such as fingerspelling, handsewing and how to use a sewing machine.

Although she never learned to talk, she could make about 50 sounds, which she used as names for people she knew. At the age of 23, she was sent home where it was assumed she would be happy with household chores. But the sudden loss of noise and activity affected her poorly; she became bedridden and near death until she was returned to Perkins, where she remained for the rest of her life.

British Sign Language   This highly complex system is the language of the deaf community throughout Great Britain and Northern Ireland, although there are regional dialects. As in many natural sign languages, BSL has a topic-comment structure: for example, "Drink—you want more?" instead of "Do you want another drink?" It includes an inflection system, with which it is possible to show person or number by the way signs move.

As in AMERICAN SIGN LANGUAGE, BSL and English are quite different, although the two-handed BSL manual alphabet is based on the English alphabet.

There are no exact figures on the number of people who use BSL, but estimates suggest that as many as 30,000 profoundly deaf people in the United Kingdom use BSL and were educated through its use. It includes a two-handed fingerspelling system that was first published in 1680.

Although the use of BSL was widespread by the mid-19th century in combination with English, it fell out of favor as oralism reached popularity in Britain. Today, BSL is becoming increasingly well accepted and is a topic of research and study by linguists.

Bulwer, John   This 17th-century English physician was very interested in manual communication as an orator but later became involved in its uses as a tool to educate deaf students.

Bulwer believed it was possible for deafmutes to learn speechreading and speech, although he believed that sign language and manual alphabets were more practical. His *Philocophus, or the Deafe and Dumbe Man's Friend,* published in 1648, was the first major English book on deafness. In it, he discussed the anatomy and physiology of speech and the etiology of deafness. He also explored the elements of phonetics, describing specific movements of each speech sound and insisting that speech is *movement* rather than *position.*

However, Bulwer was not a teacher of deaf students and never applied any of his theories. Although he hoped to establish a deaf school to teach communication methods to hard-of-hearing students, he never accomplished his goal.

Canada As in the United States, about one in 25 Canadian citizens have some type of hearing problem. Nearly 4,000 children with hearing problems are in special programs, almost half of these students are profoundly deaf. These numbers, however, are estimates since there has been no national deaf census and the figures do not include native Canadians in the far north, among whom hearing loss is reportedly endemic. About 200,000 Canadians are deaf.

The result is a small and widely scattered minority population served only by a small number of professionals, in a country with a decentralized method of administering social services. This decentralization, in which the provinces fiercely maintain sole right to administer social services for its people, virtually guarantees a crazy-quilt pattern of services for deaf people across the country. Most important, education for Canada's deaf students has no uniform, comprehensive standards or administration.

Although deaf Canadians have made strides in civil rights, including the rights to legal interpreter services and to become adoptive parents, they have not been as successful in effecting improvements in postsecondary education, audiological service delivery and research.

Canada's history has been closely linked to England and France, but the country has allied itself with the United States in its development of educational services for its deaf citizens.

The first school for deaf Canadians was opened in 1831 in Champlain, Quebec, by Ronald McDonald, who had spent a year at the American School for the Deaf at Hartford training under Thomas Gallaudet and Laurent Clerc. All schools gradually evolved from reliance on a manual to an oral educational philosophy.

American signs and AMERICAN SIGN LANGUAGE (ASL) have remained the preferred method of communication, although the small French deaf community within the country uses French-Canadian Sign Language. Across the country, there are regional differences in sign.

A bilingual dictionary of the basic vocabulary of sign language used in Canada is being compiled by the Canadian Coordinating Council on Deafness and will include the signs used in French Canada.

Because most Canadians prefer sign language, many disagree with the school-based English sign systems used as part of Total Communication in many educational programs. Many Canadians support a bilingual approach to learning language, with ASL as the first language and English signs as an added benefit to a student's curriculum.

Captioned television became available with the development in 1982 of the Canadian Captioning Development Agency, which captions a wide variety of Canadian programs in English and French. For a time, the agency also captioned French language telecasts around the world since there was no closed captioning system available to the French.

The Canadian Coordinating Council on Deafness and the Canadian Association of the Deaf are major national organizations with affiliated groups throughout the provinces.

Canadian Sign Language Just as the culture of Canada has evolved along two lines, French and English, so has the language of the deaf community. Canada's deaf community speaks two completely different sign languages: Canadian Sign Language (CSL)—used primarily by deaf people in the English Canadian community—and Langue des Signes Quebecoise (LSQ)—used primarily by deaf French Canadians.

As in many sign languages around the world, much investigation is still being done into the structural properties of the communication methods. It appears, however, that CSL may share certain properties with British Sign Language, and LSQ may be similar to the sign language used in France (Langue des Signes Française [LSF], also called French Sign Language). There is also some evidence that CSL shares some structural similarities with American Sign Language. Still, research also suggests that both CSL and LSQ have different structures from English and French.

Although the Canadian constitution stipulates that English and French are equal official languages, it is extremely rare for a deaf student to be taught both CSL and LSQ.

As with many other sign languages, CSL and LSQ depend on systematic changes in movement, space and facial expression as linguistic devices to change meaning.

canal hearing aid   Designed for mild to moderate hearing loss, this tiny device is even smaller than the in-the-ear devices and fits almost completely into the ear canal. It does not normally have a T-switch capability. Further, the ear canal must be of the right shape and size in order to use this type of hearing aid. Successful wearers are able to place the tiny unit into the ear, and utilize its even tinier controls. Cosmetically, it is the most appealing of all HEARING AIDS. See also TELECOIL.

cancer of the outer ear   Cancer of the outer ear usually appears as a small painless ulcer covered by a dry scab that slowly deepens in areas exposed for years to the sun. Treatment involves complete removal of the cancerous area and radiation therapy.

More serious—and more rare—is cancer that begins in the ear canal, where it may spread to the bone before being discovered and can therefore be more difficult to cure. See also ACOUSTIC NEUROMA; CHOLESTEATOMA; CHORISTOMA.

Capital Communications for the Deaf   CapCom, Inc. offers counseling and mediation services for people who have disability issues relating to

employment or other civil liability matters. CapCom encourages employment of people with hearing deficits, provides information on issues of deafness and the workplace and provides sign interpreters as needed in many areas nationally and internationally.

caption-capable TV sets   A type of television set with built-in decoders to receive and display closed captioned TV programs. In the past, a person would need a special set-top decoder to receive the captions. Today, sets with built-in decoders are available at all consumer electronics stores. See also AMERICANS WITH DISABILITIES ACT; CAPTION CENTER; CLOSED CAPTIONS.

Caption Center   This nonprofit service of Boston's WGBH Educational Foundation was the world's first television captioning agency.

The center began offering open captioning (captions visible on all TV sets) on programs in the early 1970s to stations affiliated with the Public Broadcasting Service (PBS). Usually, the first showing of a program had no captions, and rebroadcasts carried open captions.

Today, the center produces captions for every segment of the entertainment and advertising industries and offers an array of services, including real-time captions (live captions created as a program is broadcast) and open captions. Its development of software programs has enabled agencies and schools to caption their own programs and events.

The Caption Center maintains an ongoing commitment to conducting outreach among viewers with hearing loss, those learning English as a second language, and people of all ages learning to read. Each year, The Caption Center captions more than 10,000 hours' worth of broadcast and cable programs, feature films, large-format and IMAX films, home videos, music videos, DVDs, teleconferences and CD-ROMs. See also CLOSED CAPTIONS; NATIONAL CAPTIONING INSTITUTE; TELECAPTIONS DECODER; Appendix II.

Captioned Media Program   A free loan service of theatrical and educational films and videocassettes captioned for deaf viewers. Established in 1958, the project is funded by the U.S. Department of Education to promote the education and welfare of deaf people through the media. This branch also provides funds for several closed-captioned TV programs, including the live-captioned news on the ABC, NBC and CBS networks.

Captioned Media Program grew out of a private, nonprofit corporation established by the Junior League of Hartford and the CONVENTION OF AMERICAN INSTRUCTORS OF THE DEAF that was designed to caption films for deaf people. Because the expense and size of the job soon became too much for the small company, Congress passed Public Law 85-905, which established Captioned Films for the Deaf (now Captioned Media Program) as a government service.

All videos are open captioned (meaning that consumers don't need a decoder to view the captions). There are more than 4,000 titles currently in the library, and more than 300 titles a year are added to the catalog, including both educational and general interest titles. Educational videos include all school subjects from preschool through college, together with appropriate lesson guides. General interest videos include movie classics, travel, hobbies and recreation.

Deaf individuals, parents and teachers may borrow videos by filling out an application form (also available online). Videos may be ordered through the mail or from the Internet free of charge; prepaid return labels are included. See also CLOSED CAPTIONS; NATIONAL CAPTIONING INSTITUTE; TELECAPTION DECODER; Appendix II.

carhart notch   A loss in bone conduction hearing acuity at 500, 1,000, 2,000 and 4,000 Hz first discovered by audiologist Raymond Carhart in patients with OTOSCLEROSIS. The loss is not attributed to impairment of the COCHLEA but to blockage of cochlear fluid movement by the STAPES which have become fixed in place.

CASE   See CONCEPTUALLY ACCURATE SIGNED ENGLISH.

catarrhal deafness   Hearing loss caused by inflammation of the mucous membrane of the air passages in the head and throat together with a

blocked EUSTACHIAN TUBE. Since this is an early stage of an acute ear infection, antibiotic drug treatment is generally prescribed, together with decongestants to alleviate symptoms.

catarrhal otitis media   See SEROUS OTITIS MEDIA.

cauliflower ear   A deformity of the shape of the outer ear (pinna) caused by blows or friction that are sharp enough to start bleeding within the soft cartilage of the ear itself. It is most commonly found in boxers and can be prevented by using a protective helmet.

After a severe blow to the ear, swelling can be reduced by applying an ice pack, and blood can be drained from the ear with a needle and syringe. Repeated injuries to the ear, however, will distort its shape in a way that can only be repaired through plastic surgery.

CC   Acronym used to denote closed captioning on TV programs, videocassettes and so forth. See CLOSED CAPTIONS.

Center for Bicultural Studies, Inc.   This group promotes public education about the interaction between deaf and hearing cultures and fosters public acceptance, understanding and use of AMERICAN SIGN LANGUAGE and other natural signed languages. It disseminates information on deaf culture and American Sign Language, sponsors forums, public discussions and video projects and publishes the *TBC News.* See also Appendix II.

Center for Hearing Dog Information   A national advocacy resource and referral center for hearing ear dog programs sponsored by the American Humane Association. The center publishes a Hearing Dog Program Directory, which outlines hearing dog programs and also lists support dog training programs (dogs who assist the physically disabled) and agencies that train dog guides for the blind.

Individuals with a severe to profound hearing loss who can demonstrate a need for such a dog can qualify. Only a few programs place children with dogs because children often cannot maintain the necessary control over an animal. See also HEARING EAR DOGS; Appendix II.

central auditory imperception See AUDITORY AGNOSIA.

central auditory processing test (CAP) A type of test that assesses the ability to process the sounds children hear. A child must be able to speak in full sentences and have reasonably advanced language to take the central auditory processing test, so they must be at least over the age of five. Some children hear very well but have difficulty deciding what to do with the sound once they hear it. These children are typically intelligent but have trouble following directions in school (especially in noisy environments). They may have had many ear infections when they were younger and developed difficulty dealing with sound as a method of communication. See also CHILDREN AND DEAFNESS.

central hearing loss A type of hearing loss that results from damage or impairment to the nerves or nuclei of the central nervous system, either in the pathways to the brain or in the brain itself. Central hearing loss may result from congenital brain abnormalities, tumors or lesions of the central nervous system, strokes or from some medications that specifically harm the ear. See also HEARING LOSS; OTOTOXIC DRUGS.

cerebral palsy A general term for nonprogressive disorders of movement, posture or speech caused by brain damage during pregnancy, birth or early childhood. About 25 percent to 30 percent of people with cerebral palsy have hearing problems.

The degree of physical disability varies widely from slight clumsiness to complete immobility. About two to six infants per 1,000 develop cerebral palsy—90 percent shortly before or during birth, usually from a lack of oxygen. Sometimes, cerebral palsy can result from a mother's infection that has passed to her unborn baby or from an excess of bilirubin in the blood after birth. After birth, cerebral palsy also can result from a head injury, encephalitis or meningitis.

Although there is no cure for cerebral palsy, it is possible to treat people who have it; physical therapy can help develop muscular control, and speech problems can be treated by speech therapy.

certified hearing aid audiologist An AUDIOLOGIST certified by the AMERICAN SPEECH-LANGUAGE-HEARING ASSOCIATION as qualified to dispense hearing aids. The certified hearing aid audiologist must hold a master's degree in AUDIOLOGY, pass a national certifying examination and hold the certificate of clinical competence.

cerumen See EARWAX.

chemicals and deafness Some environmental chemicals can damage the delicate hearing mechanism. These chemicals include:

- trichloroethylene
- xylene
- styrene
- butyl nitrite
- toluene
- hexane
- carbon disulfide
- mercury
- manganese
- tin
- lead
- carbon monoxide

chicken pox A childhood infectious disease related to the herpes viruses, which has been known to cause sudden severe deafness in one ear. An attack of chickenpox, which is caused by the varicella-zoster virus, confers lifelong immunity. Afterwards, the virus lies dormant within nerve tissues and may erupt as herpes zoster (shingles) later in life.

The airborne virus is easily spread during the two days before the rash appears and for about a week afterward. Women in the last months of pregnancy are particularly vulnerable and may pass the disease on to their infants, who may have severe cases.

Chicken pox is heralded by a rash on the body, face, upper arms and legs, under the arms, inside the mouth and sometimes in the bronchial tubes. Children usually have only a slight fever, but adults may become quite ill with severe pneumonia and breathing difficulties. Complications include encephalitis (brain inflammation), which can lead to deafness.

Treatment involves rest with acetaminophen to reduce the fever and lotion to relieve the rash, although acyclovir (a drug used to treat other herpes viruses) may also be used in severe cases of chicken pox. The current vaccine against chicken pox is effective. See also VIRUSES AND HEARING LOSS.

children and deafness The lack of early detection of hearing problems in children is a major public health problem. The average age at which moderate to severe hearing impairment is detected in children is two to three years of age, but these problems can and should be identified and treated much sooner. If undetected and untreated, hearing loss in children leads to delayed speech and language development and can contribute to emotional, social and academic problems. Ideally, doctors should identify infants with hearing loss before age three months so that intervention can begin by six months of age.

Parents are usually the first to suspect a hearing loss; the earlier a loss is found, the better the chances of preventing language and learning delays. Any child who has a history of frequent ear infections and who shows signs of poor hearing, not following directions, poor pronunciation or behavioral problems should have a hearing test. If a parent or doctor suspects a hearing problem, the child's primary care provider may choose to conduct a hearing screening for a preschool age child, but infants and young toddlers will need a referral for special tests. A pediatrician should conduct ongoing exams when a child has middle ear fluid until it has cleared. If present for several months without clearing, consultation with an otolaryngologist should be considered.

If a child care provider or parent has any doubt about slower than normal sound and speech-language development in a child, these concerns should be discussed with the child's primary care provider, and hearing testing should be seriously considered. For more information, brochures are available from the American Speech-Language-Hearing Association at 800-638-8255 or through e-mail at actioncenter@asha.org

A hearing test can be done with fluid in the ears; in fact, this can provide valuable information because it will indicate how much hearing loss is caused by the fluid. No hearing test should be done on a child whose ears are filled with wax. The wax must be cleaned before any testing is done.

A pediatrician should consider a hearing evaluation in the following situations:

- Children at high risk for hearing problems, such as those with abnormalities of the skull or face, prematurity, intrauterine infection history, meningitis, genetic conditions related to hearing loss or a family history of hearing loss.

- A child who has a speech or language delay (such as no babbling in a six-month-old, no words by 18 months, or no word combinations by age two).

- A child whose parent is concerned about hearing. Hearing losses at specific frequencies may exist despite normal language.

- A child whose eardrums are hard to see because of wax or small canals. (These may need to be cleaned and evaluated by an otolaryngologist.)

There are several ways to test hearing in children:

Behavioral Testing

A behavioral test is a better measure of hearing and generally should be tried first in the overwhelming majority of children (even older infants). In sound field audiometry, the child is placed in a soundproof booth to see if she will respond to sound (even babies at one or two months of age will startle after a very loud noise). An infant who doesn't startle may have a hearing problem. However, relying on startling alone may not identify infants with smaller but still significant losses. In a type of test called visual response audiometry, older infants will turn their head toward noises that get their attention. Eventually they can learn that a stuffed animal will light up when there is noise, and they will look for the animal when they hear the noise. If they don't look, they did not hear it. Conditioned play audiometry is a type of test that teaches toddlers up to age three or four to put a toy in a box when they hear the noise. Failure to put a toy in the box is an indication that they didn't hear the noise. In an air-conduction audiometry test, children with a developmental age of four or older wear earphones and raise their hands when they hear a sound. Older children can respond to a bone vibrator, which helps to determine whether a hearing problem is in the middle or inner ear in cases where both ears are not the same. This is called bone conduction audiometry.

Brainstem Evoked Response Testing (BER, ABR, BSER)

The brainstem evoked response testing method is not a direct measure of hearing, but a measure of nerve activity; it's used with children who can't respond in the soundproof booth because in this type of test, no responses are required from the child. As the child sleeps (with or without sedation), earphones and electrodes record activity from the hearing nerve. The test, which measures high-pitched sounds better than low-pitched sounds, is often used by hospitals to test newborn infants.

Otoacoustic Emissions (OAE)

The otoacoustic emissions test is a very new method of hearing testing and also can be done in children who cannot respond to behavioral testing. This rapid test can be used for screening in the newborn nursery; it's based on the fact that the ear not only hears noise, but also makes noise. By measuring the very faint noises made by the ear, the test estimates how well the ear hears. An ear that does not hear will not make the expected noises. These noises are much too faint to be heard by our ears, but there are machines that can measure them.

Central Auditory Processing Testing (CAP)

A child must be able to speak in full sentences and have reasonably advanced language to take the central auditory processing test, so they must be at least over the age of five. The CAP assesses the ability to process the sounds children hear. Some children hear very well but have difficulty deciding what to do with the sound once they hear it. These children are typically intelligent but have trouble following directions in school (especially in noisy environments). They may have had many ear infections when they were younger and developed difficulty dealing with sound as a method of communication.

The estimates of deafness in the U.S. population vary, but it is particularly difficult to estimate the incidence of deafness among children because it often goes unrecognized or misdiagnosed in the very young. Still, the numbers of hard-of-hearing children are much greater than the numbers of deaf children. Federal government projections have estimated there are about 50,000 deaf and 325,000 hard-of-hearing children in the school-age population. More than 90 percent of the deaf children and about 20 percent of the hard-of-hearing children receive special educational services. Data on school children with hearing problems prepared by the Census Bureau in conjunction with the National Center for Health Statistics indicate that in 1982 about two out of every 100 people under age 18 had at least some form of hearing problems.

In the book *Deaf Population in the United States,* authors Jerome Schein and Marcus Delk estimate that one person in 1,000 is born deaf or is deafened before age three and that one in 500 is born deaf or is deafened before the age of 19.

In general, deaf children receive more intensive and comprehensive services while children with a milder hearing loss mainly receive speech-language therapy.

China   There are about 3 million deaf citizens in China, but services for these people are in woefully short supply. Only about 33,000 of them currently attend schools for deaf students.

The first school for deaf students opened in 1887 at Dengchou, and by 1948 there were 23 such schools, most of which were private. When the People's Republic of China was founded in 1949, the new government mandated major changes in the education of deaf children.

First, the government took control of all schools for deaf students, limited class size to 15 pupils, established a Bureau of the Deaf and Blind to administer education and began research in oral teaching methods. Since then, education for deaf children has grown to more than 30 schools with more than 9,000 staff for 33,000 students.

Students can attend combined schools for deaf and blind children, schools for deaf students only or special classes in regular schools. Still, the school enrollment rate of deaf children is very low, and the system of education is considered poor.

Deaf Chinese citizens are given the same rights as every other member of society and, in cities, receive government-paid medical care and pensions. The government has special rules for its deaf criminals: Since 1980, Chinese law states that if a deaf person violates a criminal law, he or she can be exempt from punishment or only lightly punished.

Although there were no unified language communication methods for deaf Chinese in the past, in 1963 the government adopted the Chinese Fingerspelling Alphabet Scheme, based on the Chinese pronunciation scheme and consisting of 30 separate fingershapes.

The primary association for deaf Chinese is the Chinese Association for the Blind and the Deaf, which is headquartered in Beijing and is a member of the World Federation of the Deaf.

Chinese Sign Language   The standard communication mode for the people of mainland China, Chinese Sign Language (CSL) includes 3,000 signs with 41 recurrent handshapes. Although there are three million deaf Chinese, it is unknown how many use CSL.

In general, CSL places the verb last, with the modified followed by the modifier: "Girl sleep not." It has a manual alphabet with 26 letters and four digraphic consonants used to fingerspell words. It is used primarily in schools; deaf Chinese signers rarely use fingerspelling.

Ideograms are still the main type of writing found in China, and 22 of these ideograms are used in CSL. Not surprisingly, given the isolated nature of mainland China, very few of its signs have come from foreign shores.

cholesteatoma   This chronic middle ear inflammatory disease is a rare, serious condition in which skin cells and debris collect within the middle ear, usually as a result of a middle ear infection that has caused the eardrum to burst. Cholesteatomas can either be present at birth or appear later in life; the rare congenital variety may appear anywhere in the temporal bone.

Acquired cholesteatoma may be caused by a persistent narrowing of the EUSTACHIAN TUBE, eventually pulling the upper part of the eardrum back and forming a sac in the middle ear. The acquired form may also occur because of a tiny hole in the eardrum that allows skin cells of the external ear canal to move into the middle ear.

If the cholesteatoma is not treated, it may grow and damage the small bones in the middle ear and surrounding bone structures, causing a conductive or a mixed hearing loss and serious complications, including secondary infection, LABYRINTHITIS, MENINGITIS or a brain abscess.

The cholesteatoma must be removed either through the eardrum or by MASTOIDECTOMY (removal of the mastoid bone behind the ear together with the cholesteatoma).

Chomsky, Noam (b. 1928)   This American linguist is one of the founders of generative grammar, an original system of linguistic analysis. He believes there is a universal pattern in all languages and linguists should study a native speaker's unconscious knowledge of his own language and not the speaker's actual production of language.

Unlike structuralists, who collect samples of language and then classify them, Chomsky developed transformational grammar—a set of rules that can generate structural descriptions for all the grammatical sentences of a language. He then tested results against actual language samples. Transformational grammar has continued to evolve since Chomsky first introduced it in 1957.

Chomsky, whose father was a Hebrew scholar who studied historical LINGUISTICS, teaches modern languages and linguistics at the Massachusetts Institute of Technology.

choristoma A benign tumor in the middle ear that is really a congenital misplacement of the salivary gland and usually occurs with a middle ear malformation. It is treated by complete surgical removal. Although benign, these tumors can cause a conductive hearing disorder by their physical presence—filling the middle ear, destroying OSSICLES and interfering with eardrum movement. See also TUMORS OF THE MIDDLE EAR.

classifiers Handshapes that represent or describe certain types of classes of objects or occurrences (for example, upright index fingers brought together to indicate two people meeting).

cleft palate and hearing loss A number of children with cleft palates also have mild to moderate CONDUCTIVE HEARING LOSS because of the cleft condition in the mouth area; this loss is usually medically treatable. A hearing assessment is usually given during speech tests to find out if such a hearing loss is present.

Clerc, Laurent (1785–1869) This leader in education for deaf people was born in LaBalme les Grottes, France, the son of a family noted in local politics.

Deafened at age one after an infection following a facial burn, Clerc was taken to the famous Royal National Institute for the Deaf and Dumb in Paris (now the INSTITUT NATIONAL DES JEUNES SOURDS), where he studied with the brilliant deaf instructor JEAN MASSIEU; by the age of 20 he had completed his education and was teaching classes at the institute.

At the school, Clerc met THOMAS HOPKINS GALLAUDET, who had come to learn the manual alphabet developed there. Gallaudet convinced Clerc to return with him to the United States for three years to help establish a school for deaf students.

It was on the ocean voyage to this country that Gallaudet taught Clerc English and Clerc completed Gallaudet's training in manual communication. Once in the United States, Gallaudet and Clerc raised $5,000 at presentations and special programs

they conducted throughout New England, an amount that was later matched by the Connecticut general assembly.

With this money, the AMERICAN SCHOOL FOR THE DEAF opened its doors in 1817 in Hartford, Connecticut, with seven pupils. The next year, Clerc married one of them, Eliza Boardman, and decided to remain in America. He returned to France to visit only three times.

Although Clerc could not speak, he had great political influence and could write fluently in French and English. With these skills, he was able to convince Americans that deaf children could be educated and that sign language was the best type of communication to use while teaching them. At the age of 73, Clerc retired after 50 years of teaching. He died on July 18, 1869, and was buried beside his wife in Hartford.

closed captions The audio portion of a television program that has been translated into typed dialogue that usually appears across the bottom of the screen. All TV sets built after 1993 have built-in caption decoders.

Although captioning was at first limited to previously-taped programs, in 1984 the development of computer technology had reached the point where "real time" captioning became available for live broadcasts.

Most captioning is done at the headquarters of the NATIONAL CAPTIONING INSTITUTE (NCI) in Falls Church, Virginia, and at WGBH-TV in Boston. When captioning prerecorded programs, an editor records captions on a magnetic disk that is then sent to the TV broadcaster where it is inserted into line 21 of the TV signal. It takes about 30 hours to caption a one-hour program. Captioned programs air on CBS, NBC, ABC, PBS, FOX, independent stations and many cable companies.

For live broadcasts, a court stenographer enters phonetic symbols into a computer that then translates the symbols into captions and beams them through the network to viewers about four seconds after words are spoken. While it works fairly well, captions cannot be edited and mistakes occasionally appear.

Closed captioning was introduced in 1980 and is now used in more than 70 percent of primetime programming on networks and cable TV in addition to local and national news, sports and political events. Further, a large number of video movies are now available in closed captioned versions.

A free service of TV and cable networks and home video producers, captioning is funded by corporations, foundations, the government, producers, networks and program sponsors. In addition, people interested in closed captioned programs may

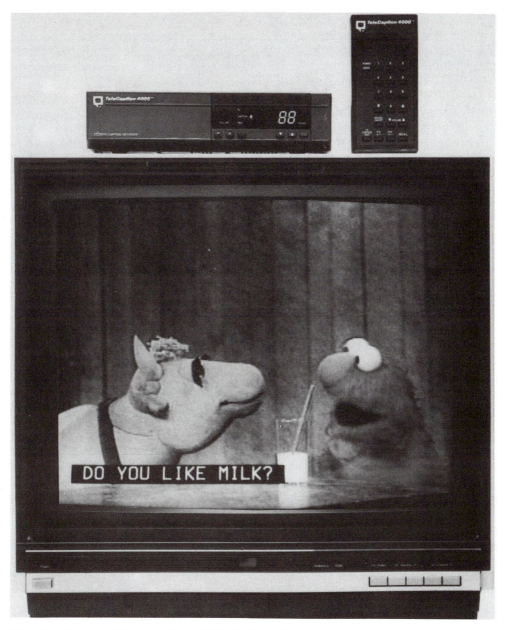

Closed captioning of *Sesame Street*/PBS television show

join NCI's Caption Club, whose membership dues are used to fund captioning of TV programs that reflect viewer's preferences.

Published TV schedules usually mark captioned programs with a "C" or "CC." The TeleCaption decoder itself provides a Program Listing Update Service (PLUS), which is a daily listing of captioned programs and sponsors. TeleCaption decoders are produced by the National Captioning Institute.

There are several different methods of producing closed captions. These include:

Prerecorded Captions

Videotaped programs may be broadcast with prerecorded captions, prepared before the airing of the program. In advance, the captioner watches a tape of the program, then writes the captions and types them into a computer together with instructions regarding when and where they should appear on the screen. Then a new tape is made combining the tape of the program and the captions.

Live Display Captions

For live TV programs in which there is a script prepared in advance, it is possible to prepare captions before the program airs. The captions are typed into a computer, and when the live program is aired, the captions in the computer are sent to a machine that adds them to the TV signal.

Real-Time Captions

For live programs with no prepared scripts (such as debates and news conferences), it is possible to create captions as the program is being aired. In this case, a captioner uses a stenotype machine similar to the one used by court reporters, which uses a type of shorthand. As the operator types out the shorthand, the computer converts the symbols into English and organizes them into captions; the captions are then sent to a machine that combines them with the TV signal. They appear on a TV set after a short delay since the operator must hear the word before it can be typed and the computer takes a few additional seconds to perform its functions. These captions are presented in a rolling fashion in order to appear as quickly as possible. There may be mistakes since there is no time to proofread what is typed.

Commentary Captions

Some sports shows use this form of closed caption, which does not follow word-for-word what commentators say but simply reports the scoreboard, play-by-play and background information. For the first two types of information, brief descriptions are typed into a computer that types out a more involved caption (the computer might take the brief "out 1" and translate it to "That's the first out for the Red Sox"). Background information is prepared ahead of time in the same way live-display captions are. (See above.)

Combination

Some shows may use several types of captioning; for example, a news show with a prerecorded or scripted segment may use live-display together with real-time for those spots that are live with no scripts. In the past, people needed a special decoder placed on top of the TV set to receive and translate closed captions on TV screens. However, federal legislation that took effect in 1993 requires that all TV sets with screens 13 inches or larger manufactured for sale in the United States must contain built-in closed caption decoders. Since then, consumers using some older top-of-the-set decoders have noticed incorrect letters in captions or missing captions.

The TELEVISION DECODER CIRCUITRY ACT OF 1990 requires built-in decoder circuitry in television receivers that meet the standards set by the Federal Communications Commission (FCC). The law took effect July 1, 1993.

The original caption decoders (TeleCaption I) went on sale in 1980. These models were sold as stand-alone decoders or were built into television sets. Five years later, the National Captioning Institute introduced the TeleCaption II. This same basic decoder design was also used in subsequent set-top models TeleCaption 3000, TeleCaption 4000 and TeleCaption VR 100. However, set-top decoder sales never reached more than about 350,000 homes. There was a huge difference between the number of decoders sold and the potential audience for captioning—22 million deaf and hard-of-hearing viewers. Many viewers who could benefit from captioning didn't buy a decoder either because they didn't know about the service, it cost too much or it was too hard to install. These factors, combined with the potential educational benefits of captioning for millions of children and adults who struggle with literacy or are learning English as a second language, prompted Congress to pass the Television Decoder Circuitry Act of 1990, which required decoders to be built into all TV sets.

On August 7, 1997, the FCC unanimously approved a new law that mandated captioning on virtually all television programming in the United States. The ruling took effect January 1, 1998, and phases in requirements separately for "old" and "new" programming.

All new (aired for the first time on or after January 1, 1998) video programming must be captioned by January 1, 2006; 75 percent must be captioned by January 1, 2004. For programming aired for the first time before January 1, 1998), 30 percent had to have been captioned by January 1, 2003, and 75 percent by January 1, 2008. With Spanish-language programming, the deadline is 2010 for new programming and 2012 for old programming. See also CAPTION CENTER, CAPTION-CAPABLE TV SETS.

cochlea   A snail-shaped part of the ear located behind the oval window. The cochlea contains fluid, thousands of microscopic hair cells tuned to various frequencies and more than 20 types of cells. This complex inner ear organ contains the ORGAN OF CORTI, which lies between two fluid channels—the scala vestibuli and the scala tympani.

The sodium-rich PERILYMPH fluid of the scala vestibuli is separated from the potassium-rich ENDOLYMPH fluid of the membranous cochlea by the paper-thin REISSNER'S MEMBRANE. Because these two fluids are separated, they maintain a vital difference in electrical charge imperative for the correct function of the cochlea's sensory cells.

The entire membranous part of the cochlea is surrounded by bone, into which there are two entrances: the round and oval windows.

Sound, traveling through the middle ear, reaches the STAPES (the third bone of the ossicles), which is attached to the oval window by a ligament that allows it to move, transferring sound vibrations to the scala vestibuli. This fluid brushes the tiny hair cells (or sensory cells) where separate pitches are registered, generating an electrical cur-

rent that telegraphs sound through acoustic nerves to the brain. Once in the brain, the current is then interpreted as sound.

There are two types of hair cells; about 12,000 outer hair cells and about 3,500 inner hair cells lying close to the core of the cochlea. These hair cells are part of the organ of Corti, which lies on the BASILAR MEMBRANE, both part of the membranous cochlea.

When the hair cells of the cochlea die, there is no way to revive or replace them. These cells can die from a variety of causes, including excess noise and the aging process. The hair cells responsible for registering high notes almost always fail first, perhaps because they are located in a more exposed area.

cochlear duct   See SCALA MEDIA.

cochlear implant   An electronic device that is surgically implanted under the skin behind the ear to stimulate the hearing nerve and enable a hard-of-hearing or profoundly deaf person to perceive some sound; the implant does not restore normal hearing. The device is designed to help people with a SENSORINEURAL HEARING LOSS ("NERVE DEAFNESS"). Cochlear implants are profoundly different from hearing aids and other assistive listening devices, which simply make sounds louder. Sounds provided by even the most powerful and effective hearing aids may not offer much useful benefit to someone with a profound hearing loss in both ears. A cochlear implant, on the other hand, is a medical device designed to bypass damaged parts of the inner ear and to stimulate the nerve of hearing electronically.

The first research on cochlear implants was conducted in France more than 30 years ago. Since then, cochlear implant technology has evolved from a device with a single electrode (or channel) to systems that transmit more sound information through multiple channels.

Cochlear implants are designed to bypass the hair cells that aren't functioning and to stimulate the auditory nerve directly. There are a number of different cochlear implants currently available, but all implant systems consist of a microphone, a speech processor, a transmitter and receiver, and electrodes that are implanted in the cochlea. The implant consists of internal and external components: The internal parts of the device are surgically implanted completely under the skin and include a receiver/stimulator positioned under the skin in a shallow bed made in the bone behind the ear. The receiver/stimulator is attached to 22 tiny electrode bands, arranged along a flexible tubing that is inserted approximately one inch into the COCHLEA (the snail-shaped section of the inner ear containing the hearing nerve endings).

The external components worn outside the body include a speech processor about the size of a calculator, a headset with a transmitting coil (a ring about an inch wide) held in place over the implanted receiver behind the ear by small magnets; and a microphone worn like a BEHIND-THE-EAR HEARING AID. The recipient wears the external microphone behind the ear, and a magnet holds the transmitter to the side of the head near the microphone. Each piece is connected to the speech processor by a thin cord. The speech processor can be worn on a belt or in a pocket; many recipients are so good at disguising the implant system that others aren't aware of it.

As sound enters the microphone, it is sent to the speech processor via the thin cable that connects the headpiece to the speech processor. The speech processor converts the sound into a special signal using sophisticated software programs. The special signal is sent back up the same cable to the headpiece and transmitted across the skin via radio waves to the implanted device. The signal then travels down to the electrodes in the inner ear, stimulating the auditory nerve, which transmits the electrical signal to the brain where it is interpreted as sound.

Cochlear implants have significantly improved the communication skills of some adults who have lost their ability to hear after they learned to speak. More typically, speechreading ability improves. As of 2002, about 59,000 people around the world had received implants. In the United States, about 23,000 people had implants; about 13,000 were adults and 10,000 were children.

The simplest version has a single channel (electrode), but multichannel implants with more than 20 electrodes (each implanted further along the cochlear duct) have considerably enhanced performance. These electrodes are used with a device that encodes frequencies, providing some pitch discrimination. Implants may transmit only certain features of the speech signal (feature-extraction) or the input signal may be transmitted to the electrodes without extraction-specific speech cues (non-feature specific).

Although early expectations were limited to hopes that patients would be able to hear enough sound to increase speechreading, many patients can now understand spoken words without speechreading. Unfortunately, it isn't yet possible to predict who will benefit from a cochlear implant to that extent nor how well one will work for any particular person. When tested, people with similar devices score from 0 percent to 90 percent on speech comprehension tests.

However, there are some risks: besides the usual danger inherent in any surgery, it is possible that the implant could damage the inner ear, destroying residual hearing. There is also risk of skin infection at the surgical site and possible damage to the facial nerve or vestibular system. However, incidence of damage to date has been slight.

Cochlear implants remain a controversial choice in the treatment of hearing problems. As yet, it is unclear how much help the implants can provide to hearing or learning spoken or sign language with children deaf from birth and with those who lost their hearing before acquiring speech or language. Experts stress the implant is not for everyone and research on its value is continuing.

However, new research with implants used in pre- and postlingually deafened children suggests that they can achieve some awareness of sound with this device. Recent research suggests some children deaf since birth can understand some words when using the multichannel implant system. The long-term changes due to implant and tissue interaction are unknown.

Young children can also be candidates for implants. In the United States, 12,000 babies a year are born with some degree of hearing loss. Among those, it is believed that about a third would benefit from a cochlear implant. Cochlear implants together with intensive post-implantation therapy can help young children acquire speech, language, developmental, and social skills. The best age for implantation is still being debated, but most children who receive implants are between two and six years old. Earlier implantation seems to perform better.

Good candidates for implant surgery include those whose cochlea is completely ineffective but whose hearing nerve endings still respond to direct stimulation. In these cases, sound activating the implanted electrode stimulates the hearing nerve, and the person can hear noise that is usually described as different from the original sound. This difference is because the implant can't match the normal complex process of the ear as it converts sound into nerve impulses. Candidates for a cochlear implant include adults and children who meet the following general criteria:

Adults (18 years of age and older)

- Severe-to-profound sensorineural hearing loss in both ears
- Hearing loss acquired after learning oral speech and language
- Limited benefit from appropriate hearing aids; in other words, a score of 30 percent or less on sentence recognition tests in the best-aided listening condition
- No medical contraindications
- A desire to be part of the hearing world

Children (ages two through six)

- Profound sensorineural hearing loss in both ears
- Little or no useful benefit from hearing aids
- No medical contraindications
- High motivation and appropriate expectations (both child and family)
- Placement in an educational program that emphasizes development of auditory skills after the implant has been fitted

Extensive testing is needed to determine if a patient might benefit from the cochlear implant because the implant is designed only for those who receive little benefit from hearing aids. Candidates are usu-

ally at least two years old. Becoming a cochlear implant patient involves an evaluation, including otologic, audiologic, radiographic and psychological tests.

The first visit usually includes a medical exam to make sure there is no active infection or other problem within the middle or inner ear that would interfere with the surgical placement of the implant. Extensive hearing tests must be performed to determine the degree of hearing with and without a hearing aid together with special tests to evaluate potential benefits from hearing aids. A special hearing test determines how well a patient could handle a hearing aid. Speech tests are required for all children and some adults. Other tests that stimulate the inner ear ensure that the hearing nerve is intact and able to carry impulses to the brain. This test usually takes about an hour and is only performed on adults. CT scans can show the condition of the cochlea, and a psychological evaluation will make sure the patient understands the process, and has appropriate expectations for success. Children may be evaluated for any other factors (such as learning disabilities) that could affect performance of the implant.

Cochlear implant surgery is performed under general anesthesia. An incision is made behind the ear to open the mastoid bone, leading to the middle ear. The operation takes from $1^1/_2$ to 5 hours depending on the specific cochlear implant being used, and the hospital stay varies from one night to several days. The patient returns to the implant clinic one to two months after surgery to be fitted with the external portions of the device (signal processor, microphone, transmitter). Technicians teach the patient how to care for the system, and how to listen to sound through the implant. Cochlear implant programs differ in the amount of time required to fit the device and the amount of training they offer. In addition, patients are usually required to return to the clinic at regular intervals for checkup and assessment.

The total cost of the cochlear implant varies depending on the area of the country in which the surgery is done, but it is much more expensive than a hearing aid.

Because cochlear implants are medical devices, they are regulated by the Food and Drug Administration (FDA), and because of this, the many insurance companies will provide benefits that cover some or much of the cost. Whether a device is approved or still under investigation may make a difference as to who can receive the implant, how often return visits to the clinic are required and whether insurance companies will pay for the procedure. It will also make a difference in how much is known about the safety and benefits of a particular device. Each manufacturer of cochlear implants has brochures and other patient information.

The technology behind cochlear implants is changing rapidly. With advancements in technology and continued follow-up research with people who have already received implants, researchers are evaluating new opportunities and additional possible candidates for cochlear implants. See also Appendix II.

Cochlear Implant Association   A nonprofit organization that provides information and support to COCHLEAR IMPLANT users, health professionals and the general public. CIAI distributes educational materials, organizes national and international meetings and conventions, promotes cochlear implant technology and deafness research and advocates on all governmental levels for the rights and services of deaf people. See also Appendix II.

cochlear Ménière's disease   An atypical form of MÉNIÈRE'S DISEASE in which sufferers experience hearing loss, DIZZINESS and TINNITUS—but not the spinning sensation of VERTIGO, as in the classical form of the disorder.

Cogan's syndrome   This inflammation of the cornea, which occurs for no known reason, can also damage new bone formation around the ROUND WINDOW and destroy the ORGAN OF CORTI and cochlear nerve cells, resulting in vertigo, tinnitus and severe SENSORINEURAL HEARING LOSS. Treatment with steroid drugs is often effective in suppressing disease activity; in some patients drugs may be tapered off and stopped, while others require maintenance level treatment.

Cogswell, Alice (1805–1830)   The inspiration behind the establishment of the first permanent school for deaf students in the United States, Alice Cogswell was born in 1805 in Hartford, Connecticut, the third daughter of Dr. MASON FITCH COGSWELL and his wife, Mary.

When Alice was two years old, she contracted cerebrospinal meningitis and lost her hearing before she had completely learned to speak. Whatever speech she had at that point was almost gone by the time she was four, and she could hear very little. Although bright and eager to learn, she fell behind other children her age in spite of the efforts of her family to teach her.

Fortunately for Alice, her neighbors were the THOMAS HOPKINS GALLAUDET family. Alice played with the Gallaudets' children and communicated with them using her own code of gestures.

One day, when Gallaudet spelled "hat" for Alice on the ground, using his hat as an illustration, Alice immediately understood that objects had written names and demanded to learn the names of other objects. This was the beginning of real communication between Gallaudet and a deaf child and the start of a lifelong interest for Gallaudet.

When Gallaudet subsequently opened the American Asylum for the Deaf and Dumb in 1817 (now the AMERICAN SCHOOL FOR THE DEAF), Alice was first in line to attend, carrying a slate with her to communicate with those who did not know sign language.

Alice, who believed she could not live without her father, died 13 days after he had succumbed to pneumonia in 1830. She was 25 years old.

Cogswell, Mason Fitch (1761–1830)   Cofounder of the AMERICAN SCHOOL FOR THE DEAF, this Connecticut surgeon and Yale University professor first became interested in deafness when his daughter Alice became deaf at the age of two from cerebrospinal meningitis, a childhood illness associated with a prolonged high fever.

Cogswell's neighbor was young THOMAS HOPKINS GALLAUDET, who noticed Alice's struggles to communicate with neighbors and began to teach her. Unable to find a school for the deaf in 18th-century America and inspired by Gallaudet's success, Cogswell sent Gallaudet to Europe to learn how to teach deaf children. When Gallaudet returned with a French expert in deaf education, Cogswell—together with Gallaudet and 10 Hartford city fathers—founded the American School for the Deaf in Hartford. See also CLERC, LAURENT; COGSWELL, ALICE.

Coiter, Volcher (1534–1600) A Dutch physician who first traced the path of sound waves from the ear canal through the EARDRUM and middle ear bones into the COCHLEA.

A student of anatomy for many years in some of the most celebrated universities of Italy, Coiter also served as personal physician to Count Palatine Ludwig VI.

He is best known for his book, *De auditus instrumento,* published in 1566 and the first devoted entirely to the ear. The book contained 17 chapters dealing with the various parts of the organ of hearing from anatomical and physiological points of view. His theories were generally accepted by his contemporaries.

Comité International des Sports des Sourds (CISS)
This group was organized in 1924 by representatives from six nations (Belgium, Czechoslovakia, France, Great Britain, the Netherlands and Poland) and is similar to the International Olympic Committee in that it regulates olympic-style competition for deaf athletes.

Formerly named the Comité International des Sports Silencieux, CISS is made up of many national sports federations of deaf people and is supervised by an executive committee made up of one deaf person from each of eight different countries. All business at its international meetings and congress is conducted in GESTUNO (international sign language), and no interpreters are used.

It is staffed by volunteers and earns money through dues, fines and competition fees. Officers of CISS are chosen by the executive committee from among federation members. See also WORLD GAMES FOR THE DEAF.

compliance The ability of the EARDRUM to accept and transmit sound vibrations from the EXTERNAL EAR CANAL to the MIDDLE EAR. Disorders of the eardrum or the middle ear decrease this ability.

Conceptually Accurate Signed English (CASE)
Another term for PIDGIN SIGN ENGLISH or SIGN ENGLISH.

conditioning tests One of several hearing tests designed for infants. In the *visual reinforcement test,* a loud sound is paired with presentation of something visually interesting, such as a flashing light or a puppet. After a number of repetitions, the baby will be conditioned to respond to the sound alone. The sound can then gradually be reduced in intensity and used for testing. Practice sessions may be needed in this test.

In the *conditioned orienting response test,* a sound is sent through one loudspeaker; if the infant turns toward the speaker, a light is flashed. The difference with the conditioned orienting response test from other conditioning tests is that the infant is rewarded for localizing the sound.

In *conditioned play audiometry,* a child is taught to respond to a sound presented through an earphone or loudspeaker by manipulating a toy—for example, putting a peg in a pegboard when a sound is heard. These tests are reliable only if the child is able to respond to the test, usually after the age of two and one half. Adult tests can usually be used after age five.

Sounds used in these tests are either two-syllable sounds, bursts of noise or pure tones. See also AUDIOMETRY.

conduction tests See AUDIOMETRY.

conductive hearing loss People with this type of medically treatable hearing loss usually have normal inner ears but specific problems in the outer or middle ear that prevent sound from getting to the inner ear in a normal way. See also HEARING LOSS.

Conference of Educational Administrators Serving the Deaf (CEASD) A nonprofit organization committed to improved management in programs for deaf students and educational options for deaf people.

The organization was founded in 1869 as the Conference of Superintendents and Principals of American Schools for the Deaf. The dream of EDWARD MINER GALLAUDET, then president of the

Columbia Institution for the Deaf and Dumb (now GALLAUDET UNIVERSITY), was to unite school principals behind his philosophy of communication in the classroom.

Today, the group tries to promote a continuum of educational opportunities for deaf people in North America and to encourage efficient management of schools and programs for deaf people.

The organization holds annual meetings for its members, who must have administrative roles in educational programs for deaf students. In odd-numbered years, its meeting is held at the same time as the CONVENTION OF AMERICAN INSTRUCTORS OF THE DEAF. At these shared meetings, CEASD dedicates one day for its own business, sharing the convention schedule's presentations for the rest of the meeting.

In addition, CEASD (together with the ALEXANDER GRAHAM BELL ASSOCIATION FOR THE DEAF and the Convention of American Instructors of the Deaf) provides certification programs for teachers of deaf students through a confederation called the COUNCIL ON EDUCATION OF THE DEAF.

Conference headquarters are located in Silver Spring, Maryland at Halex House (the building owned by the NATIONAL ASSOCIATION OF THE DEAF). Both CEASD's office and executive director are shared with the Convention of American Instructors of the Deaf. It also shares administrative responsibility with the convention for its journal, AMERICAN ANNALS OF THE DEAF.

congenital nerve deafness   Occurring at or soon after birth, this type of hearing loss may be caused by too little oxygen during a long and difficult delivery. Other causes include KERNICTERUS—a form of jaundice caused by an incompatibility of Rh blood factors between the infant and its mother—and, rarely, an inherited failure of the cochlea to develop properly.

Congenital nerve deafness cannot be cured or improved by surgery, although hearing aids can be helpful to take advantage of whatever residual hearing remains.

Convention of American Instructors of the Deaf
Founded in 1850, the convention is one of the oldest American professional organizations interested in education for deaf students.

Its initial meeting in New York, organized by instructors at the New York Institution for the Deaf, marked the first time that a convention for deaf educators was held anywhere in the world. Among other things, conference attendees adopted the *American Annals of the Deaf* as their official publication. Today, the convention and the CONFERENCE OF EDUCATIONAL ADMINISTRATORS SERVING THE DEAF manage the journal as equal partners. For more than 150 years the *Annals* has focused on the education of deaf students and on information for professionals who teach them. The *Annals* also incorporates the broad interests of educators in the general welfare of deaf children and adults.

The purpose of the convention is to promote the education of deaf students "along the broadest and most advanced lines." The organization is located in Silver Spring, Maryland in Halex House, owned by the NATIONAL ASSOCIATION OF THE DEAF, and shares its office and executive director with the Conference of Educational Administrators Serving the Deaf. Contact: Convention of American Instructors of the Deaf, P.O. Box 2025, Austin TX 78768; telephone (voice and TDD): 512-441-2225. See also Appendix VII.)

Cornett, R. Orin   **(1913–2002)**   Inventor of CUED SPEECH, Dr. Cornett was also a vice president at GALLAUDET UNIVERSITY. Born in Driftwood, Oklahoma, on November 14, 1913, Cornett earned a B.S. in mathematics from Oklahoma Baptist University in 1934, followed by an M.S. from the University of Oklahoma in 1937 and a Ph.D. in physics and applied mathematics from the University of Texas in 1940. Between 1935 and 1945, Dr. Cornett taught physics, mathematics, and electronics at Oklahoma Baptist University, Penn State University, and Harvard University. In 1959, he became the director of the Division of Higher Education at the U.S. Office of Education. While working there, he reviewed Gallaudet's funding and in the process, learned that most deaf persons have below-grade-level reading skills.

He became interested in deafness in 1965 when he became aware that most persons born deaf are never able to read well enough to enjoy reading, or even to look up a word in the dictionary and learn its meaning. He became convinced that the underlying cause of the reading problem was the lack of any reasonable way to learn spoken language, without which they could not use speech for communication, become good speechreaders, or learn to read (as opposed to being taught the recognition of each written word). Dr. Cornett decided that deaf people needed a convenient way to represent the spoken language accurately, through vision, in real time. He became vice president for long-range planning at Gallaudet University in August 1965 and during his first year, developed cued speech as a way to help children with hearing problems to become good readers.

Dr. Cornett remained vice president of long-range planning at Gallaudet University until 1975, when he became research professor and director of Cued Speech Programs, a position he held until 1984.

He adapted cued speech to more than 50 languages and major dialects and wrote and published audiocassette lessons in 34 of these languages and dialects.

Dr. Cornett retired from Gallaudet University in 1984. He died of a heart attack on December 17, 2002, at his home in Laurel, Maryland.

Corti, Alfonso (1822–1888) With the aid of a powerful compound microscope, Corti traced the BASILAR MEMBRANE attached to the lamina and detected thousands of tiny hair cells that rest on the membrane.

Now known collectively as the ORGAN OF CORTI, these cells make up the actual hearing organ and are linked to the brain through the auditory nerve.

cosmetic surgical reconstruction A procedure performed to correct a malformation of the external ear (also called PINNA or auricle). The most common cosmetic reconstruction of the external ear is to treat excessively protruding ears caused by hypertrophic development of the conchal cartilage or insufficient folding of the antehelix ridge. In the worst cases, the ears can extend at a 90 degree angle from the scalp.

If cosmetic surgery is to be performed, it is usually done while the child is young. In the operation, a surgeon cuts the skin behind the ear, excises a portion of the exposed cartilage and moves the antehelix closer to the mastoid bone, holding it in place with stitches.

Cosmetic surgery is also beneficial in the treatment of macrotia (an overdeveloped external ear), which can affect one or both ears.

It is also possible to totally reconstruct the ear. Generally, there is a rudimentary ear already present, which is cut in half horizontally to form the new ear. A piece of tubular skin graft or rib cartilage is placed between the two halves, inserted under the skin over the mastoid bone.

cotton swabs Despite frequent warnings against their use in the ear, these small sticks tipped with cotton are often used to dislodge EARWAX within the ear canal. In actuality, the swabs can push the wax farther into the ear canal, potentially damaging the eardrum. A punctured eardrum with a hole larger than 1.5 mm will produce a CONDUCTIVE HEARING LOSS by interfering with the eardrum's vibration. Larger holes can cause even greater hearing loss; for example, perforation of less than 20 percent of the eardrum causes a 15 dB hearing loss. Destruction of the entire eardrum can result in a maximum of 45 dB loss. Swabs such as these are particularly dangerous when used to clean the ears of infants, whose uncontrolled movements can force the swab deep into the ear with disastrous results.

An infant's outer ear may be cleaned with a wet washcloth, but nothing should ever be placed into the ear canal. Accumulated earwax in danger of blocking hearing may be removed by a physician; however, most earwax is normal and is a natural way for the ear to protect itself.

Council on Education of the Deaf Founded in 1960, this group, representing more than 10,000 teachers, sets standards for teachers of deaf students, conducts evaluations of teacher training programs and issues certificates for teachers of deaf students. There are about 15,000 teachers serving more than 46,000 deaf and hard-of-hearing students in classes throughout the United States and Canada.

The council coordinates the efforts of three groups involved in deaf education: the CONFERENCE OF EDUCATIONAL ADMINISTRATORS SERVING THE DEAF, the CONVENTION OF AMERICAN INSTRUCTORS OF THE DEAF and the ALEXANDER GRAHAM BELL ASSOCIATION FOR THE DEAF.

The professional certification of teachers of deaf students had first been studied separately by the Alexander Graham Bell Association and the Conference of Educational Administrators Serving the

Deaf. The two plans that had been developed by these organizations were administered separately, as a teacher registry (Bell) and as a certification program (CAID) until 1935, when they were joined into a single program. See also Appendix II.

Council on Professional Standards The primary certification and accreditation board of the AMERICAN SPEECH-LANGUAGE-HEARING ASSOCIATION (ASHA) located at the association's headquarters in Rockville, MD. Originally established as a certification board in 1959 as the American Board of Examiners in Speech Pathology and Audiology, the group was renamed in 1980 to better describe its larger role as both a certifying and accrediting organization. The council concerns itself not only with the certification of individuals, but with the accreditation of college and university programs and the clinical programs that employ speech-language pathologists and audiologists. See also Appendix II.

Court Interpreter's Act This 1978 act of Congress ensures that people with hearing problems will be given an interpreter if they are involved as the defendant in proceedings brought by the federal government in a district court. It was later amended and broadened by the 1979 BILINGUAL, HEARING- AND SPEECH-IMPAIRED COURT INTERPRETERS ACT. The law requires that either an oral or manual interpreter must be provided at public expense whenever a defendant has a hearing problem that inhibits the ability to communicate or understand testimony.

Before the act was passed, interpreters were allowed but not required, and the decision to have an interpreter was left up to the individual judge. In many occasions, however, judges did not ask for an interpreter, and individuals with hearing problems did not receive communication assistance. Because of this, subsequent appellate court rulings stipulated that without the ability to communicate with lawyers and confront witnesses, hard-of-hearing people are deprived of their constitutional right to due process under the law.

The act requires that the clerk of each U.S. district court maintain a current list of all court-certified interpreters within that court's jurisdiction. The director of the administrative office of U.S.

courts is responsible for outlining qualifications for interpreters.

An interpreter may be appointed at the request of the judge, the hard-of-hearing person's attorney or the person himself. Hard-of-hearing people may waive the right to a court-appointed interpreter and use their own interpreters, who will still be paid by the court. The interpreter can interpret simultaneously, consecutively or in summary (although the latter is not recommended).

In court actions outside of federal court, a hard-of-hearing defendant or witness may ask for help from the court clerk in locating an interpreter, but the interpreter may not necessarily be provided at public expense. The presiding judge will determine who should pay for the interpreter.

Further, privileged communications between defendant and attorney through the interpreter are confidential, and the interpreter cannot be required to testify about them. See also INTERPRETERS AND THE LAW; LEGAL RIGHTS.

CRIS-CROS hearing aid Because of feedback problems, a person with severe hearing loss in both ears may be unable to wear HEARING AIDS at ear level. (Feedback occurs when the amplifier leaks sound back into the microphone because it is too close to the receiver.) In this case, a CRIS-CROS aid uses two CROS HEARING AIDS behind the ear, each unit encompassing the microphone for the other side.

CROS hearing aid Named for "contra-lateral routing of signals" and also called a "crossover" system, this is a special HEARING AID for people with normal hearing in one ear and moderate to severe hearing loss in the other.

This system features a microphone, amplifier and controls beside the poorer ear in a partial mold that feed the amplified signal to the receiver or earphone in the better ear, thereby eliminating "head shadow" (the head blocking sound from the better ear). The amplified sound from the hearing aid on the one side is added to the normal sound entering the healthy ear. The two sides are usually linked by a built-in FM radio signal system, although there are wired models available.

This system may help make speech easier to understand for people with a high frequency loss in both ears. It also allows the listener to understand from which direction sounds are coming.

The benefit of this type of hearing aid system is that it can prevent feedback, which occurs when amplification leaks sound into the microphone located near the receiver.

cued speech This method of communication was developed in 1966 by Dr. R. ORIN CORNETT as a speechreading support system that, in English, uses eight hand configurations and four hand positions near the mouth to supplement visible speech. As such, it's closer to an oral than a manual approach.

The hand cue signals a visual difference between sounds that look alike on the lips, such as "p" and "b." These cues enable the deaf person to see the phonetic equivalent of what others hear.

Each cue (hand placement or configuration) identifies a special group of two to four speech sounds. The combination of cues and mouth movements makes all the essential speech sounds appear different from each other, so that the spoken message is clarified.

The hand configurations and locations are called cues, not cued speech, which is the combination of the cues with speech (the cues are not readable alone).

Each hand configuration identifies a group of consonants; vowel sounds are shown by position of the hand in one of four ways, all within a few inches of the mouth (the side of the face, throat, chin and corner of the mouth).

Cued speech can also be used to indicate approximate voice pitch for each syllable uttered, which is important in tonal languages (such as Thai, Cantonese and Mandarin). For example, in Cantonese, the syllable "ma" can mean "mother," "scold," "horse" or "right?" depending on the pitch.

Tone cueing is also helpful in speech therapy. In order to cue tone, a person changes the inclination of the cueing hand to indicate changes in pitch.

Cued speech has been adapted to many languages, and audiocassette lessons designed for self-instruction by hearing persons are available. (See Appendix XII.) The system is generally the same in all languages.

Cued speech was developed primarily because some congenitally deaf persons do not become good readers because they don't have an easy way to learn spoken language as young deaf children, according to Dr. Cornett. Proponents believe cued speech makes spoken language visually clear and solves the communication problem and also helps youngsters learn a spoken language more easily. It is an easily learned system, taking only about 12 to 20 hours to master. It is most successful when used consistently from early childhood.

Initial research suggests that cued speech does help make the spoken language clear, but the long-term effectiveness of the language is not known. One of the recent advances used in conjunction with cued speech is the AUTOCUER, a device invented by Dr. Cornett, which contains a miniature computerized speech processor that automatically analyzes speech input and produces cue-equivalents through light signals.

There was a great deal of initial interest in cued speech after it was introduced in the 1960s, but it was overshadowed by the spread of TOTAL COMMUNICATION at about the same time. Cued speech tries to clear up some of the problems with speech reading. However, it has not been widely adopted in schools, and is not widely popular among the deaf population. It is popular in Australia and Canada, however. See also NATIONAL CUED SPEECH ASSOCIATION.

cytomegalovirus (CMV) One of the family of herpes viruses, this infection is fairly common in pregnant women; if a woman becomes infected for the first time while she is pregnant, she can pass the infection on to her baby since the virus can cross the placenta. Approximately 80 percent of adults have CMV antibodies in the blood, indicating prior infection. It usually produces no symptoms.

About 11 percent of babies born to mothers infected with CMV during pregnancy will have a bilateral, SENSORINEURAL HEARING LOSS of varying severity. Hearing loss in these infants most often is profound, although there are milder losses in some babies.

Some studies suggest CMV has replaced rubella as the most common viral cause of prenatal

dactylology   A term that generally refers to FIN-GERSPELLING, although it has been used sometimes to include signs.

DAF   See DELAYED AUDITORY FEEDBACK.

Dalgarno, George (1626?–1687)   This 17th-century Scottish theoretician's interest in techniques for teaching deaf students grew out of his fascination with the idea of a universal language for all people.

The headmaster of a private grammar school in England, Dalgarno discussed his theories and techniques for teaching deaf students to speak in *The Deaf and Dumb Man's Tutor,* in which he explained that the senses were connected in complex ways. He believed that a person blind from birth could learn quicker than a deaf person. However, with maturity, a deaf person would surpass a blind person in learning because, Dalgarno thought, sight was more essential to education in the long run than hearing. Although he implicitly believed that a deaf person could learn to speak and speechread, he believed that writing and his manual alphabet (a variation of the ROCHESTER METHOD, which he called DACTYLOLOGY) were more practical.

Espousing a natural language approach and early language stimulation, Dalgarno believed that a deaf infant could learn as quickly as a hearing baby if given the proper stimulation.

Danish Mouth-Hand System   See MOUTH-HAND SYSTEMS.

Danish Sign Language   Considered to be the primary language of deaf people in Denmark, Danish Sign Language has about 6,000 signs and is used together with the INTERNATIONAL HAND ALPHABET intro-duced by the WORLD FEDERATION OF THE DEAF in 1975. This manual alphabet is now used in Norway, Denmark and Finland. In addition to fingerspelling, a MOUTH-HAND SYSTEM has become an integral part of DSL.

Deaf Danish students were first taught in 1807 using methods based on the French manual method of ABBÉ CHARLES-MICHEL DE L'EPÉE. Danish students were using their own signs, but teachers supplemented these with French signs when necessary; this influence by FRENCH SIGN LANGUAGE is still noticeable in the Danish sign vocabulary.

Although the oral method of education was introduced in 1881, DSL was never banned from Danish schools. Today, the five deaf schools all emphasize a manual educational method.

In addition, a combination of spoken Danish and sign language is called Signed Danish. It is used, as in many other sign systems around the world, primarily when communicating between deaf and hearing people and in interpreting.

D.E.A.F., Inc.   The Developmental Evaluation Adjustment Facility, Inc., is a multiservice agency serving deaf people in New England. Acting as a sister organization to GLAD in California, the agency offers independent living services, an evaluation unit, education and training and also sponsors the telephone relay (TDD) service for Massachusetts. In addition, D.E.A.F. sponsors Project Alas, a service for deaf Latinos and their families. See also Appendix II.

deaf and dumb   An archaic term coined by Aristotle meaning that a person can neither hear nor speak. The term is not in favor today because of its negative implication that deaf people are also "dumb" in a literal sense.

Deaf and Hard-of-Hearing Entrepreneurs' Council
A group that encourages, recognizes and promotes entrepreneurship by people who are deaf or hard-of-hearing.

Deaf Artists of America   A group organized to bring support and recognition to deaf artists by collecting, publishing and disseminating information about deaf artists. It also provides cultural and educational opportunities and services to members and exhibits and markets deaf artists' works.

The group offers two directories—one of visual artists and one of performing artists. The directory of visual artists (such as painters, sculptors and graphic designers) includes names, addresses, telephone numbers, education, type of artist and availability, along with several photographs of artwork. The directory of performing artists lists information on individual artists and performing arts groups. It includes names, addresses and telephone numbers of actors, dancers, mimes, poets and storytellers with information on their availability, fees and willingness to travel.

deaf-blindness   The twin difficulties of the inability to see and hear cause special problems for the individual as well as the person's teachers and rehabilitators. The exact term used to describe people who are both deaf and blind is controversial. People who are both deaf and blind sometimes prefer their condition to be described as "deafblind" or "deaf-blind." Some people feel that removing the hyphen to create one word separates the condition from deafness and from blindness, reflecting the unique nature of the condition. Others assert that hyphenating the words achieve this distinction. Because deaf-blindness is rare, there has been relatively little help from agencies in this country. The first federal program for deaf-blind people was legislated only in 1968.

This legislation authorized and funded the rehabilitation facility called the National Center for Deaf-Blind Youth and Adults and regional educational programs for deaf-blind students, aimed at helping states educate deaf-blind children.

Although the particular problems of deaf-blind citizens were not widely known, the 1964 rubella epidemic brought the problem to the attention of the U.S. Congress—of the 30,000 infants who suffered visual or auditory systems problems because of this epidemic, about 1,500 were born blind and deaf. In 1966, there were 564 deaf and blind students in this country, but only 177 were enrolled in school. A realization of the impending influx of deaf-blind students prompted Congress to appropriate special funds for their education in 1968.

Deaf-blind people have a loss of two senses in common, but there is wide variation among their other abilities, just as in the hearing and sighted population.

One of the problems faced by deaf-blind people is the definition of deaf-blindness: Different facilities and educational programs define it differently. Further, blindness itself is defined differently across the country. Many groups support this definition: Deaf-blindness involves visual and auditory problems so great that they prevent accommodation in programs for those who are only visually impaired or hard of hearing.

The number of deaf-blind people in the United States is hard to calculate, but a national study commissioned by the Department of Education in 1980 estimated between 42,000 and more than 700,000, depending on how deaf-blindness is defined.

Most people who are deaf-blind are over age 65 because as individuals get older, the risk of impairments increase. More women than men are deaf and blind, which may be related to a woman's longer lifespan. The study also revealed the so-called rubella bulge (the excess number of children born blind and deaf during the 1964–65 rubella epidemic), who were from 14 to 16 years old at the time of the study.

In the absence of epidemics, between 250 and 300 deaf-blind children can be expected to be born each year because of genetic problems, accidents and diseases.

Only 1.7 percent of deaf-blind people are institutionalized, which means that for every person institutionalized, more than 50 are living in the general population.

Despite this national study, many gaps in understanding this population remain. There is no available data on socioeconomic status, education, race, employment or civil status of deaf-blind people, which inhibits efforts to reach this population.

Education

Teaching a deaf-blind child is certainly difficult, but it is not impossible. According to the National Needs Assessment of Services for Deaf-Blind Persons, the major obstacle to success is the low opinion of the abilities of deaf-blind people held by parents, teachers and society.

When the Elementary and Secondary Education Act of 1968 was passed, it authorized the establishment of centers for deaf-blind children. But it was not until the passage of the Education for All Handicapped Children Act of 1975 (PL 94-142) that education for all deaf-blind children could be guaranteed, since any local agency could deny education to a student it considered too difficult (or costly) to teach. From 1968 to 1980, enrollment for deaf-blind students increased from 110 to 6,000.

According to research, even children born blind and deaf can be taught to communicate, especially if provided with early intensive intervention soon after birth. Without early efforts to stimulate deaf-blind infants, they develop stereotypical, asocial behavior in an effort to provide the stimulation they don't get from their environment. To counteract this, parents must provide continual, consistent stimulation of taste, feel, smell, movement and temperature together with enhancing whatever residual sight or hearing the child has.

Although deaf-blind children are just as intelligent as sighted and hearing children, their communication problems mean they acquire knowledge more slowly and often show self-stimulatory behavior. This behavior, which appears almost autistic, can include waving fingers, rocking and rubbing their eyes.

History

The first deaf-blind student successfully educated was LAURA DEWEY BRIDGMAN, who was taught by 19th-century educator Samuel Gridley Howe, director at the Perkins Institute for the Blind in Massachusetts. Eight-year-old Laura first learned the names of objects by feeling raised letters that spelled out their names and were pasted on the objects. She later learned the manual alphabet, although she never learned to speak.

Her educational success was followed by HELEN KELLER's, who was taught by another Perkins school graduate, Anne Sullivan. Keller later attended Perkins and met the elderly Laura Bridgman.

The first school with a formal program for deaf-blind students was Perkins, which established a department for the education of deaf-blind students in 1931. This was followed by seven other schools for deaf-blind students within the next 30 years.

Deaf Entertainment Foundation (DEF)   An organization that recognizes and encourages excellence among deaf artisans and that promotes the realistic portrayals of the deaf and hard-of-hearing world. The Deaf Entertainment Guild Directory (DEG) lists more than 150 talented people (the largest publication of its kind), including deaf, hard-of-hearing and hearing people who are fluent in American Sign Language.

Deafness, Speech and Hearing Publications, Inc. (DSHP)   A joint venture of the AMERICAN SPEECH-LANGUAGE-HEARING ASSOCIATION and GALLAUDET UNIVERSITY in Washington, D.C., this group was formed to condense information from published sources about the processes and disorders of human speech and hearing. It published a quarterly journal, *dsh Abstracts.*

Formerly called the National Index on Deafness, Speech and Hearing, the DSHP published research abstracts in January, April, July and October. Since 1983, *dsh Abstracts* selected relevant citations from the National Library of Medicine's computerized bibliographic database (MEDLINE), which reviews 3,000 domestic and foreign biomedical journals monthly.

Early in 1985, Gallaudet and ASLHA decided to discontinue subsidizing *dsh Abstracts* and disbanded DSHP; the last issue appeared in October 1985.

Deafness and Communicative Disorders Branch
This office is part of the Rehabilitation Services Administration in the Office of Special Education and Rehabilitative Services of the federal Department of Education.

Designed to promote better rehabilitation services for deaf, hard-of-hearing, speech-impaired and language-disordered people, the office offers technical assistance to administration staff, public and private agencies and individuals and funds interpreter training programs.

Deafness Research Foundation (DRF) The nation's largest voluntary health organization devoted primarily to furthering research into the causes, treatment and prevention of hearing loss and other ear disorders.

Founded in 1958, this group provides grants for fellowships, symposia and research, provides information and referral services and publishes *The Receiver.*

Second only to the federal government in its research support into hearing loss and ear problems, the DRF also maintains an otologic fellowship program to aid talented third-year medical students interested in research. Since the foundation began, it has awarded more than $21 million through more than 1,750 research grants. See also Appendix II.

DEAFPRIDE A nonprofit, community-based advocacy organization that works for the human rights of all deaf people and their families. DEAFPRIDE helps groups organize and work together for change in the District of Columbia and throughout the country.

DEAFPRIDE also provides interpretative services for residents of the Washington, D.C., metropolitan area, the agencies that employ them and the programs that provide social, health, legal and educational services, including a 24-hour emergency service for medical and legal emergencies.

The organization is working for a changed society where deaf people are understood as persons with their own language and culture and who have equal access to everything society has to offer. The organization has a special focus on deaf people who have the least access to resources and education. See also Appendix II.

DEAFTEK.USA An international nonprofit organization focused on job opportunities for deaf and hard-of-hearing people. DEAFTEK was established in 1978 by the Deaf Communications Institute of Framingham, Massachusetts. No longer in operation, the institute was an independent organization that focused on telecommunications services and offered a range of other communications services in addition to DEAFTEK. See also Appendix II.

decibel A measure of the intensity of sound. Zero decibel (dB) is the softest intensity of sound or speech that can be heard by a normal person; 100 dB is the most intense sound an audiometer can produce.

degree of hearing loss An indication of how much hearing loss has been sustained. Specific terms are used to define this loss.

Hearing Impairment A hearing loss of any degree in one or both ears.
Mild Loss Loss of some sounds.
Moderate Loss A loss of enough sounds so that a person's ability to understand his surrounding environment is affected, including some speech sounds.
Significant Bilateral Loss Loss of hearing in both ears with the better ear having some difficulty hearing and understanding speech.
Severe Loss Many sounds are not heard, including most speech sounds.
Profound Loss An inability to hear almost all sounds, generally over 90 dB.
Deafness In this sense, the ability to hear is disabled to an extent that precludes the understanding of speech through the ear alone with or without the use of a hearing aid. (This definition was adopted in 1974 by the CONFERENCE OF EDUCATIONAL ADMINISTRATORS SERVING THE DEAF.)

delayed auditory feedback (DAF) Also called delayed side tone, this is a speech signal delayed on the return to the speaker's ears. Research shows that when a person's own speech is delayed to his ears by 200 msec, the delay will cause a change in vocal rate and intensity as the person continues to speak simultaneously with the DAF. This theory can be used in tests to diagnose FUNCTIONAL HEARING LOSS.

diabetes and hearing loss This metabolic disorder results in a decrease or absence of insulin, the hormone responsible for the absorption of glucose into cells, where it is used for energy. Because diabetes tends to degenerate blood vessels and peripheral nerves, compromising blood supply to the ear and the internal auditory canal, it can result in a degeneration of cochlear and vestibular nerves and cause a SENSORINEURAL HEARING LOSS.

digital hearing aid A type of aid that allows an external computer to program the hearing aid to match the hearing ability of the wearer. The aid also has the capability to reduce noise and adjust itself and features advanced signal processing techniques and better ways to process speech signals.

The problem with these aids to date is that they consume more power and take up more space than conventional HEARING AIDS. To offset these problems, a hybrid hearing aid has been developed that offers conventional amplifiers and filters that are adjusted automatically by a digital control. These hybrids are small enough to be worn on or in the ear.

diplacusis A condition in which a given frequency produces a different pitch in each ear; this common problem is called binaural diplacusis. The disorder is diagnosed by having the patient adjust the frequency in one ear to equal the pitch to a reference pitch in the other ear.

Although it is normal for a person with normal hearing to have slight differences in pitch between the two ears, people with a cochlear or retrocochlear hearing problem may experience up to an octave difference in pitch.

A related condition, called monaural diplacusis, results in hearing a group of tones when only one tone is actually present.

Often, an individual is unaware of having diplacusis unless he or she is a musician.

direct audio input (DAI) A recent technological advance designed to lessen the problem of hearing aid sound distortion, the DAI features a cord attached to a behind-the-ear aid either by a special outlet or by a connector called a "shoe," which may be added to the hearing aid. This cord is attached to a plug to connect to any type of sound source, such as TV, radios, tape recorders and FM ASSISTIVE LISTENING DEVICES.

The direct connection eliminates many of the background noises that often disturb the users of HEARING AIDS.

discomfort level The level at which pure tones and/or speech become too loud for comfort to the listener. See also AUDIOMETRY.

discrimination The percentage of a word list with or without background noise that is understood by an individual as part of a hearing test. See also AUDIOMETRY.

dispensing audiologist An AUDIOLOGIST who sells HEARING AIDS. Generally, they have more training than a hearing aid dispenser. See also HEARING AID DEALERS.

distortion break The level at which sounds become unnatural as HEARING AIDS are turned up.

dizziness This sensation of unsteadiness is a mild form of VERTIGO, which is characterized by a feeling of spinning either of oneself or the surroundings.

Although most attacks of dizziness are harmless, they may occur because of a disorder of the inner ear, hearing nerve or the brain.

In LABYRINTHITIS, a viral infection can inflame the fluid-filled canals within the inner ear, affecting balance; in severe cases, even a sudden movement of the head can cause dizziness and fainting. In the inner ear degenerative syndrome called MÉNIÈRE'S DISEASE, dizziness and vertigo are common symptoms.

In more rare cases, a tumor or MENINGITIS affecting the hearing nerve can cause dizziness. Any disorder of the brain stem that connects with the hearing nerve—such as reduced blood supply or tumors—can also result in dizziness.

In cases of dizziness caused by disorders of the inner ear, some physicians may recommend antiemetic or antihistamine drugs.

Doerfler-Stewart test An auditory test used to determine FUNCTIONAL HEARING LOSS or psychogenic hearing loss by testing a patient's ability to respond to spondee words (two long or accented syllables) spoken in the presence of a masking noise presented through earphones. In cases of a functional hearing loss, the patient will be unable to respond consistently to words at varying intensity levels. See also AUDIOMETRY.

Down's syndrome   A disorder caused by a chromosomal problem and resulting in mental retardation and physical deformities. People born with this syndrome often have irregularities in the middle and inner ears and are susceptible to middle ear infections (OTITIS MEDIA) that can cause CONDUCTIVE HEARING LOSS.

Down's syndrome is caused by an excess chromosome, usually number 21. About one in 650 babies is born with the syndrome, and the incidence of affected babies rises sharply with maternal age, to about one in 40 in mothers over age 40.

In addition to hearing problems, most people with Down's syndrome have a typical facial appearance, including sloping eyes with extra folds of skin, a small face and features and a small oral cavity. The degree of mental retardation varies, although many of these children are educable.

Although medical techniques have improved the prognosis for people with Down's syndrome and have extended their life expectancies, many still do not survive beyond early middle age.

drugs and deafness   See OTOTOXIC DRUGS.

dual party relay service   See RELAY SERVICE.

Dutch Sign Language   Formally known as Sign Language of the Netherlands (SLN), this sign language has five separate dialects, each related to a school for deaf students. There are about 25,000 deaf Dutch people who use sign language.

Dutch Sign Language is based on signs invented in 1827 and later formally taught in a school based on the educational principles of French deaf educator ABBÉ CHARLES-MICHEL DE L'EPÉE. Developed from French Sign Language, some features are similar to British and American Sign Languages. However, most other Dutch schools were oral in approach, and these students developed their own signs independent of their schools.

It is only recently that Dutch educators have begun to accept SLN based on new research findings. The language is different from Signed Dutch.

dysacusis   Meaning "faulty hearing," the term includes any hearing problem not caused primarily by a loss of auditory sensitivity.

From the word *acusis* (or "acousis"), referring to hearing, and *dys*, meaning ill or painful, the word is also spelled *dysacusia* and *dysacousia*. It is caused by a malfunction or injury of the central nervous system, the auditory nerve or the organ of Corti and is not helped by amplifying speech. Therefore, dysacusis is not measured in decibels.

It must be emphasized that deafness/hearing loss and dysacusis are not necessarily mutually exclusive; for example, a person may have both HEARING LOSS measured in decibels and also a dysacusis in the form of a loss of discrimination.

Dysacusis may also be used as a broader term meaning loss of all kinds of hearing—two or three of which may be present in the same person. On the other hand, *hard-of-hearing* implies specifically one kind of problem—loss of sensitivity.

There are several types of dysacusis, including discrimination loss for words, syllables or PHONEMES; reduced intelligibility for sentences; AUDITORY AGNOSIA; phonemic regression; and binaural DIPLACUSIS and monaural diplacusis.

dysphasia   Speech or language problem. It is thought that children with dysphasia hear sounds but can't make sense of them, or, if they can make sense, they are unable to put their responses into words. There may be problems with perception, sound discrimination, auditory memory, comprehension, word-finding, reading and writing.

Unlike adults with APHASIA (often following a stroke), there is no loss of previous function; instead, children fail to develop normal language.

Sometimes, deaf children are wrongly labeled aphasic or dysphasic, especially those who don't make progress in oral-only programs. Because there are not any clearcut tests for developmental dysphasia, careful and repeated evaluations are necessary.

ear See INNER EAR; MIDDLE EAR; or OUTER EAR.

earache The most common cause of this severe, stabbing pain is an infection of the middle ear (OTITIS MEDIA). Otitis media occurs most often in young children and the stabbing pain is usually accompanied by a fever and a temporary loss of hearing. If the eardrum breaks, the pain and pressure is relieved immediately.

Another common cause of earache is otitis externa (also called SWIMMER'S EAR), which is the inflammation of the outer ear canal, usually caused by an infection. This infection may affect the whole canal or only parts of it and may form an abscess or boil. There may be irritation or itching, discharge and temporary mild deafness as well.

Much more rare is earache resulting from herpes zoster, which can cause blisters in the ear canal and can produce pain for weeks or months after the infection has ended.

Earaches that come and go could also occur from a host of problems, including tooth pain, tonsillitis, throat cancer and pain in the lower jaw or neck. In fact, almost any disorder that affects areas near the ear can cause an earache since the same nerves that serve the ear also supply many nearby areas.

Earaches may be treated with painkilling drugs, and antibiotics are often prescribed for infection. Pus in the outer ear may need to be removed or drained via an operation (MYRINGOTOMY) if it is located in the middle ear.

ear canal See EXTERNAL AUDITORY CANAL.

eardrops Eardrops are prescribed for certain conditions in the outer and middle ears but cannot affect the inner ear. Eardrops cannot restore hearing in cases of nerve damage, but they can treat itch, discomfort or ear infection in the outer or middle ears. Eardrops should only be used upon recommendation by a physician.

eardrum An important part of the hearing mechanism, the eardrum (also called the tympanic membrane) separates the OUTER (external) EAR from the MIDDLE EAR and vibrates with sound or speech. The eardrum is thin and slightly transparent; its inner layer consists of mucous membrane, and its outer layer is skin.

Blood vessels supplying the eardrum are extremely tiny, but inflammation can engorge them and can make them so diffuse that the whole membrane becomes reddish and opaque.

eardrum, perforated A hole (perforation) may appear in the EARDRUM as a result of gradual erosion from chronic OTITIS MEDIA (ear infection). Rupture of the eardrum usually is the result of otitis media when pus builds up and—left untreated—bursts the eardrum.

The eardrum may also be perforated by inserting a sharp object into the ear, a blow on the ear, a loud noise, skull fracture, barotrauma (damage from excessive air pressure) or tumor.

The perforation is usually treated with antibiotics to take care of any infection. Except in the case of a chronic otitis media, this is usually the only treatment required. If a perforation does not close within six months, a TYMPANOPLASTY, also called a myringoplasty, may be performed. See also AERO-OTITIS MEDIA; COTTON SWABS.

Ear Foundation, The A national, nonprofit organization founded in 1971 and committed to leading the effort for better hearing through public and professional educational programs, support services and applied research. The foundation is particularly interested in problems of ear-related disorders, specifically hearing loss and balance disturbances. From its inception, the foundation has been dedicated to the continuing education of ear specialists and to the development of auditory and vestibular research.

The foundation also administers THE MENIERE'S NETWORK, a national network of patient support groups that provide people with Ménière's disease the opportunity to share experiences and coping strategies. See also Appendix II.

ear infection   See OTITIS MEDIA.

ear infection vaccine   The pneumococcal conjugate vaccine (Prevnar), which is designed to prevent meningitis and other serious diseases in infants, toddlers and preschoolers, also can reduce the risk of middle ear infections (OTITIS MEDIA) caused by the same bacteria by about 10 percent.

The American Academy of Pediatrics recommends the vaccine for all children less than two years of age. Children 24 months to 59 months are eligible for the vaccine if they are at high risk for serious pneumococcal disease, including Native Americans, Alaskans, premature infants, and children with poor immune systems.

ear lobe   This fleshy hanging lower portion of the outer ear, also called the lobule, is the only part of the external ear that does not contain any cartilage.

ear massage   Although it is untrue that pressing on the skull behind the ear or on the neck can improve hearing, gentle massage can restore hearing caused by a problem with the EUSTACHIAN TUBE.

However, ear massage can also cause disarticulation of the middle ear bones and is not recommended.

When the eustachian tube doesn't equalize pressure in the MIDDLE EAR cavity (such as during an airplane flight), rubbing the ear gently, yawning, swallowing, chewing and so forth can fill the middle ear with the needed air.

earmold   Part of the HEARING AID system, the earmold is a plastic insert that, when fitted into the ear or ear canal, conducts the amplified sound into the ear.

Earmolds come in many shapes, depending on the type of hearing aid and the physical shape of the person's ear. For example, earmolds in canal and in-the-ear aids encase all the hearing aid's components. Earmolds for behind-the-ear and eyeglass hearing aids are placed in the ear and are connected to the hearing aid by a piece of clear plastic tubing. Body type aids have an earmold that allows a button-shaped receiver to snap into a metal ring on its back, with a cord connecting the earmold to the rest of the aid.

When a hearing aid is selected and fitted, the AUDIOLOGIST or dispenser will make an impression of the ear to customize the earmold. Earmolds are made of various types of material, including hard plastic or several varieties of soft, pliant materials. Hypoallergenic earmolds are also available.

An earmold should fit snugly into the ear without pain or a "plugged up" feeling; a loose fit could cause feedback or whistling. Modifications can alleviate problems with earmolds; for example, a hole bored in an earmold can alleviate pressure in the ear canal, and a larger vent can alter the response of the hearing aid so that it is more appropriate in certain types of hearing loss.

ear muffs   See EAR PROTECTORS.

earplugs   See EAR PROTECTORS.

ear protectors   There are two types of ear protecting devices: earplugs, which fit inside the ear canal, and ear muffs, which fit outside the ears. Earplugs and earmuffs worn together provide the most effective protection against noise.

Earplugs

Earplugs to be used for protection against noise should not be purchased over the counter, such as the earplugs designed for swimming. In order to be effective in screening out excess noise, earplugs must fit snugly in the ear canal so that no air can get through. In addition, a person's ears may not be the same size, requiring earplugs of two different dimensions.

Custom-fit earplugs are made to fit only one person's ears, usually by an AUDIOLOGIST or hearing aid dispenser. One type of earplug has a valve that allows soft sounds—such as voices or speech—to pass through, but closes for loud sounds.

In fitting the earplugs, the dealer makes an impression of the ear canal and sends the dimensions to a manufacturer, where the soft rubber earplug insert is made. These fitted earplugs should only be used by adults, since the ear canals of children and teenagers change rapidly.

Earplugs must fit properly in order to shut out sound and must be kept clean to avoid infection. Most types give about 30 decibel protection against excess noise.

Earmuffs

Earmuffs can provide even more effective sound protection than earplugs and are preferable if there is a draining ear or chronic infection. In addition, some ear canals simply don't accept earplugs without pain.

Earmuffs completely cover the ear; the earpieces are made of sponge material and are held in place by a tension headband. Earmuff protectors generally cost more than earplugs, but they are harder to lose, and some believe they are more comfortable for daily wear than earplugs. Those who wear glasses, however, may find that the glasses interfere with the earmuffs' seal.

Other Protectors

Dry cotton is almost useless in preventing excess noise. Some types of disposable ear protectors are made of cotton wax and other specially treated material, and these are somewhat effective.

ear squeeze   See AERO-OTITIS MEDIA.

ear structure   Ears collect and decipher everything from whispers to screams, and can distinguish not only one musical note from another but even the same note played on different instruments. Superbly crafted to handle our environment, ears contain a sort of gyroscope to help maintain balance, and can protect themselves against noise and selectively tune out unwanted sounds—even during sleep.

The outer and middle ears amplify some sound waves because of the way the ear canal narrows as it proceeds inward, funneling the noise. Once the sound reaches the eardrum, it is transmitted and amplified by the vibrations of the eardrum's skin. Next, the middle ear's three bones (OSSICLES) receive sound through the drum and push it through the oval window into the inner ear.

Once inside the inner ear, the COCHLEA (a small-shaped system of canals located behind the oval window) takes over to interpret pitch. The cochlea contains fluid and about 20,000 tiny hair cells tuned to various pitch frequencies. When the middle ear's stirrup pushes the sound through the oval window, it makes the cochlea vibrate, and the fluid travels to the tiny hair cells where separate pitches are registered. Hair cells responsible for high notes are located near the base of the cochlea; lower-frequency cells are near the apex.

The cochlea generates tiny electrical currents, sending the sound through acoustic nerve connections to the brain, where it is decoded and presented as one of the 350,000 separate sounds a human can recognize. See also INNER EAR; MIDDLE EAR; OUTER EAR.

ear trumpet   A mechanical HEARING AID first created in the 17th century but popularized at the turn of the 20th century, used to increase sound levels by 10 to 15 decibels.

Many of these devices were designed to hide a hearing problem: Men could wear one under beards and sideburns or carry one concealed in the head of a cane. Women could wear an "aurolese phone," a cup-shaped sound collector that was concealed by elaborate hairdos popular at that time.

Ear trumpets were usually cone- or dome-shaped devices and made of metal, rubber, and plastic.

Related to the ear trumpet were the speaking tube and the hearing fan. Speaking tubes were popular in Europe and included a bell-shaped plastic or rubber speaking end connected to a small eartip by two feet of tubing. Hearing fans, which were really a bone-conduction hearing aid, featured a thin rubber fan held between the teeth, kept taut by strings. Sound passed through the fan to the teeth, through bone to the inner ear.

ear tube   A small tube that is inserted through the EARDRUM during a surgical incision (MYRINGOTOMY) made in the eardrum to treat a chronic middle-ear effusion in children.

The tube serves to equalize the pressure on both sides of the eardrum, which allows the fluid to drain out of the ear. About six to 12 months after the operation, the tube usually falls out on its own as the eardrum heals.

Water should be kept out of the ear in children with an ear tube, and swimming is usually forbidden. See also SEROUS OTITIS MEDIA.

earwax   A yellow or brown secretion called cerumen, earwax is produced only by glands in the outer ear canal. Any wax deeper inside the canal has been pushed there by a finger or a cotton applicator. The normal function of wax in the ear is to protect the skin of the ear canal by keeping it soft and moist.

Among people who have very narrow or hairy ear canals and among people who work in dirty or dusty environments, wax can build up until it completely blocks the ear canal. When wax is pushed into the ear canal and presses on the EARDRUM, it may sometimes cause ear noises and even dizziness, both of which disappear when the wax is removed.

Earwax is a normal part of the body's function and should not be stopped. Removing earwax with a COTTON SWAB is dangerous; probing can remove protective layers of keratin, opening the way for possible infection of skin cells. There is also a danger that the swab could be pushed through the eardrum, causing problems ranging from severe pain to total deafness. Often cotton swabs push wax farther into the ear canal, which eventually causes impacted earwax. To be kept clean, the ear only needs soap, water and a washcloth.

echolocation   The technique of locating objects by emitting bursts of sound and interpreting the echoes; used by sonar and animals such as bats.

Education and Auditory Research (EAR) Foundation   A national nonprofit association of doctors, educators and concerned citizens dedicated to providing information and resources to people who suffer from hearing problems. The EAR Foundation offers support services promoting the integration of people with hearing and balance problems into mainstream society. The foundation also provides practicing ear specialists with continuing medical education courses and related programs specifically regarding rehabilitation and hearing preservation. Finally, the group tries to educate young people and adults about hearing preservation and early detection of hearing loss, enabling them to prevent at an early age hearing and balance disorders. See also Appendix II.

Education for All Handicapped Children Act   See LEGAL RIGHTS.

education of deaf children   Deafness itself does not affect either a person's intellectual capacity or the ability to learn. Since most deaf children have hearing parents, it is important to begin exposing these children to communication as early as possible. But often, a child's hearing loss—or his parents' acceptance of it—might not come until the second year of the child's life. Even if the parents are willing to learn American Sign Language at that point, it takes time to learn before they become proficient. Crucial early interaction with some form of language has been lost.

Because deaf children of hearing parents are not exposed to a continuous language flow, they miss out on an enormous amount of language stimulation. Language delays can be offset by exposing deaf children to early, consistent visible communication methods (sign language, fingerspelling or cued speech) together with amplification and aural/oral training, if desired.

Only a small percentage of deaf children have deaf parents, but those who do have the great advantage of learning AMERICAN SIGN LANGUAGE (ASL) from the beginning. Studies show that these children progress in language development and acquisition at the same rate as hearing children learn English and outdistance their deaf peers who did not learn ASL from infancy.

Type of School

The first problem facing parents of a school-age deaf child is where to get the best education. In the past, deaf children were educated primarily in residential schools, which provided maximum exposure to the latest technology in deaf education but limited the child's family relationship.

Today, the trend is growing in favor of MAINSTREAMING the child at least part of the day at the local public school, enabling the child to live at home and remain in touch with the neighborhood. This change reflects the popularity of the mainstreaming movement and also the Education for All Handicapped Children Act of 1975, which mandates a free public education for all "handicapped" children in the least restrictive environment and sets specific guidelines to protect their rights. The act also requires each child to receive nondiscriminatory testing and an individualized educational plan that is renewed each year. (See also LEGAL RIGHTS.)

As a result, parents have many more educational options today than they did prior to the 1960s. There are four major choices: residential school, special day school, special day classes, or regular classes supplemented by special services. Each of these options is described below.

Residential schools. These schools board deaf students full time, although most programs allow the students to spend weekends at home with their families. These schools offer instructional, recreational and social programs designed for their deaf pupils. Students who live nearby may attend these residential schools as day pupils.

Day school programs. Deaf students in these programs go to a school exclusively for deaf youngsters but return home in the afternoon like other school children.

Self-contained day classes. Many neighborhood public school systems offer special classes for deaf students. Under this program, deaf students may join hearing students for physical education and art or be "mainstreamed" (put in classes with hearing students) with interpreters for some classes. Usually, these special programs provide a resource room to help deaf students get information for classes they attend with hearing students.

Regular classes. This choice, known as mainstreaming, allows deaf students to attend regular classes with hearing students for most or all of the day. Often, the deaf child may be provided interpreters, tutors and resource room teachers.

In addition, some school districts may design their own programs for deaf students, utilizing some or all of the above methods.

In high school, deaf students can choose to enter a vocational training program or take academic courses with an aim to attending college, either at a regular university or a college for deaf students, such as GALLAUDET UNIVERSITY in Washington, D.C., or the NATIONAL TECHNICAL INSTITUTE FOR THE DEAF in Rochester, New York. In addition, there are many community colleges and technical schools in the United States with special programs for deaf adults.

Manual vs. Oral Approach

In addition to the type of school, parents must make another important—and historically far more controversial— decision. There has been no issue in deaf education more bitterly disputed over the past 200 years than the question of how students and teachers should communicate in the classroom.

The problem was made more difficult by a misunderstanding of American Sign Language by linguists in the first part of the 20th century, who insisted only spoken language was a real language. Today, linguists accept that American Sign Language is indeed a language with its own syntax and grammar and all the richness and complexity of any other language.

The manual approach was brought to this country by educator THOMAS HOPKINS GALLAUDET, who, thwarted in learning the oral English method, studied the French manual method instead. Trained at the famous Paris Institute (Institut National de Jeunes Sourds) in this method, Gallaudet introduced the manual approach to America at the first public school for deaf students in Hartford, Connecticut.

Other methods from Europe soon followed. In 1867, Bernard Engelsmann, a teacher of deaf Viennese students, introduced the German method—the oral approach—in a school for deaf children in New York City, now known as the Lexington School.

In 1878, Zenas Westervelt introduced the ROCHESTER METHOD at a school for deaf students in Rochester, New York, based on a system in which deaf students are taught to speak and fingerspell English simultaneously while written English is also being emphasized.

Gradually, schools in this country began to rely on the oral approach of communication until almost all preschool and elementary classes for deaf children were oral-only and forbade the use of signs or fingerspelling. Schools emphasized oral education based on the theory that any type of manual communication would interfere with English and speech development and would keep the deaf child isolated from the larger hearing world.

But as the skills of deaf students—who have the same intelligence range as hearing children—lagged behind, educators began to question whether all-oral schools were failing large numbers of deaf people. This growing doubt was fueled by studies showing that deaf children of deaf parents out-performed deaf children of hearing parents in academic achievement, social adjustment, reading and written English skills. These studies seemed to show that not only did ASL not inhibit English fluency but apparently enhanced its acquisition. Today, few schools use an oral approach.

Manual approach supporters also argue that many children do not have the aptitude for oral instruction and that the time spent on trying to speak could better be spent developing the child's mental abilities. Further, some advocates of a manual education believe that deaf people prefer to associate with other deaf people and therefore have no need to be able to speak.

Some oral approach supporters, on the other hand, still believe that training in speech and speech reading help the child adjust to a speaking world. By learning to speak, they reason, the deaf child will not be confined to the deaf community or to those willing to use sign or a pad and pencil. They further point out that a person who can speechread and speak may find it easier to land a job. In general, oral supporters believe that orally-trained youngsters are likely to do better as more teachers are trained in this field.

All organizations of deaf educators believe that deaf children should be given the opportunity to learn to speak, but there is often heated debate as to what constitutes "fair opportunity."

Total Communication

Today, programs for deaf students are moving toward a more inclusive form of education called TOTAL COMMUNICATION, which supports a deaf child's right to be exposed to any form of communication that is effective. This includes speech, speechreading, gestures, reading, writing, FINGERSPELLING, manual codes of English, ASL and use of residual hearing.

Most programs today use a manual code of English together with spoken English.

How much the child's inability to hear will affect school performance depends on many things—the degree and type of hearing loss, the age of onset, additional handicaps, the quality of the school and support the child receives.

Typically, deaf children from ages one to three begin their education in a clinical program featuring extensive support from parents. Because 85 percent to 90 percent of deaf children are born to hearing parents, these programs often emphasize the implications of deafness and teach parents how to cope with problems. At age three, the child can attend preschool sessions with other deaf children, and by age four many deaf youngsters attend special nursery and kindergarten classes full time.

In order to learn, deaf children must devise a way to communicate. A child's hearing may be helped by hearing aids, but hearing may still be quite limited. In order to develop a consistent, two-way means of communication, many deaf children and their parents learn sign language.

EEG audiometry   See ELECTROENCEPHALOGRAPHY AUDIOMETRY.

eighth cranial nerve   This nerve, also called the auditory, hearing or cochlear nerve, is really two separate nerves, one responsible for transmitting sound and the other with sending balance information to the brain from the inner ear. The two parts of this nerve are intertwined as they pass through the bony canal leading from the inner ear to the brain.

This nerve is the only connection between the hair cells of the COCHLEA and the cochlear nucleus of the brainstem and is essential for good hearing. The nerve is about 25 millimeters long and contains about 32,000 nerve fibers.

electrocochleogram An electrophysical hearing test that measures impulses in the cochlear nerve by inserting a thin electrode through the EARDRUM into the promontory of the basal turn. This indicates how well the COCHLEA is functioning. See also AUDIOMETRY.

electrodermal response audiometry (EDR) A special hearing test procedure that measures sweat changes on the hands or feet in response to sound or speech and records these changes on a graph.

This test is one of the nonspecific electrophysiologic hearing tests used to estimate the auditory threshold in people who cannot respond voluntarily to auditory stimuli—such as newborns, infants and people with nonorganic hearing loss. See also ELECTROPHYSIOLOGIC AUDIOMETRY.

electroencephalogram (EEG) The measure of the brain's constant low-voltage electric signals. During the 1930s, scientists discovered that sudden loud sounds caused sudden changes in the EEGs of sleeping research subjects. These changes in the EEG were called auditory evoked potentials, since they were evoked, or caused, by a sudden sound.

When several sounds were presented at the same time, however, the evoked potentials became too small to differentiate on the EEG. It was not for another 20 years before the averaging computer was invented, allowing researchers to identify the brain's slight response to a series of sounds.

These auditory evoked potentials can provide information about how the brain responds to sound and also about how healthy the ear is. See also AUDITORY BRAINSTEM RESPONSE TEST.

electroencephalography audiometry A special hearing test that measures brain waves changes in response to sound or speech; it is particularly useful in testing the very young.

In this test, a brief pure tone causes a small variation in the baby's brainwave, which can be measured through the scalp by an electroencephalogram (EEG). During the test, an OTOLOGIST repeats a stimulus up to 100 times and then uses a computer to average the brain's response to these tones, eliminating the effects of background noise. This averaged response establishes the auditory threshold almost as accurately as the more standard audiometric tests in older children. See also AUDIOMETRY.

electromagnetic induction A process used in HEARING AIDS that replaces normal reception of sound by the hearing aid microphone with a direct connection in telephones and many public buildings that have been equipped for that purpose. The benefit of electromagnetic induction is that it significantly reduces amplified background noise.

electronystagmography A test to determine the presence of damage to the body's balance system, which can help determine damage to the inner ear. It records the electrical changes caused by eye movement. This technique has been used successfully for more than 50 years. For this test, electrodes are placed on the face above, below and beside the eyes. The patient is then placed in a variety of situations, and resulting eye movements are electrically recorded. See also AUDIOMETRY.

electrophysiologic audiometry Hearing tests that measure changes in the electric properties of the body as a response to auditory stimuli. Because the client cannot control these responses, electrophysiologic AUDIOMETRY is considered to be a completely objective test of hearing sensitivity.

There are two types of electrophysiologic audiometric tests. The first type measures specific auditory response systems, which respond only to auditory stimulation, including the COCHLEA, the AUDITORY NERVE and certain auditory pathways within the brainstem and the brain. Electrodes are placed on the promontory of the middle ear or in the external ear canal, and instruments pick up the evoked potentials of these systems, which are amplified and extracted from background brain activity.

The second type of test measures nonspecific electrophysiologic response systems, which respond to more than auditory stimulation and are only indirectly related to the auditory stimulation. The cortex, central autonomic centers or spinal autonomic mechanisms are excited by auditory stimuli, which in turn stimulate neural activity or motor reflexes that alter the electrical activity of other mechanisms, including electric recordings of heart rate, electric potential or resistance of the skin as influenced by sweat glands and ongoing electroencephalic activity.

The first electrodermal response tests were developed in the late 1940s to record changes in the electric properties of the skin as influenced by sweat glands. Sweating is an autonomic response that is set in motion when the listener is aroused in anticipation of a coming event. Using classical conditioning, a listener is conditioned to anticipate sensing a shock upon hearing a sound. Although popular up to the 1960s, it fell from favor by the 1970s. It was least effective among very young infants and retarded children.

The heart's response to auditory stimulation is usually identified by computing the difference in electric activity of the heart before and after an auditory stimulus.

By the mid-1960s, scientists began studying evoked response audiometry using a computer to extract an auditory evoked response from ongoing brain activity. Today, it is possible to get a reliable estimate of auditory sensitivity in the very young by using brainstem evoked response audiometry or electrocochleographic audiometry (which uses electric responses from the cochlea to estimate auditory thresholds and gain information about the integrity of the cochlea.) See also AUDITORY BRAINSTEM RESPONSE TEST.

El Mudo   See NAVARRETE, JUAN FERNÁNDEZ DE.

employment of deaf people   Deaf people work in the same jobs as hearing people, and their deafness in itself does not prevent them from doing most jobs. In fact, according to the National Information Center on Deafness at GALLAUDET UNIVERSITY, more and more deaf people have been moving into professional, administrative, managerial and technical careers. Today, they are working as physicians, dentists, lawyers, physicists, engineers and computer analysts and programmers in addition to other technical and professional positions. Prior to the 1970s, however, most deaf people were employed mainly as factory workers, craftspeople and unskilled laborers.

The movement of deaf workers into all job levels can be credited to improved educational opportunities, antidiscrimination laws, a better understanding of deafness by the general public and an increased assertiveness in the deaf community.

Unfortunately, salaries have not kept pace with the upward movement of deaf employees; the average salary of deaf workers has been somewhat less than the salary of hearing workers in similar jobs, although this gap is closing due to antidiscrimination laws.

Like their hearing colleagues, deaf employees vary in skills and working ability. Traditionally, many have been trained in skilled trades such as auto repair, printing, mechanics, electronics, machining and welding. However, better educational services have increased access to professional jobs, enabling deaf individuals to work as computer analysts, statisticians, chemists, geologists, librarians and teachers. All too often deaf workers are underemployed because they work at jobs that do not make full use of their skills. This is not caused by prejudice as much as a consequence of faulty assumptions about how deafness affects job performance. For example, many employers overestimate the need to use a telephone for certain jobs.

encephalitis   An inflammation of the brain itself, encephalitis can cause a large variety of symptoms of brain injury, including central hearing problems. The impairments are usually neurological, not audiological, although sometimes there is a cochlear impairment.

Encephalitis is usually caused by an infective organism; viruses are the most common, although the disease can be caused by many different kinds of organisms, including bacteria, protozoa or worms, or by chemicals. There are two types of viruses that cause encephalitis: viruses (like rabies) that invade the body and do no harm until they are carried by the blood to the brain cells, and other viruses (herpes simplex and zoster, yellow fever) that first harm nonnervous tissues and then invade brain cells. The most common viral cause is herpes simplex Type I (which also causes cold sores). In the United States, mosquitoes carry St. Louis encephalitis, and increasingly cases of encephalitis are caused by infection with HIV (human immunodeficiency virus), responsible for AIDS. Chemicals that can lead to encephalitis include lead, arsenic, mercury, ethyl alcohol, chlorinated hydrocarbons, morphine and barbiturates.

Children often contract the demyelinating encephalitis type, which develops as a complication of viral diseases such as measles or chicken pox, or as a result of vaccination against these diseases. In this case, damage is not done to the cell itself but to the sheath (myelin) around the nerve cell.

Meningoencephalitis is an inflammation of the brain, the meninges (outer layer of the brain) and the spinal cord; symptoms include fever, headache, vomiting and neck and back stiffness.

Common symptoms of most types of encephalitis include fever, headache, drowsiness, lethargy, tremors and coma. Convulsions may occur in patients of any age, but they appear most often in infants. Other symptoms include uncoordinated movements, weakness and unusual sensitivity of the skin to stimuli.

Encephalitis can be diagnosed from a spinal tap (insertion of a needle into the lower part of the back to extract a small sample of cerebrospinal fluid, the liquid that surrounds the entire central nervous system) and from the results of CT scans and EEG (which records electrical activity of the brain). The cause of encephalitis can be determined by a culture for the particular virus involved or by isolating the virus through a brain tissue biopsy. Sometimes, however, the cause of the disease remains unknown and makes treatment difficult. But even if the virus is discovered, there is often no treatment. There are no specific antiviral agents other than those used in the treatment of herpes simplex.

Treatment may be used to relieve some symptoms that remain after the brain inflammation subsides. Intensive medical treatment is required to monitor heart and respiratory function and to manage fluid and electrolyte balances. Survival depends on the type of virus and the age and health of the patient.

The most common problems following encephalitis include hearing loss, speech problems, paralysis and mental retardation. Any form of encephalitis in young children may damage the brain and prevent proper development.

Human infection from equine encephalitis (carried by mosquitoes) can cause irreparable brain damage in half of those who contract it. The only prevention lies in vaccinating horses and controlling mosquitoes. See also VIRUSES AND HEARING LOSS.

endolymph   A viscous fluid contained in a small canal called the SCALA MEDIA. It is a triangular structure made up of the spiral lamina, the spiral ligament and the BASILAR MEMBRANE, located in the labyrinth of the inner ear.

endolymphatic hydrops   See MÉNIÈRE'S DISEASE.

ENT physician   Abbreviation for "ear, nose and throat" physician; a doctor who has earned a medical degree with further study in the ear, nose and throat field combined with residency at a hospital.

These physicians are also known as head and neck surgeons or as otorhinolaryngologists (oto—ear, rhino—nose, laryngo—throat). They are highly trained in ear pathology and surgical procedures, but they may not necessarily be experts in aural rehabilitation (therapy that helps a person with hearing loss communicate better).

Epée, Abbé Charles-Michel de l' (1712–1789)
Born in 1712, de l'Epée was a French cleric who, upon meeting two deaf daughters of a Parisian family, saw the children's deafness in spiritual terms and wanted to teach the girls about the Catholic church in order to save their souls. Making up his methods as he went along, the cleric eventually taught the girls to read and write.

Following this experience, he opened a school in Paris in 1760 for deaf students; this became the first school that taught only deaf children and the first large community of deaf people anywhere in the world. Today it is known as the INSTITUT NATIONAL DES JEUNES SOURDS.

As he worked with his pupils, de l'Epée discovered that many of these children—especially those whose parents were deaf—communicated with each other by using systematic gestures. Suspecting that these gestures might be the "mother tongue" of deaf people, de l'Epée collected these signs and added his own "methodical" signs for gender, tense and number.

Although de l'Epée recognized the importance of speech and taught it to some of his pupils, he realized that in his classes (some as large as 60) signing was more practical. He believed that it was better to give many deaf children some idea of language—albeit a silent one—rather than teach only a small number to speak. His critics argued that SIGN LANGUAGE condemned deaf people to isolation, but de l'Epée believed it was important to allow deaf students to have their own identity. This tension between the value of sign versus the ability to speak is the core of a controversy over educational methods for deaf students that has lasted for more than 200 years. See also SICARD, ABBÉ ROCH-AMBROISE CUCURRON; SPEECHREADING.

Episcopal Conference of the Deaf   This group, affiliated with about 50 Episcopal congregations in the United States, promotes ministry to deaf people though the Episcopal Church.

Originally called the Conference of Church Workers Among the Deaf, the group was founded in 1881 at St. Ann's Church for the Deaf in New York City to support church members working with deaf people. The organization holds annual meetings and publishes a newsletter, *The Deaf Episcopalian.*

The Episcopal Church was the first religious group in the United States to establish a congregation specifically for deaf members—St. Ann's Church for the Deaf in New York City, founded in 1852 by Thomas Gallaudet, the eldest son of THOMAS HOPKINS GALLAUDET.

Soon, a second church for the deaf was established in 1859 in Philadelphia (All Souls Church)

with help from St. Stephen's Church, which had been holding special services for deaf members. All Soul's Church also became known for allowing the ordination of the first deaf Episcopal priest in 1876 in the United States.

epitympanum   Also called the attic, a smaller but continuous extension of the middle ear cavity that contains the bulk of the incus (anvil) and malleus (hammer).

eustachian tube   The canal that connects the middle ear and the back of the nose. It acts as a drainage passage from the middle ear and maintains hearing by opening to regulate air pressure.

From the middle ear, the tube runs forward, downward and in toward the middle of the head, ending at the back of the nose just above the soft palate. The lower end opens during swallowing and yawning to allow air to flow up to the middle ear and equalize air pressure on both sides of the eardrum.

A person with a blocked eustachian tube who undergoes rapid change in air pressure may suffer from barotrauma (pressure damage to the eardrum or other structure). When a head cold blocks this tube, pressure cannot be equalized, causing severe pain and interference with hearing. See also AERO-OTITIS MEDIA; EUSTACHIO, BARTOLOMEO.

Eustachio, Bartolomeo (1510?–1571)   Roman anatomist and great pioneer of otology who described the air passage from the throat to the ear now known as the EUSTACHIAN TUBE.

Eustachio studied in Rome, becoming the personal physician to the duke of Urbino. When he returned to Rome as the personal physician to the pope, he soon became famous as an anatomist, physician, philosopher and linguist.

His discoveries span the entire field of anatomy, although his greatest contribution was the description of the shape and course of the structure that bears his name. Although the existence of the eustachian tube had been vaguely known, it was left to Eustachio to explore it fully.

Exact English   See MANUALLY CODED ENGLISH.

expressive skill The ability to express oneself in the language of signs and FINGERSPELLING.

external auditory canal Also known as the ear canal or meatus, this inch-long curved tube extends from the floor of the external ear inward to the EARDRUM (tympanic membrane) and can be partly straightened by pulling on the external ear itself.

The outer third of the ear canal is cartilage and lined with fairly thick skin. There are fine hairs and modified sebaceous and ceruminous glands embedded in this skin. The sebaceous glands open into the hair follicles, and the ceruminous glands are found deeper under the dermis. These glands produce EARWAX (cerumen), which protects the inner portions of the ear against dirt and insects. The canal cleans itself by shedding skin cells.

The inner two-thirds of the canal is bone covered by very thin skin with no hairs or glands.

external auditory meatus See EXTERNAL AUDITORY CANAL.

external ear See OUTER EAR.

external ear diseases and hearing loss In general, blocks in the external ear canal that cause hearing loss involve IMPACTED EARWAX, a foreign body lodged in the canal or a narrowing of the canal because of disease.

Impacted earwax blocking the ear canal can prevent sound from reaching the middle ear, causing a mild conductive hearing loss, especially in higher frequencies.

Foreign objects that block the ear canal (usually found in children) do not usually cause a serious hearing loss unless they totally block the ear canal or perforate the eardrum. Foreign objects that disrupt the LABYRINTH can cause a sensory hearing loss.

If the ear canal is sufficiently inflamed and swollen due to chronic bacterial, viral or fungal infection or allergic reaction, a temporary hearing loss can result if the chronic infection causes a narrowing of the ear canal.

PERICHONDRITIS (infection of the connective tissue covering the cartilage of the external ear) may destroy the cartilage and deform the ear, narrowing or closing the ear canal. Narrowing of the ear canal could also occur after surgery or a bad burn.

Cancer is also sometimes found in the external ear, and the resulting tumor can destroy the adjacent tissue and spread to nearby lymph nodes. See also CANCER OF THE OUTER EAR.

external otitis See SWIMMER'S EAR.

eyeglass hearing aid Typically, eyeglass hearing aids enclose all the components of the hearing aid—microphone, amplifier and receiver—that inside a case fits into an eyeglass frame. They are useful for those whose hearing loss ranges from mild to severe. BONE CONDUCTOR HEARING AIDS are also available in the eyeglass model. In most states, they are fitted by a licensed specialist (either a dealer, dispenser or dispensing audiologist). See also HEARING AIDS.

facioscapulohumeral muscular dystrophy (FSH MD)   One of the mildest forms of muscular dystrophy, some recently reported patients with FSH MD have SENSORINEURAL HEARING LOSS in both ears. However, not enough cases have been documented to clearly define the incidence of hearing loss associated with this condition.

This is an autosomal dominant condition, which means it can be transmitted genetically to other offspring in 50 percent of all cases. See also GENETICS AND HEARING LOSS.

Falloppio, Gabriele (1523–1562)   One of the foremost Italian anatomists of his time, Falloppio of Modena was the founder of the Italian School of Anatomy and was among the first to describe the anatomy of the ear, ACOUSTIC NERVE and tympanic cavity.

fast auditory fatigue   A hearing problem that occurs in patients with a tumor on the auditory nerve in which continuous loud sounds decrease in intensity.

During a continuous sound, a normal listener hears the tone loudly at first, then less loudly because of adaptation, but the tone remains audible and at a fairly steady loudness after the first 15 or 20 seconds.

However, if the auditory nerve is partially compressed—by a tumor, for example—the loudness continues to fall until the tone is inaudible. If the intensity is increased, the tone becomes audible again but then fades out again. See also ACOUSTIC NEUROMA.

feedback, acoustic   A loud squeal from the amplifier of a HEARING AID caused by a loud sound escaping around an ill-fitting earpiece and then being picked up and amplified. The squeal is unpleasant and may drown out the sound the wearer wishes to hear.

A hearing aid can deliver much louder sound without squeal if the earpiece fits well, but even so, some sound inevitably escapes through the back of the receiver. A very sensitive instrument with high maximum output squeals too easily.

It is possible to lessen squeal in a number of ways: making sure the earpiece fits well in the ear, reducing the volume of the hearing aid, moving the microphone farther away from the receiver or adjusting the tone control. See also HEARING AIDS.

fenestra cochlea   See ROUND WINDOW.

fenestra ovalis   An opening in the inner wall of the MIDDLE EAR into which the footplate of the STAPES is imbedded; also called OVAL WINDOW.

fenestration   This name for an operation on the ear literally means "opening a window." Fenestration was once the treatment of choice for OTOSCLEROSIS, a familial form of deafness corrected only by surgery.

In 1938, American otologist Julius Lempert discovered and first performed a fenestration, which can relieve deafness by creating a new route for sound to travel from the outer ear to the cochlea. By removing most of the bone in the middle ear, Lempert extended the outer ear canal and created a new OVAL WINDOW (or fenestra) through which sound waves could be sent to the inner ear. After a fenestration, sound by-passes the entire chain of bones (OSSICLES) in the middle ear, and although the otosclerosis is still present, the new window is located in the horizontal semicircular canal of the LABYRINTH—an area rarely affected by otosclerosis.

For 20 years, fenestration was the only surgical way to treat otosclerosis, but it was never performed casually since afterwards hearing can never again be completely normal. Although patients had a good chance for some improvement of their conductive hearing at first, most patients experienced a deterioration in hearing afterwards. Since both the eardrum and ossicles (which usually help magnify sound waves) were removed, patients experienced a hearing loss of at least 25 decibels. Many experienced unpleasant side effects, including facial paralysis, VERTIGO and suppurative (draining) ear infections. The patient must be careful of his ears for the rest of his life. Even a small amount of water in the ear can cause a serious infection; baths, showers and hair-washing can be a major problem.

Because of this, fenestration has not been the treatment of choice in otosclerosis since 1951, except for a few patients. These would include someone whose disease has progressed to the point of solidifying the entire oval window, people who have already had more than one STAPEDECTOMY (an operation to free the fixed stapes) because of closure of the oval window from otosclerosis or people born without an oval window or stapes.

For everyone else—and for those for whom fenestration did not work—stapedectomy gives more satisfactory results.

fenestra vestibuli   See OVAL WINDOW.

fetal alcohol syndrome   This combination of birth defects is caused by excessive alcohol consumption by a pregnant mother. It has been reported that fetal alcohol syndrome causes either a sensorineural or conductive deafness in 64 percent of children born with the disorder.

Although even small amounts of alcohol may be harmful to a developing fetus, fetal alcohol syndrome appears only in the presence of persistent alcohol use—two mixed drinks or two to three bottles of beer or glasses of wine a day.

Symptoms of fetal alcohol syndrome include an abnormally short baby with small eyes, vertical folds of skin extending from the upper eyelid to the side of the nose and a small jaw. There may be a small brain, cleft palate, heart defects and joint de-

formities. About one-fifth of affected babies die during the first weeks of life. See also PRENATAL CAUSES OF HEARING LOSS.

fingerspelling   This system of communication involves spelling out words in an alphabetical language by using the letters of the manual alphabet—with handshapes and positions corresponding to each letter of the written alphabet.

Manual alphabets are found throughout the world, although the systems in Continental Europe and the Americas are quite different from the one used in Great Britain, where manual English uses both hands.

Manual alphabets differ from sign languages in that they are not a natural language but a method invented by educators and derived from a written language.

Fingerspelling can either be used by itself or together with sign language, when it is generally employed to spell out proper names or technical words. The alphabet can be modified for use with deaf-blind people by making handshapes and movements on the palm of the receiver of the message.

It is thought that the earliest manual alphabet was developed by PEDRO PONCE DE LEÓN in the 1500s and first published by JUAN PABLO BONET in 1620, and its roots can still be seen in many of the one-handed alphabets used today throughout the world. Even countries that do not use the Latin alphabet—such as Israel, which uses the Hebrew alphabet, or Russia, which uses the Cyrillic alphabet—still use a manual alphabet related to Bonet's.

Unrelated to Bonet's alphabet is the British two-handed system, which is used throughout the British commonwealth countries. A third type is the Swedish manual alphabet invented by Per Borg and exported to Portugal. It is the parent alphabet of the Swedish and Portuguese manual alphabets used today.

Still, other types of manual alphabets developed in countries without written alphabetic systems, such as Japan and China. Japan uses a fingerspelling system based on syllables instead of single sounds, and although a Chinese manual alphabet is being developed, most deaf Chinese draw the outline of the Chinese characters in the air or on palms.

In the American manual alphabet, conversations can be entirely fingerspelled, but among deaf individuals, fingerspelling is more often used in conjunction with AMERICAN SIGN LANGUAGE for proper names and terms for which there are no signs. Fingerspelling alone is used more often among people who are both deaf and blind, presented either at close distance or inside the hand.

It takes only a few hours to learn the individual hand shapes, but becoming fluent as a fingerspeller is quite difficult. The drawback to the method is its relative slowness; for people very experienced in its use, the average fingerspelling rate is about 60 words a minute, which is only about 40 percent as fast as the normal speaking rate.

Although very rarely used as the primary mode of communication in schools for deaf students today, fingerspelling combined with spoken English is known as the ROCHESTER METHOD.

Finnish Sign Language There are two major dialects of Finnish Sign Language (FinnSL), one used by the Finnish-speaking majority and the other by the Swedish-speaking minority. (Finland has three official languages: Finnish, Swedish and Lappish). About 5,000 of the 8,000 deaf Finns use one of the two forms of FinnSL.

By far, the majority of Finns speak the Finnish dialect; 16 of the 17 schools for the deaf are Finnish. Signing is not forbidden in any of the Finnish schools for deaf students, and teachers use Signed Finnish, a pidgin type of FinnSL using the syntax of Finnish and the vocabulary of FinnSL. As is typical in many other countries, congenitally deaf Finns can use Signed Finnish, but they ordinarily do not communicate among other deaf Finns in anything other than FinnSL.

There are 37 handshapes in FinnSL: 31 are distinctive, although six of these are rarely used. Handshapes are classified into three groups: fist, one-finger and multi-finger. Further, every multi-finger handshape must include at least one finger that appears in a one-finger handshape. There are 12 locations of signs and 24 movements. In addition, the international manual alphabet has replaced the Swedish manual alphabet for spelling out place-names and proper names.

Fitzgerald Key A printed system to help deaf children learn to speak, read and write syntactically correct English sentences. The Fitzgerald Key was developed in 1929 at the Texas School for the Deaf by Edith Fitzgerald, a deaf supervising teaching.

Its set of six words and symbols help children analyze the relationships between units of connected language, enabling them to write good sentences and correct their own errors. Under the system, a child places individual words under the headings of subject, verbs and predicates, indirect and direct objects, phrases and words telling where, other word modifiers of the main verbs and "when" words and phrases. The system is still widely used today. See also EDUCATION OF THE DEAF.

flat hearing loss A hearing loss that is about the same at all important frequencies.

Flourens, Marie-Jean-Pierre (1794–1867) This 19th-century French experimental neurologist was the first scientist to find evidence that the vestibular labyrinth is the organ of equilibrium. His experiments with pigeons showed, among other things, that hearing was not affected by destroying the nerves to the vestibular organs, but it was destroyed by cutting the cochlear nerve.

fluoride and hearing Fluoride is chiefly used in this country to combat tooth decay, but it is believed to strengthen the bones of the body as well.

Research suggests that the COCHLEA—the strongest bone in the body—may also benefit from fluoridation of public water systems. These studies suggest that just as tooth decay decreases in areas of fluoridated water, the incidence of OTOSCLEROSIS (softening and overgrowth of bone within the middle or inner ear) decreases in those same areas.

However, if otosclerosis is already present, fluoride does not appear to have any effect.

footplate In the ear, the base of the stirrup, or STAPES, that rests on the oval window.

Fourier analysis A mathematical principle in which any complex sound may be represented as the sum of a series of pure tones (a single frequency) whose frequencies increase in the ratio of the natural numbers 1, 2, 3 and so on.

France This country, with its long history of education for deaf students, has about 3.5 million people with hearing problems; between 50,000 and 100,000 of these use sign language as their primary means of communication. With a deafness rate at 47 out of 100,000 France has one of the lower proportions of deafness in the world.

One of the most famous schools for the deaf is the INSTITUT NATIONAL DE JEUNES SOURDS founded in 1790 as a school favoring the manual education philosophy. It was to this school that THOMAS HOPKINS GALLAUDET came to learn sign language and, together with French instructor LAURENT CLERC, returned to America with the manual method.

Since the early 1960s in France, physicians emphasized the early identification of hearing problems together with immediate use of hearing aids and preschool education beginning in infancy. The four largest public national institutes for the deaf are primarily residential and were founded in the 19th century or before; most private schools for the deaf are religious institutions and today make up the Federation of Institutions of the Deaf and of the Blind of France. This private group of 40 schools, mostly residential, stresses vocational training. Finally, there is a group of private nonresidential centers that teaches students from preschool age up. These centers use more innovative techniques than the older schools and take a medical approach to deaf education.

Although the history of education for deaf students stressed vocational training, there were a few students who chose instead a more academic curriculum. Today, one private institution prepares students to take the special "baccalaureate," an exam required of 18-year-olds for many jobs and for acceptance to a university. Very few deaf students pass the exam, however, and even fewer go on to university training.

The oral approach in education became accepted in France following the Congress of Milan of 1880 and endured in all schools until the late 1970s.

FRENCH SIGN LANGUAGE (FSL) began making a return to popularity in the wake of the WORLD FED-ERATION OF THE DEAF Congress in Washington, D.C., in 1975, where French delegates were impressed at how AMERICAN SIGN LANGUAGE was accepted. As organizations have gathered to fight for the use of FSL, demand for classes and interpreter services has risen dramatically. The National Association of France of Interpreters for the Hearing Impaired was created in 1979. See also EPÉE, ABBÉ CHARLES-MICHEL DE L'; SICARD, ABBÉ ROCH-AMBROISE CUCURRON.

free field test A method of measuring auditory sensitivity by lowering sound intensity to the threshold of perception and then measuring the actual intensity of the sound after the patient has been removed from the field. See also AUDIOMETRY.

French Sign Language The primary method of communication among deaf French people and the first sign language to earn acceptance as a separate, complete language of its own. Called LSF (Langue des Signes Française), this language was made famous by the ABBÉ CHARLES-MICHEL DE L'EPÉE, leading educator of deaf students in the 19th century.

By the 18th century, LSF was a fully integrated sign language among the deaf French populace; at the beginning of the 19th century l'Epée and the ABBÉ ROCH-AMBROISE CUCURRON SICARD borrowed signs from LSF, added some of their own and created their "methodical signs." This system, which included signs representing French grammatical structure, was the first attempt at applying the structures of a spoken language to a sign language.

It was during the 19th century that the great debate between oralists and manualists took place; as the debate between the French manualists and the German oralists raged, disciples of the French method were sent all around the world. As a result, traces of LSF can be found internationally, especially in the sign languages of the United States. In fact, some say more than half the signs of ASL have been borrowed from the French.

By the 1820s, French educators were arguing that deaf students should be educated in LSF, not the artificial "methodical sign" language. For the next 50 years, LSF was used in schools as a primary communication method. With the Milan Congress of 1880 came the triumph of the oral approach over sign, however, and sign language was banned in French schools by the government. But in the late 1970s, the sign language movement gathered steam again around the world.

Today in France, LSF is taught by deaf people outside the educational system, as deaf schools have not been quick to welcome back sign language. It is estimated that up to 100,000 deaf people in France use LSF.

Research suggests that LSF is grammatically similar to ASL; handshapes are quite similar between the two. Like AMERICAN SIGN LANGUAGE, there are three categories of LSF verbs: verbs that don't use personal pronouns, verbs that change direction with the use of personal pronouns ("you give me") and classifier verbs. Many similar facial expressions are also shared between the two to indicate negative sentences, questions and conditional and relative clauses. See also FRANCE; MANUALISM; ORAL APPROACH.

frequency The number of sound waves that pass a fixed point in a certain period of time. It is also a measure of the number of cycles or vibrations during a period of time. Frequency is generally expressed as a HERTZ (Hz), named after the 19th-century German physicist HEINRICH HERTZ. One hertz is equal to one cycle per second; one kilohertz (kHz) is 1,000 hertz; and one megahertz (mHz) is 1,000,000 Hz.

frequency range A term used to describe the measure of power that exists in certain pitch ranges and how far the amplification ability of a hearing aid extends into the high and low pitches. For example, if a person has a high-frequency hearing loss, that person would need an aid that boosts high frequencies. See also HEARING AIDS.

functional hearing loss (nonorganic) Functional hearing loss exists when there is no physical reason for the patient's apparent inability to hear. It is also known as psychogenic hearing loss or hysterical hearing loss.

Instead, the person's hearing loss is primarily a result of psychological or emotional factors; the hearing mechanism itself may be completely normal. Sometimes, there is some slight damage in the ear, but the recorded hearing loss is much less than the patient reports.

Functional hearing loss is often caused by anxiety resulting from emotional conflicts and is beyond the control of the patient. In many cases, a functional hearing loss may occur at the same time as a true organic hearing problem. Called functional overlay, the problem in this case is to recognize the two different components of the hearing problem using a patient history and otologic exams.

A person with unilateral functional deafness may have a complete absence of bone conduction on the side of the bad ear and normal acuity on the side of the good ear. Such a person may even claim not to hear a shout on the bad side in spite of good hearing on the opposite side. It is these inconsistencies that help establish a functional loss.

furuncle Another name for a boil in the skin, this is a staphylococcus infection of a hair follicle that can occur in the outer ear canal. A boil in this location can be particularly painful because the skin of the ear canal is closely attached to the cartilage beneath it. There is usually swelling, redness and tenderness without fever.

Treatment includes the application of heat (hot water bottle or electric heating pad) to help the ear drain together with eardrops and a careful cleaning of the outer canal to prevent infection of other follicles.

Gallaudet, Edward Miner (1837–1917) This leading educator of deaf people established the first college for deaf students in the United States and fought to introduce a combined educational system integrating oral methods with the MANUAL APPROACH dominant at that time throughout the country. At a time when the rest of the world had changed to oral instruction in the wake of the Milan Congress of 1880, he clung resolutely to his belief in retaining the "natural" language of deaf people, although he did recognize the strong appeal ORAL APPROACH held for many people.

The son of a deaf mother and THOMAS HOPKINS GALLAUDET, cofounder of the first public school for deaf students in the United States, Edward Gallaudet felt a profound sensitivity toward deaf people. His understanding of their educational potential made him a leader in the field.

Although young Edward did not start out intending to focus on education of deaf children as a career, he changed his mind after his father died. He began teaching at the AMERICAN SCHOOL FOR THE DEAF in 1855 but, unhappy at the school, he left and was on the verge of heading to Chicago when he received a letter from philanthropist Amos Kendall of Washington, D.C.

Kendall, a multimillionaire, wanted Gallaudet to take over the Columbia Institution for the Deaf. Gallaudet saw this as his chance to establish his dream: a university for deaf students.

He began his job there in 1857 when he was only 20 years old, and in 1864 he asked Congress to allow the institution to grant degrees after a six-year course of study.

Gallaudet went to Europe in 1867 to study the ORAL APPROACH just being introduced in the United States, and upon his return, he submitted a plan to introduce oral instruction in combination with the MANUAL APPROACH then being taught at the school.

He strongly believed in an equal emphasis on the manual approach and offered oral instruction as a separate course at the school. Other courses were taught manually, with additional classes in speechreading and speech.

In his career of educating deaf students, Gallaudet became an implacable opponent of oralist ALEXANDER GRAHAM BELL. Although the two initially disagreed politely, over time their enmity deepened. In 1895, Gallaudet accused Bell of fanaticism over the oral approach, calling him an outsider before a CONVENTION OF AMERICAN INSTRUCTORS OF THE DEAF. Bell and Gallaudet did not speak for the next five years.

Gallaudet lived to see the 100-year celebration of the American School for the Deaf, the institution founded by his father. He died in Hartford, Connecticut, in 1917.

Gallaudet, Thomas Hopkins (1787–1851) This Connecticut theologian was a pioneer in U.S. education for deaf people and opened the American School for the Deaf, the first permanent school for deaf students in the United States at Hartford, Connecticut.

The eldest of 12 children, Thomas Gallaudet was born in Philadelphia, the son of a merchant family of deep religious convictions. A brilliant child, Thomas entered Yale at age 14 and graduated first in his class three years later; within five years, he had apprenticed with a law firm, studied literature and earned a master's degree from Yale. He graduated with a divinity degree from Andover Theological Seminary in 1814 and intended to become an itinerant preacher until a chance meeting with a young deaf girl changed his life forever.

While visiting his parents in 1814, the 27-year-old Gallaudet met ALICE COGSWELL, nine-year-old deaf daughter of Dr. MASON FITCH COGSWELL, a prominent Hartford physician. Gallaudet began trying to teach young Alice some reading and the manual alphabet and succeeded in breaking through the communication barrier by teaching her the word "hat." With the enthusiastic backing of her father, who did not want to have to send young Alice to Europe to be educated, Gallaudet was persuaded to learn the European methods of teaching deaf students so he could return and set up a school in Connecticut.

When Gallaudet's informal census of deaf children suggested there were about 80 in Connecticut, he guessed there might be at least 400 in New England and perhaps 2,000 in the entire country.

It is probable that when Gallaudet set out, he intended to study both the British method of oral instruction and the French manual style in order to develop a combined approach to education. But when Gallaudet arrived in Great Britain, the developers of the British method—the THOMAS BRAIDWOOD family—were unwilling to share their methods. Gallaudet spent some time studying educational philosophies in Scotland and then went to Paris to interview ABBE ROCH-AMBROISE CUCURRON SICARD, head of the Institut Royal des Sourds-Muets (now called the Institut National de Jeunes Sourds) who welcomed Gallaudet. At the school Sicard allowed Gallaudet to observe methods used at each level and personally taught him the manual method used at the school. Gallaudet also studied sign language with JEAN MASSIEU and LAURENT CLERC at the school.

With Sicard's permission, Gallaudet took Clerc, one of Sicard's best pupils and a master teacher himself, back to Connecticut with him in 1816 to help organize a school for deaf students. In order to garner support for the school, Gallaudet, Clerc and Mason Cogswell toured New England, presenting demonstrations at town meetings, churches and public gatherings. Clerc's presence at Gallaudet's side was proof of the possibility of educating a deaf person and their fund-raising tours were very successful.

Within six months after returning to America, Gallaudet opened the country's first permanent school for the deaf in Hartford, Connecticut. The school featured the manual (French) method of education. Soon Gallaudet's Asylum for the Educa-

tion and Instruction of the Deaf and Dumb (now the AMERICAN SCHOOL FOR THE DEAF) began enrolling students from other states.

Because the school was on its way to becoming a national institution, Gallaudet was granted financial aid from the U.S. Congress to continue his programs.

By the middle of the 19th century, there were schools for the deaf in 12 states and a national college for the deaf in Washington, D.C., run by Gallaudet's son, EDWARD MINER GALLAUDET.

Most of the schools that began during the 1800s used the French method of manual instruction, a trend established with Gallaudet's American School for the Deaf in Hartford.

Gallaudet College, renamed after Thomas (formerly the Columbia Institution for the Deaf), was officially chartered by an act of Congress in 1864 and signed into law by Abraham Lincoln. It has now operated for more than 100 years as the only liberal arts college for deaf students in the world.

Gallaudet's position as leader of the movement for deaf education was helped by his talents as preacher, orator and writer, which were useful in his push for educational reform from the pulpit and the podium.

He died on September 10, 1851, in Hartford, but his interest in education for deaf students was continued by his deaf wife Sophia Fowler, a graduate of the Hartford School, and by two of their children. Their oldest child, Thomas Gallaudet, was a minister to a deaf congregation at St. Ann's Church in New York City; EDWARD MINER GALLAUDET was the first president of Gallaudet College, now GALLAUDET UNIVERSITY, in Washington, D.C.

Gallaudet Preschool Signed English system   An invented sign system based on the spoken English language and including English spelling, pronunciation and meaning. The signs used in this system feature letter initialization and compounding. See also MANUALLY CODED ENGLISH.

Gallaudet Research Institute   This eight-unit research group, located at GALLAUDET UNIVERSITY in Washington, D.C., is the largest institute in the world dedicated to investigating the immediate and long-range concerns of deaf people.

The institute has a multiple mission of research, teaching and service and supports broad-based research involving collaborations among scientists from many disciplines. The group brings together individuals from around the world to discuss deafness-related research and shares its information through conferences, seminars, lectures, training and consultation.

As part of its dedication to service, the institute offers a wide range of resources through its eight units, including:

- genetic counseling
- communications networks for teachers and administrators
- technological device referral
- monograph series
- demographic statistics
- projections/recommendations on needs of deaf elderly people
- "working paper" series in a wide variety of topics
- advice and consultation for researchers
- published proceedings of major deafness-related events
- technical assistance to businesses developing new devices for people with hearing losses

Firmly believing in the importance of outreach and service, institute staffers often give lectures and presentations to various groups, consult on deafness-related topics, serve on advisory boards, review and edit manuscripts and participate in peer review for funding agencies. A national advisory committee helps guide the institute's choice of research priorities, and the Office of the Dean of Graduate Studies and Research administers the institute.

The eight units in the institute are:

Center for Assessment and Demographic Studies

This unit analyzes national databases containing information on deaf and hard-of-hearing people and advises governmental agencies on national policy. Since 1968, this unit has conducted its own annual survey of hard-of-hearing children. In addition, the unit monitors hard-of-hearing stu-dents receiving special services and studies national test standardizations for hard-of-hearing students.

Center for Studies in Education and Human Development

This unit was established in 1981 to conduct research in the field of deafness. Today, ongoing research studies include how deafness affects parent-infant interaction, the earliest stages of language development and reading and writing processes. In addition, scientists are trying to develop models of the best educational environments for deaf children.

Center for Auditory and Speech Sciences

Researchers in this unit investigate ways of improving the speech perception of deaf and hard-of-hearing people through auditory, visual or tactile means. Through auditory experiments, researchers try to discover the exact types of distortions hearing problems impose on the perception of specific speech sounds. Researchers are currently developing tactile devices to aid speechreading and are investigating certain types of hearing deficits common to the elderly.

Genetic Services Center

This center was established by the institute in 1984 to explore the more than 200 known genetic forms of hearing problems as well as certain other kinds of deafness acquired through environmental means. The primary function of this center is to provide genetic evaluations and counseling sessions to help deaf people and their families understand the causes and effects of hearing loss. Staffers also consult with and train AUDIOLOGISTS, geneticists, parents, consumers and the medical community.

Technology Assessment Program

Established in 1985, this program produces information for industrial, government and consumer groups interested in improving access to technology for people with hearing problems. The unit collaborates with several technical centers to develop devices that can, for example, alert deaf drivers to approaching emergency vehicles, convert speech to text, allow deaf people to communicate in sign language or speechread over telephone lines and provide deaf-blind people with robotic finger-spelling as an alternative to braille or personal interpreters.

Culture and Communication Studies Program

This unit analyzes and compares the processes involved in acquiring language and forming cultural identities in the United States and other countries. Presently, the program's cross-cultural studies involve Spain, Italy, Mexico and some countries of Central and South America.

Mental Health Research Program

The cause and effect of mental health problems among people with hearing problems is explored by this unit, which is also working to develop better ways of testing and treating these problems. Researchers are currently studying differences in cerebral organization among hearing and deaf children, personality characteristics of deaf college students and depression among deaf adults. The program also provides information on coping strategies for people who lose their hearing in adulthood and psychologists are involved in translating standard psychological tests into AMERICAN SIGN LANGUAGE.

Scientific Communications Program

This program was created in 1987 to intensify the institute's efforts to communicate results of deafness-related research to others. In addition to its publication *Research at Gallaudet* and the institute's annual report, the group publishes research monographs, conference proceedings and working papers to help publicize results of selected studies. See also Appendix II.

Gallaudet University   Located in Washington, D.C., Gallaudet University is the only liberal arts university specifically for deaf students in the world.

The school was established in 1864 on land donated by Amos Kendall, a well-known journalist, politician and philanthropist, who had become interested in the welfare and education of deaf children. Called the Columbia Institution for the Deaf and Dumb and Blind when it was incorporated by Congress in 1857, it was granted a charter in 1864

to operate a collegiate division at the request of its first superintendent, EDWARD MINER GALLAUDET. Gallaudet was the son of THOMAS HOPKINS GALLAUDET, who founded the first public residential school for deaf children in the United States.

The National Deaf Mute College opened with 13 male students, one professor and one instructor; in 1887 it admitted six women as part of a two-year experiment. Although criticized for this decision, Dr. Gallaudet allowed the women to remain, letting them live in the president's house until the experiment was considered successful and a woman's dormitory could be built.

A Normal Department was begun in 1891 to train hearing teachers of deaf students, and three years later the school's name was changed to Gallaudet College to honor Edward Miner Gallaudet's father, Thomas.

Today, Gallaudet has a student body of more than 2,200, including a limited number of hearing undergraduate students. The school includes two campuses: the original 99-acre Kendall Green campus in northeast Washington and a newer nine-acre Northwest Campus seven miles from Kendall Green. Students are accepted upon recommendation from local school districts or special schools and must have graduated from high school and have passed the Gallaudet entrance exam. Of the more than 1,400 students who take the exam, usually only half qualify for admission; of these, about 70 percent must take up to one year of preparatory work before they can be admitted to the first-year class.

About two-thirds of the student body have a profound hearing loss and more than one-fourth have a severe loss. Almost all students lost their hearing before school age; since 1970, most students have been congenitally deaf.

In 1988 the university elected King Jordan as its first deaf president after a one-week mass protest and demonstration initiated by the deaf community, faculty and students. The successful protest is considered by deaf people to be a historic event, and profoundly important to the deaf community.

Gallaudet continues its commitment to education, research and service and houses the world's most complete collection of materials related to hearing loss, deafness and deaf people. Its library archives contain written, visual and audio materials on deafness dating back to 1546.

Gallaudet's MODEL SECONDARY SCHOOL FOR THE DEAF opened on 17 acres on the northwest part of the Kendall Green campus in 1976, and a KENDALL DEMONSTRATION ELEMENTARY SCHOOL began in 1980 on six acres in the northeast part of campus.

Gallaudet's 288 faculty members, of whom 35 percent are deaf and hard-of-hearing, teach in more than 40 undergraduate and graduate programs offered through the following schools: College of Arts and Sciences, School of Communication, School of Education and Human Services, School of Management and School of Preparatory Studies. Educational programs are also offered through the College for Continuing Education.

The university grants bachelor of science or arts degrees in 26 major fields of study; its graduate school offers hearing students a two-year program leading to a master of science in audiology and both hearing and deaf students a master of arts in education, rehabilitation counseling, school counseling, educational technology and linguistics.

The Ph.D. degree in the administration of special programs is offered by the graduate school in conjunction with the Consortium of Universities in the Washington area, of which Gallaudet is a member. About one-third of these doctoral candidates have hearing problems.

Gallaudet also offers extensive noncredit courses, workshops, seminars, internships and an associate of arts degree in interpreting for hearing people who wish to become certified sign language interpreters.

The university maintains an active student government and publishes a school paper *(The Buff and Blue)*, an annual literary magazine *(Manus)* and a yearbook *(Tower Clock)*. Plays are produced twice a year and are presented in signs and voice; they are open to the public. The college has three sororities and three fraternities and a varied sports program that includes football, soccer, rugby, track, volleyball, basketball, baseball, field hockey, tennis and golf.

Gallaudet also maintains the NATIONAL CENTER FOR LAW AND DEAFNESS, the International Center on Deafness, GALLAUDET RESEARCH INSTITUTE, the NATIONAL INFORMATION CENTER ON DEAFNESS and the Management Institute.

The university's Center on Deafness also features educational extension centers in cooperation with local colleges and universities. These include Ohlone College in Fremont, California; Northern Essex Community College in Haverhill, Massachusetts; Flagler College, St. Augustine, Florida; Kapiolani Community College, Honolulu, Hawaii; Johnson County Community College, Overland Park, Kansas; Eastfield College, Dallas, Texas; Gallaudet University Regional Center, Washington, D.C.; and University of Puerto Rico in San Juan. See also GALLAUDET UNIVERSITY ALUMNI ASSOCIATION; Appendix II.

Gallaudet University Alumni Association   Representing more than 4,000 deaf people, the Gallaudet University Alumni Association members include about half of all alumni from the four-year college.

Founded in 1889 in Washington, D.C., the association meets twice a year and is open to graduates, past attendees of the college and people who have received an honorary degree from the school. It is an associate member of the WORLD FEDERATION OF THE DEAF and maintains more than 55 chapters throughout the United States and Canada. Local chapters raise money for student loans, scholarships and awards, athletic uniforms, and so forth and have provided money for memorials, endowment funds and travel for students participating in leadership conferences.

In addition, the association publishes the *Gallaudet Alumni Newsletter* twice a month, coordinates reunions and special events on campus and assists in recruiting, fundraising and public relations.

genetics and deafness   Most cases of genetic deafness occur at birth and do not improve over time. About half of all cases of deafness in children are inherited.

There are several ways that genes can influence a person's ability to hear. Each child receives half of his or her genetic material from each parent. All cells in the human body have 23 pairs of chromosomes (a total of 46); because the chromosomes are paired, each segment in one chromosome has a corresponding segment in its partner. The genes (a chemical coding system of the actual units of inheritance) are also paired, one on each chromosome. Each gene provides information for the development and functioning of various organ systems.

There are many different gene locations that affect hearing and many different varieties of genes; different forms of deafness may involve different gene locations. Recessive genes must be contributed from both parents if a trait it controls will result. A gene is dominant if the trait is expressed when only one gene of the pair is present. The different types of genetic mechanisms that can result in a hearing loss are:

Autosomal Recessive

Deafness genes with an autosomal recessive pattern account for between 75 percent and 85 percent of hereditary deafness. (Autosomes are the chromosomes other than the two sex chromosomes). Both parents usually have normal hearing, but each carries a recessive gene for deafness; when a child inherits both of these recessive deafness genes, the child will be deaf. Usually, there is no family history of deafness. If both parents have this recessive gene, the risk of having a deaf child is one in four (or 25 percent for each pregnancy). The odds of having a child who does not carry even one of the abnormal genes is also one in four. The remainder (one in two) will carry one recessive gene, like the parents, and one healthy gene and so will not be deaf.

Autosomal Dominant

Only one deafness gene must be inherited to cause deafness in this pattern of inheritance, which accounts for about 20 percent of hereditary deafness. In this pattern, usually at least one parent is deaf, and the deafness appears in each generation, affecting about the same number of boys and girls. The risk of parents having another deaf child is 50 percent. None of the hearing children will be carriers because if they had the deafness gene, they would be deaf themselves. The children of any hearing children would have no higher risk of having a deaf child.

In the rare case that both parents are deaf from the same type of autosomal dominant gene they would have a 75 percent chance of having a deaf child with each pregnancy and a corresponding 25 percent chance of having a child without the gene.

With this type of inheritance, the deafness gene is sometimes created from a mutation in a sperm or egg cell without any prior family history. Once the gene has mutated, it will have the same effect on future generations as if it had been passed down through the family. Often, the severity of this type of inherited deafness varies so much within a family that it can be hard to be sure of the pattern without careful study. For example, one person might be profoundly deaf while another is only mildly hard of hearing.

X-Linked Inheritance

This is an unusual cause of deafness in which the abnormal gene is located on the X chromosome. Out of all the chromosome pairs in the human body, one pair determines the sex of the child; a female has two X chromosomes (a XX pattern) and a male has one X and one Y chromosome (an XY pattern). When the 46 chromosome pairs divide in making sperm, half of the resulting sperm cells will have an X, half a Y.

In an X-linked genetic hearing disorder, the abnormal gene is located on the X chromosome. Females are usually protected by having another normal gene on their other X chromosome. But the male, having only one X, isn't protected if he receives the abnormal gene. Thus, females are carriers and have a one in two chance of giving the abnormal gene to any one son, who will be deaf, or to a daughter, who will be a carrier. Affected males cannot pass the deafness on to their sons because they only give them the Y chromosome, but all their daughters will be carriers because their daughters must receive the damaged X chromosome from their fathers.

Chromosomal Disorder

This problem can cause a hearing disorder when the 46 chromosomes are being reduced to 23 in the formation of egg or sperm. The best-known example of a chromosomal disorder is Down's syndrome, which is often associated with some degree of hearing loss. These genetic accidents are not usually passed on.

There are about 200 different types of genetic hearing problems, ranging in degree from mild to profound. A large proportion of hearing problems that occur at birth or during the first few years of life are hereditary, as are many kinds of progressive hearing losses that occur later in life.

Although some kinds of hearing loss are associated with other physical characteristics or medical problems (changes in the eye or hair color, kidneys or heart), most types of genetic hearing problems don't involve other physical changes.

Because hearing problems are so often genetic, it's common to refer a family with a deaf member to a genetic counselor or a genetic team. A medical geneticist can often tell whether someone's hearing problem has been inherited. Genetic counseling for hearing loss always includes a detailed family history, a medical history of the deaf person and a pregnancy history of the mother of that person. The individual or family is then seen by the medical geneticist for a physical exam to uncover clues in the appearance that might suggest a basis for the hearing problem. In cases where it is possible to determine the cause of the hearing problem and how a gene has passed through the family, the team meets with the individual or the family and explains how the hearing loss was inherited and what the implications and possibilities are for future generations. This knowledge can be very important because the earlier a child is diagnosed, the better the issues around the deafness can be addressed. If there is more than one person in the family with a hearing loss, the problem is almost always genetic.

Hearing Loss Genes

Recently, scientists have found mutations in several genes linked to deafness. The gene called Connexin 26 may be responsible for as many as 40 percent of cases of inherited hearing loss. Most of these children are born to parents with normal hearing. About 40 percent of children with this genetic mutation will have a profound hearing loss. Another gene (GJB2) mutation is the predominant cause of inherited moderate-to-profound deafness in the midwest. Although there are many deafness-causing mutations in the GJB2 gene, one mutation (called 35delG) causes the most cases of deafness. Couples who have had one child with GJB2-associated deafness have a 17.5 percent chance of having a second deaf child.

Hearing Gene

Scientists have also recently discovered a gene that plays a significant role in the development of cells essential to hearing. This discovery raises hope for the development of treatments for hearing loss because of disease, trauma and aging. The gene (Math 1) sends a signal that triggers certain ear cells to mature into hair cells in the inner ear. Hair cells are responsible for both hearing and balance, and loss of these cells is a common cause of deafness. Once these cells have been destroyed (either through trauma, disease or aging), they cannot be recreated. With these findings, doctors may one day be able to generate new hair cells in those with hearing loss. See also Appendix IV.

German measles   See RUBELLA.

German Sign Language   In Germany, almost all prelingually deaf Germans use Deutsche Gebardensprache (DGS), a sign language with many dialects arising from various schools for deaf students.

A traditionally oral country, there has been little research into DGS, which has not generally been used in educational settings, although it is a natural communication mode among deaf people outside the classroom. When manual approaches are mentioned in schools, the reference is to Signed German.

Although similar to AMERICAN SIGN LANGUAGE in some ways, DGS—as many other European sign languages—uses more lip movements. FINGER-SPELLING, using a manual alphabet similar to the American one, is also used with DGS, although older DGS users do not know the manual alphabet. More popular is a manual system called PMS (Phonembestimmtes Manualsystem), which represents phonemes instead of letters. This system is used in schools for deaf students to teach articulation.

gestuno   The first "international" SIGN LANGUAGE, developed by members of the WORLD FEDERATION OF

THE DEAF in an attempt to overcome the problem of communication at international meetings.

Gestuno is a collection of about 1,500 signs chosen for ease of use to build a basic international vocabulary. The problem of syntax was simply ignored.

The problem with this international sign language is that few people are willing to learn the new signs, the communication it allows is often too limited, and there are not enough occasions to use it to make learning gestuno worthwhile for most people.

gestural language See SIGN LANGUAGE.

Ginkgo biloba A tree whose leaves have been used by Chinese herbalists for thousands of years to treat a variety of physical problems, including deafness and TINNITUS (ringing of the ears). Western herbalists today use ginkgo leaves for a variety of problems, explaining that the leaf can help expand blood vessels and improve blood flow in vessels and arteries (especially in the lower legs and feet). It also appears to boost blood flow to the brain. Herbalists believe that the leaves of the ginkgo tree may help reverse deafness caused by reduced blood flow to the nerves involved in hearing.

The leaves are available in dry bulk, in capsules or as a tincture. Standardized *Ginkgo biloba* extract (GBE) is available in health food stores. WARNING: Ginkgo should not be used by anyone with a clotting disorder or by pregnant or nursing women. It should not be given to children without a doctor's supervision and should only be used in medicinal amounts in consultation with a health care professional. Some people are unable to tolerate ginkgo even in small doses.

GLAD An acronym for Greater Los Angeles Council on Deafness; this nonprofit group, founded in 1969, is a comprehensive service center and umbrella agency for more than 45 California groups and agencies in the field of deafness, including social, recreational and service clubs for the deaf community and educational, professional, health and religious organizations. It serves more than 1,500 hearing and deaf members.

GLAD sponsors community workshops and educational lectures and links traditional social service agencies with the deaf community. It also offers employment referral services, interpreter referrals, telephone/TDD relay services, peer counseling and advocacy. Under a grant from California's rehabilitation department, GLAD also offers the first sign language interpreter pool free of charge to deaf people. With this pool, deaf people in California have access to more than 200 qualified interpreters.

The council consults with police, hospitals, school districts and the state legislature in support of deaf services. Located as it is in the heart of the entertainment business, the council also works with producers on projects that involve deaf subjects or actors to ensure that deaf characters are honestly portrayed and that deaf actors are hired as often as possible to play deaf roles.

The council produces an extensive resource book, the *Directory of Resources Available to Deaf and Hearing Impaired Persons in the Southern California Area* and the journal *GLAD News Magazine* and maintains a bookstore carrying volumes on deafness. The council is a member of the NATIONAL ASSOCIATION OF THE DEAF.

glue ear See MUCOUS OTITIS MEDIA.

grammar The structure of language. Grammar consists of a number of elements: *morphology* (how sounds go together to form words or (in a signed language) how the elements of position, shape and movement combine to form signs); *syntax* (how words or signs are organized in sentences); *semantics* (how to interpret the meaning of words, signs and sentences); *pragmatics* (how to participate in a conversation).

Greece The outlook for deaf people in Greece is not encouraging, since less than half the deaf citizens in the country are given any education at all. Of those who are, only 10 percent get more than elementary instruction.

Although it is estimated that there are at least 1,480 deaf children in the country, only 640 receive some form of special education, and there is no state provision for their education.

The National Foundation for the Protection of the Deaf and Dumb provides six educational facilities for deaf children, serving about 400 residential and day students (most in elementary schools). There are two other schools for deaf children. The schools all favor an oral approach, with an emphasis on speechreading and auditory training and no signing in class. Despite this, Greek Sign Language, with its roots in American and French sign languages, is used by more than 30,000 adult deaf Greeks.

Since there is no provision for deaf teacher training, specialists either are educated abroad or are trained simply as regular classroom instructors. There are currently no adult or higher education programs specifically for deaf people.

group amplification systems   See ASSISTIVE LISTENING DEVICES.

hair cells   More than 15,000 microscopic hair-like cells are located inside the inner ear in an area smaller than a fingernail. They cover the ORGAN OF CORTI—the actual part of the ear that allows a person to hear.

There are about 3,400 inner hair cells in the human cochlea that extend in a row from the base to the apex of the cochlea. In much the same way, close to the lateral surface of the organ of Corti are three or four rows of about 12,000 outer hair cells. These inner and outer hair cells incline toward each other, and cilia emerge from the upper surface of the inner and outer hair cells to penetrate the tectorial membrane, which forms a roof over the organ of Corti.

When a sound wave makes the eardrum vibrate, the vibrations are carried across the middle ear by the hammer, the anvil and the stirrup, which passes the vibrations through the oval window to the fluid in the tubes of the inner ear. This makes the hairs of the organ of Corti vibrate—and the more hairs that vibrate, the louder the sound. The shorter, thinner hair cells pick up high sounds, and the longer, thicker hairs pick up low sounds. The auditory nerve picks up the messages from these hairs and sends them to the brain, where the sound is processed.

Excessive noise can overload the tiny, irreplaceable hair cells and can seriously impede the ability to hear.

hammer   See MALLEUS.

hard-of-hearing   A term used to describe mild to moderate hearing loss. This term is preferred over *hearing-impaired* by the deaf community.

head injury and deafness   Severe head injury can cause sensorineural and conductive deafness in one or both ears.

Sensorineural deafness resulting from severe head injury can be associated with a transverse fracture of the temporal bone, which causes a complete destruction of the hearing and balance mechanism on the affected side.

This type of deafness is usually permanent, although the dizziness that can accompany it will usually subside over a period of several weeks and the unsteadiness and swaying toward the affected side may subside after several months. Sometimes a transverse fracture of the temporal bone results in a hearing loss that is incomplete, but this is uncommon.

It is possible to have hearing damage following a head injury that doesn't fracture the temporal bone, especially from a blow to the back or side of the head—although the blow is usually severe enough to cause loss of consciousness. Deafness from this type of injury is usually similar to that which comes from excess noise. An injury of this type is often accompanied by dizziness, often made worse by a change in position of the head.

Although there may be hearing loss on the side of the injury, there may also be a mild hearing loss on the opposite side due to a concussion in the inner ear.

Conductive deafness resulting from injury is caused by blood that collects in the middle ear and external canal; occasionally there is disruption of the ossicular chain (hammer, anvil, stirrup) and a ruptured eardrum. As the blood is absorbed, however, hearing usually returns to its original level, and the eardrum heals. Occasionally, conductive deafness following head injury can be permanent, but because it is conductive, the maximum degree of hearing loss is usually about 60 dB. This means that if speech is loud enough, the person can not only hear well but can understand what is being said. Surgery can sometimes restore the hearing. See also CONDUCTIVE HEARING LOSS; SENSORINEURAL HEARING LOSS.

hearing   The sense of hearing is a complex, coordinated process involving the transmission of sound waves through the ear mechanisms into the brain, which can then interpret the message.

First, the sound waves strike the OUTER EAR (or PINNA), the part of the ear visible on the side of the head. The outer ear is designed to help gather these sound waves and funnel them down the ear canal to the paper-thin EARDRUM (tympanic membrane), which divides the outer ear from the MIDDLE EAR.

When the sound waves strike the eardrum, it vibrates and moves a chain of three small bones on the other side, called the ossicular chain (or OSSICLES), which consists of the hammer (MALLEUS) the anvil (INCUS) and the stirrup (STAPES). These tiny bones—the smallest ones in the body—are full size at birth and are located in the middle ear cavity. Together, the three bones transfer the energy of the sound wave from the outer ear through the middle ear and into the INNER EAR.

As the sound vibrates the eardrum, which vibrates the ossicles, it also moves the last bone in the ossicular chain, the stirrup (stapes), which is also attached to a tiny membrane called the OVAL WINDOW. The oval window is the entrance to the inner ear, which contains the organ of hearing called the COCHLEA. As the stirrup moves, it makes the oval window vibrate, disturbing the fluid-filled channel of the cochlea on the other side of the oval window.

As the cochlea moves, it stimulates the thousands of microscopic hair cells inside the organ, which send electrical impulses to the brain.

There are also other structures in the ear that may not contribute to hearing but serve very important purposes nevertheless. Located in the middle ear is the EUSTACHIAN TUBE, which helps maintain the balance of air pressure on both sides of the eardrum and connects the middle ear cavity to the back of the nose just above the soft palate. The upper end of this tube is usually surrounded by bone and is open; the lower end is usually collapsed and surrounded by soft tissue. About every third time we swallow or yawn, this tube opens, allowing air to flow up to the middle ear and equalizing the air pressure in the middle and outer ear. (The ear-popping feeling during airplane rides occurs if this equalization process is large and rapid, causing pressure to build up on one side of the eardrum, pushing it inward or outward.)

Within the inner ear, the three small loops of the SEMICIRCULAR CANALS, connected to the cochlea, help maintain balance. Problems within these tiny semicircular canals may cause DIZZINESS, VERTIGO and other balance problems.

hearing aids   Devices that consist of a group of tiny components worn on one or both ears to improve hearing by making sounds louder and speech easier to understand for people with certain types of hearing loss.

The first hearing aids were simple cone-shaped devices, ranging from a rolled-up tube to an elaborate EAR TRUMPET, which provided a small boost in sound. After the invention of the vacuum tube came the first "powered" hearing aids in 1921, but they were cumbersome units with large parts and heavy batteries.

Today, a hearing aid system consists of a tiny microphone that picks up sound waves and converts them into electrical signals. These impulses are fed into an amplifier, which boosts the signal to increase the output of sound and then sends it to a receiver, which converts the amplified signals back into sound and transmits them into the ear through an EARMOLD.

If it is properly fitted, the earmold provides support for the hearing aid, directing amplified sound into the ear canal. A poorly fitting earmold can cause whistles and squeals, irritation and soreness. Ready-made earmolds are available, but many wearers prefer custom-fitted molds.

Although a hearing aid can amplify sound, it does not necessarily improve clarity and cannot make hearing completely normal. Hearing aids require practice and skill to be used effectively. They are worn by both deaf and hard-of-hearing people; even profoundly deaf people can benefit from powerful behind-the-ear aids.

People with mild hearing losses may get enough improvement simply with a tiny unit that fits directly into the ear; people with more severe problems may need a larger, more powerful system, usually worn on the body. These are sturdier, less subject to distortion and easier to regulate. Still, most profoundly deaf individuals do not wear body types.

Modern hearing aids do much more than simply amplify sound: They can filter background noise, change tonal quality and control the loudness of environmental sounds. Strides in miniaturization have resulted in a much smaller, less visible aid that is of benefit to people who don't want people to know they wear an aid. In all but four states, all hearing aids may be fitted and sold only by licensed specialists, who may be called "dealers," "specialists," "dispensers" or "dispensing audiologists."

Listed below are the hearing aids that are currently available:

Behind-the-ear aids include a microphone, amplifier and receiver inside a small curved case worn behind the ear and connected to the earmold by a short plastic tube. Some models have a tone control, volume control and telephone pickup device. This model is useful for people whose hearing loss ranges from mild to severe.

Eyeglass models are much the same as behind-the-ear aids, except that the case fits into an eyeglass frame instead of behind the ear. Bone conduction hearing aids are also available in the eyeglass model.

On-the-body aids feature a larger microphone, amplifier and power supply inside a case carried inside a pocket or attached to clothing. The external receiver attaches directly to the earmold and its power comes through a flexible wire from the amplifier. Although larger than other aids, on-the-body hearing aids are also more powerful and easier to adjust than smaller devices. They are not popular but are still in use.

Monaural hearing aid systems include any hearing aid that provides sound to one ear alone.

Binaural hearing aid systems include two complete hearing aids, one in each ear. Some wearers find that the binaural system increases direction sense and helps separate sounds from unwanted background noise.

CROS (contralateral routing of signal) or *crossover* systems features a microphone beside the impaired ear that feeds the amplified signal to the better ear, thereby eliminating "head shadow" (the head blocking sound from the better ear). This system may help make speech easier to understand for those with a high frequency loss in both ears.

BI-CROS systems utilize two microphones (one above each ear) sending signals to a single amplifier. Sound then travels to a single receiver, which transfers it to the better ear via a conventional earmold.

By federal law, hearing aids may not be sold directly to consumers because they are considered to be medical devices and are regulated by the U.S. Food and Drug Administration.

The first step in obtaining a hearing aid is to have an accurate diagnosis and hearing evaluation done by an OTOLOGIST (ear specialist), OTOLARYNGOLOGIST (a specialist in ear, nose and throat diseases) and an AUDIOLOGIST. These two specialists can determine whether a hearing aid will help and can identify the type that will do the most good. This is particularly important since aids can be expensive and are not generally covered by private insurance. The cost of a hearing aid includes a hearing test, ear impressions for in-the-ear styles, the hearing aid itself and office visits for fittings and follow-ups. Until recently, there has been little price competition, but that may change with new methods of buying hearing aids on the Internet. It is also possible to compare retail prices on the web by checking the sites of audiologists.

There are a number of styles of aids that are encased within a plastic shell and are worn entirely inside the ear. These include the custom in-the-ear (ITE) model, which can completely fill the ear canal, the thinner low-profile model, the half concha, the even smaller "helix model" (for high-frequency losses), the in-the-canal (ITC) and the tiniest style—the completely in-the-canal hearing aids. The completely in-the-canal aid is so tiny that it must be removed from the ear by pulling on a thin cord that rests at the bottom of the bowl of the ear. In-the-ear aids can be of particular importance for older people who may have psychological problems in adjusting to the idea that they are losing their hearing. In those who lost their hearing as they age, wearing a hearing aid is often interpreted as a sign of aging.

Linear Hearing Aids

These conventional hearing aids produce the same amount of amplification regardless of the loudness of the sound in the environment. Consumers with this type of hearing aid have to manually adjust the volume in very quiet or very noisy situations.

Nonlinear Single Channel Aids

More-advanced technology produced a "nonlinear" aid with more amplification given to soft sounds than for loud sounds. Once sounds cross a certain level, the aid automatically adjusts the volume. This type of aid squeezes a wide range of loudness into a narrower range, which is why they are also called compression hearing aids.

Nonlinear Multichannel Aids

This newer type of aid is designed with a consumer's personal hearing needs in mind, based upon how loud certain sounds need to be interpreted for various frequencies. In hearing aids with only one channel, a loud noise of low frequencies (such as might be found during a party environment) would trigger the hearing aid to lower the amplification for all frequencies, which would help keep the sound from being too loud but would also make some high-frequency sounds (such as consonants) too soft to hear. In that same situation, a multichannel aid would decrease the amplification for low frequencies without changing the amplification for high frequencies. If fitted correctly, they can greatly improve speech clarity (especially in noisy listening environments).

Multiple/automatic Program Aids

Some hearing aids have several different programs that can be selected by the touch of a bottom (either on the aid or on a separate remote control) to select amplification that is best suited to different environments, such as listening in a restaurant, in one-on-one situations or for music. Other aids have automatic volume regulation so that the consumer doesn't have to bother with volume control. (However, some people don't like aids that take away too much of the control.)

Digitally-Programmable Hearing Aids

This is one new type that can provide consumers with a way to amplify different tones. Although most hearing-impaired people have difficulty with certain tones within the hearing spectrum, most aids amplify all tones equally. Digital aids can be adjusted to screen out background noise and amplify certain tones, depending on the environment (from noisy to quiet). Some of the newest digital hearing aids break down sound into more than twice as many channels as other aids on the market, providing a more personalized hearing experience. They are set by hearing health care providers using an external computer.

Digital Aids

These represent a major breakthrough in hearing aids—hearing instruments that are fully digital. Actually these aids are tiny computers that have a computer chip inside doing the amplifier work, instead of the traditional analog circuitry. These new aids greatly increase the amount of sound processing possible in the same amount of space. These new aids offer minimal distortion, so that they have a clearer, crisper sound. The newest digital aids have the ability to analyze the sound environment and adapt the amplification accordingly, enhancing speech clarity automatically without the necessity of volume controls.

One of the main problems with hearing aids is that they amplify not only the desired sound but extraneous noise as well. Particularly when the source of sound is far away (as on a stage or in a large building), other environmental noises can get in the way. Hearing aids favor sounds in the frequency range of speech; therefore, sounds that lie outside this range may be altered by a hearing aid.

In cases in which the hair cells, which convert vibration to nerve impulses, do not function, a hearing aid will not help. In this case, a COCHLEAR IMPLANT may be helpful. This device converts sound to electrical impulses transmitted directly through wires to the auditory nerve. Although sounds may not be clear, the implant can enhance sound and improve speech comprehension.

hearing aid dealers   Hearing aids may legally be sold and fitted by either a hearing aid dealer (or dispenser) or a "dispensing AUDIOLOGIST" (an audiologist who also sells hearing aids).

The hearing aid dealer will be responsible for making the impression for the EARMOLD and making sure the aid fits properly. The dealer will also explain the general care and use of the aid and will be able to perform both minor and major repairs. Generally, the dealer can offer suggestions about using a hearing aid or about possible changes in hearing aid models and the settings in which they can be used.

Before audiologists moved into the dealership field, hearing aids were sold by people who were not required to have additional training in the field. Most learned the trade by apprenticing to an experienced dealer; for many years, no licensure or registration was required. Some hearing aid dealers call themselves audiologists, but this title should be used only by people who have earned at least a master's degree in audiology.

Today, most states have laws that prohibit anyone from selling a hearing aid before the client has been examined by a physician who can rule out the possibility of a medical problem. (Waivers are permitted for people whose religious beliefs preclude physician visits.) In addition, a license is required for dealers in most states. In order to be licensed, a person combines study with training under a licensed person and then must pass state examination.

As audiologists move into the hearing aid dispensing field, state licensing exams are already being designed with an emphasis on audiological education.

hearing aid helpline   This toll-free telephone number is operated by the National Hearing Aid Society for anyone who suspects a hearing loss and is uncertain what to do or who needs information about hearing loss and hearing aids. The helpline may be used by consumers to locate qualified, competent hearing aid specialists and answer questions about hearing instruments, dispensing and service.

Callers can also obtain a consumer information kit, which includes a regional edition of the membership directory of the Hearing Aid Society plus a 22-page booklet covering topics such as how hearing works, signs of hearing loss and types of hearing aids.

Information is available on ASSISTIVE LISTENING DEVICES, requirements for entering the hearing aid profession, statistics on hearing loss and hearing instruments, federal regulations pertaining to the hearing instrument industry and so forth. The helpline does not provide medical advice, recommend specific products or quote prices.

Although direct financial assistance is not available through the helpline, the helpline can provide a list of possible financial resources. All services and materials provided are free. Callers may use the helpline numbers (1-800-521-5247; in Michigan, 1-313-478-2610) Monday through Friday, 9:00 A.M. to 4:30 P.M. EST.

hearing ear dogs   Certain dogs can be trained to respond to specific sounds (a doorbell, a crying baby, a smoke alarm, an alarm clock) by making physical contact with the owner and leading him or her to the source of the sound.

The dogs, which can be any breed or size, are usually obtained at humane shelters by a nonprofit training center. At these special centers, the dogs complete a six-month program in basic obedience, specialized skills, using both voice and hand signals, and "sound keying"—zeroing in on specific noises. Most dogs are trained to alert in different ways depending on the type of sound so that the owner can distinguish a crying baby from a ringing doorbell.

After training is completed, the dog is taken to its new home, where dog and potential owner go through an intensive one-week course together. After three months of satisfactory performance by the dog, ownership is transferred and certification is granted. The dog's blaze orange collar and leash entitle dog and master to the same legal rights accorded to blind people and their dog guides.

Hearing dog programs are completely supported by donations and community service organizations; no applicant is denied a hearing dog because of inability to pay. See also AMERICAN HUMANE ASSOCIATION; CENTER FOR HEARING EAR DOGS; Appendix XI.

Hearing Education and Awareness for Rockers (H.E.A.R.)   An organization that educates the public about the real dangers of hearing loss resulting from repeated exposure to excessive noise levels. The group offers information about hearing protection, hearing aids, assistive listening devices, ear monitor systems and testing as well as other information about hearing loss and tinnitus. Further, it operates a 24-hour hotline information, referral and support network service. H.E.A.R. also conducts a hearing screening program in the San Francisco Bay area and launches public hearing awareness campaigns, programs for schools and seminars and distributes earplugs to club and concertgoers. See also Appendix II.

hearing evaluation   See AUDIOMETRY.

hearing-impaired   A term for hard-of-hearing or deaf persons that many in the deaf community find objectionable due to its negative connotations. The preferred term is *hard-of-hearing* or *deaf*.

Hearing Industries Association (HIA)   This group is the professional association for hearing aid manufacturers and suppliers of component parts. See also Appendix II.

hearing instrument specialists   Individuals qualified to dispense hearing aids who are licensed by the state in which they practice. Specialists may also be board certified, which involves passing a more rigorous examination than the one given by individual states. There are thousands of hearing instrument specialists in the United States, many of whom belong to the INTERNATIONAL HEARING SOCIETY. (To qualify for membership, hearing instrument specialists must participate in continuing education courses.) The IHS also provides additional training to achieve board certification. See also HEARING AID DEALERS.

hearing loss   An estimated 25–28 million Americans have some form of hearing loss, which can occur at any age and range from mild to severe. Although surveys by the National Center for Health Statistics can estimate numbers of people with hearing problems, there have been no recent surveys on deafness.

While total congenital deafness is rare, occurring only about once in every 1,000 live births, hearing loss in young children is much more common. As many as one-fourth of five-year-olds starting school may have some type of hearing loss, usually because of earlier ear infections.

Partial deafness (from mild to severe) is usually the result of ear disease, injury or breakdown of the hearing mechanisms with age. About one-fourth of people over age 65 need a hearing aid.

It is now possible to detect the presence of hearing loss in a newborn, evaluate its severity and, depending on the type of loss, correct it. A baby who is deaf from birth cannot respond to sounds and, although its crying is normal, the baby will not babble or make other sounds.

In adults, hearing loss brings an inability to hear soft sounds and distorts high tones. Speech may begin to be difficult to understand in the presence of background noise. In addition, the person may experience ringing in the ear (TINNITUS), dizziness and loss of balance (VERTIGO) or even auditory hallucinations.

There are two main types of hearing loss: conductive and sensorineural.

Conductive Hearing Loss
Conductive hearing loss refers to a problem with the transference of sound from the outer to the inner ear, usually because of damage to the eardrum or the three bones of the middle ear (the OSSICLES, also called the hammer, anvil and stirrup).

In an adult, conductive hearing loss may be caused by earwax blocking the outer ear canal or by OTOSCLEROSIS (a disease in which the stapes become fixed). In a child, it is most commonly caused by ear infection with effusion (a collection of sticky fluid in the middle ear). Sometimes conductive hearing loss may be caused by damage to the eardrum or middle ear due to sudden pressure changes (barotrauma, or AERO-OTITIS MEDIA) or by a punctured eardrum.

Conductive hearing loss in children with chronic media can be treated with a MYRINGOTOMY (an operation to drain the fluid from the middle ear). Excessive earwax can be removed with a syringe and warm water, and a PERFORATED EARDRUM that does not heal on its own after a few months can be repaired during an operation called a TYMPANOPLASTY. For otosclerosis, OTOLARYNGOLOGISTS may perform a STAPEDECTOMY (replacement of the stapes).

Sensorineural Hearing Loss

Sensorineural hearing loss is a general term used to describe hearing problems from a number of conditions. It occurs when sounds that reach the inner ear do not reach the brain because of damage to the AUDITORY (hearing) NERVE or the structures of the inner ear. Its effects are permanent and irreversible in almost all cases. This type of hearing loss tends to progress slowly as a person ages and can affect one or both ears.

Sensorineural hearing loss may be mild (15–30 dB loss), causing a person to strain to hear; moderate (35–55 dB loss), requiring frequent repetition and misunderstandings; or severe (60–90 dB loss), leaving the ability to hear only very loud sounds, if anything.

People with sensorineural hearing loss usually have problems understanding speech (word discrimination) even when the speech is loud—which is one reason why hearing aids often do not help. In general, difficulty understanding speech occurs because the person has trouble hearing certain frequencies of sound (or pitch). For example, a hearing problem for high-pitched sounds would mean it would be also hard to hear some consonants (such as t, k, s) because these sounds do not carry voice. People with sensorineural hearing loss may also have a problem with RECRUITMENT (an abnormally rapid increase in sound loudness). Probably because of sensory cell damage, this means a sound that is not heard at one level becomes painfully loud after only a tiny increase in volume.

Every year, about 5,000 infants are born with sensorineural hearing loss caused by genetics, birth injury (Rh incompatibility or loss of oxygen during labor) or damage to the developing fetus because of maternal infection (RUBELLA, herpes or other viral diseases).

After birth, damage to the delicate hearing mechanisms of the inner ear (including the COCHLEA and LABYRINTH) may be caused by prolonged exposure to loud noise, which damages the sensory cells and nerve fibers, particularly if the exposure lasts for a long time. Other diseases causing this type of deafness include MÉNIÈRE'S DISEASE, certain drugs or viral infections. In addition, any disease that affects the flow of blood to the inner ear can also cause hearing problems, including diabetes, emphysema, heart problems, atherosclerosis and some kidney disorders.

Sensorineural hearing loss due to problems with the auditory (hearing) nerve or the hearing centers in the brain may be caused by stroke, head injury or damage from a benign tumor on the nerve (ACOUSTIC NEUROMA).

Among the elderly, the most likely cause of sensorineural hearing loss is related to changes in the ear due to aging (PRESBYCUSIS) which even today is not well understood by scientists.

In still other cases, the cause of sensorineural deafness is simply not known.

Central Hearing Loss

A third, much rarer form of hearing problem is central hearing loss caused by damage to the nerve centers in the pathways to the brain, or in the brain itself. With this type of hearing loss, sound levels are not affected, but understanding of language becomes difficult. Central hearing loss can be caused by high fever, excess exposure to loud noise, OTOTOXIC DRUGS, head injury, circulation problems or tumors.

Classification

Hearing loss can be classified three ways: by type, configuration and degree. Both degree and configuration refer to the range and volume of sounds that cannot be heard; type describes the part of the auditory system that has been affected.

The degree of hearing loss is the volume needed above the normal level for sounds to be heard, and is the most common way to describe a person's hearing problem (such as "profoundly deaf").

But there is more to deafness than just the degree. The configuration of hearing loss is the range of pitch or frequency at which the loss occurs, which influences the ability to hear speech.

Normally, speech varies in loudness and pitch; vowels are strong low-frequency sounds that can penetrate background noise fairly well. On the other hand, consonants tend to be both higher and weaker in pitch, fading out at a distance and obscured by background noise.

In general, hard-of-hearing people hear some frequencies better than others, which can be a problem in understanding speech that involves a broad range of frequencies—especially the higher ones.

People with mild hearing loss may lose track of conversations or have problems hearing across a crowded room. Moderate to severe loss can make speech quite difficult to understand even in the quietest room. Percent of hearing loss is strictly a medical and legal way to handle compensation. It does not deal with problems of clarity of pitch perception, loudness growth and so forth.

Treatment

Although medical and surgical techniques to correct conductive hearing loss have improved, medical correction for sensorineural deafness is more difficult. There is no treatment for central deafness, although special auditory training may provide some help.

There are various treatments for conductive deafness, depending on the cause of the problem. Otosclerosis (fixation of the hearing bones) can be treated with surgery (stapedectomy). A hole in the eardrum or missing hearing bones can be corrected with reconstructive surgery.

Sensorineural hearing loss due to Ménière's disease or other medical problems can sometimes be improved by treating the underlying condition. While there is little help for profound sensorineural hearing loss, current research on COCHLEAR IMPLANTS that provide electrical stimulation to the inner ear may lead to important improvements in the ability to correct this problem. See also AERO-OTITIS MEDIA; GENETICS AND HEARING LOSS; HEARING; PRENATAL CAUSES OF HEARING LOSS.

hearing tests   See AUDIOMETRY.

Heinicke, Samuel (1727–1790) This 18th-century German educator is considered to be the father of the ORAL APPROACH and founded one of the first state-supported public schools for deaf students in the world.

Although others believed that speaking was important in the education of deaf children, it was Heinicke who was convinced that speech is necessary in order to develop abstract thought. He was a contemporary of ABBÉ CHARLES-MICHEL DE L'EPÉE, the founder of the MANUAL APPROACH, with whom he maintained a lifelong debate over the superiority of communication modes.

Born in Nautschutz, Germany, Heinicke joined the Saxon army after a quarrel with his father. While in the army he spent most of his time studying. Eventually, he became a tutor and in 1754 began to teach one of his pupils, a deaf boy, the manual language.

With the onslaught of the Seven Years' War in 1756, Heinicke fled the Prussian troops and eventually settled in Hamburg, where he found work as a private secretary, tutor and schoolteacher. Twenty years after teaching his first deaf student, he began to teach a second, this time abandoning the manual alphabet in favor of speech. In 1775 he published the first textbook ever written for the instruction of deaf students, and his fame as a deaf teacher grew; two years later, he was asked to establish a school for deaf students in Leipzig, Germany.

This new school, the Electoral Saxon Institute for Mutes and Other Persons Afflicted with Speech Defects, opened in 1778 as the first school for deaf students in Germany. It exists today as the Samuel Heinicke School for the Deaf.

Heinicke continued to refine his beliefs in the oral approach for deaf students during his 12 years as administrator at the school. Although he kept his methods to himself, he is known to be the world's first oralist who believed that no hearing child ever learned to speak by first learning letters. Instead, Heinicke taught deaf students the way hearing children learn to speak: first came words, which were then broken down into syllables.

Because Heinicke believed that deaf people have an inner drive to speak just the way hearing people do, he believed teaching speech was not a difficult task. Heinicke was convinced that certain tastes cause the mouth to form the correct position for certain vowels and that by substituting the sense of taste for the lost sense of hearing, Heinicke believed deaf students could be taught to articulate. In his work he used a special artificial throat and tongue designed to help students produce sounds.

Heinicke condemned the practice of operating on the tongue of a deaf child to correct speech defects since he believed that a deaf child's inability to speak was because he could not hear, not because his tongue was malformed.

Although Heinicke allowed the occasional use of signs in order to explain concepts, he required his students to speak out loud to each other in his presence.

De l'Epée and Heinicke both established schools for deaf students in their respective countries, paving the way for the idea of a free public education for deaf students and emphasizing the importance of special education for everyone who needed it. Yet although both de l'Epée and Heinicke believed in the importance of educating deaf children, they differed profoundly over how to accomplish this goal.

Heinicke maintained an ongoing debate with de l'Epée over the superiority of communication methods, and was severely shaken when two universities decided that de l'Epée's manual approach was superior. Heinicke was particularly distressed to learn that the University of Leipzig, with which his school was affiliated, sided with de l'Epée in the controversy. Critics of his method persisted, and Heinicke continued to defend his methods. It appeared that the oral approach was waning and the manual approach was gaining momentum, but Heinicke's theories were eventually resurrected, refined and popularized many years after his unexpected death of a stroke in Leipzig, Germany, on April 30, 1790.

Helen Keller National Center for Deaf-Blind Youth and Adults

The only national facility providing comprehensive services for diagnostic evaluation, rehabilitation and personal adjustment training and job preparation and placement for deaf-blind people.

The center also conducts extensive field service through regional offices, affiliated programs and national training teams, offers services to elderly deaf-blind people and maintains a national register of deaf-blind people. The organization designs and improves sensory aids and publishes *The Nat-Cat News.* See also Appendix II.

helicotrema   An opening in the BASILAR MEMBRANE at the apex of the cochlear canal through which the SCALA TYMPANI meets the SCALA VESTIBULI. Low-frequency vibrations of the oval window create waves in the perilymph of the scala vestibuli through the helicotrema, passing on into the scala tympani.

helix   The curved border of the pinna (outer ear).

Helmholtz, Hermann Ludwig Ferdinand von (1821–1894)

A brilliant physiologist, anatomist, mathematician and physicist, von Helmholtz developed a resonance theory that each sound wave entering the ear induced vibrations in a basilar fiber that responded to the wave's frequency. It was these vibrations, he believed, that stimulated the ORGAN OF CORTI, which transferred the vibrations to the auditory nerve. Later scientists found, however, that while the individual fibers do not resonate, the BASILAR MEMBRANE itself can create the resonance effect.

heredity and deafness   See GENETICS AND HEARING LOSS.

herpes simplex type II   A sexually transmitted disease that can be passed on to the fetus if the mother becomes infected while she is pregnant. Babies born to mothers infected during pregnancy or with an active lesion during birth can contract herpes, which can cause a subsequent hearing loss.

The virus can cause death in affected infants, but modern drug treatments are saving more babies, although the survivors may have hearing loss. See also PRENATAL CAUSES OF HEARING LOSS; VIRUSES AND HEARING LOSS.

herpes zoster   See VIRUSES AND HEARING LOSS.

hertz (Hz)   A unit of vibration frequency adopted internationally to replace the term *cycles per second.* The term was named after German physicist HEINRICH RUDOLF HERTZ.

Hertz, Heinrich Rudolf (1857–1894)

This German physicist proved that light and heat are electromagnetic radiations, and he measured the length and velocity of electromagnetic waves in the laboratory. In honor of his achievements, the unit of vibration frequency, cycles per second, was named for him.

Hertz was also the first to broadcast and receive radio waves and proved that electromagnetic waves had the same properties of susceptibility to reflection and refraction as light and heat waves. See also FREQUENCY; HERTZ.

high-risk questionnaire This assessment, applied to all newborns, consists of a number of factors that identify an infant at risk of a hearing loss. Because most newborns are born with normal hearing, it would not be cost-effective to test all infants for hearing loss. In order to select which newborns will be tested, a high-risk register for the identification of hearing loss has been developed.

If the child has one or more of the listed factors, physicians will recommend an AUDITORY BRAINSTEM RESPONSE TEST. This is a hearing test that can be given to infants since it measures brain wave activity in response to sound. Still, only about half of newborns with one or more of the high-risk factors can be diagnosed with the auditory brainstem response test.

High-risk newborns fall into at least one of the following categories:

Risks Before Birth

Positive family history for deafness, genetic biochemical abnormality associated with deafness, blood incompatibility between mother and child, virus infection, certain OTOTOXIC DRUGS or unusual bleeding during the first trimester.

Labor Complications

Premature delivery, fetal distress, prolonged labor, difficult delivery or birth injury.

Neonatal Difficulty

Apnea, jaundice, multiple anomalies (whatever the cause), drugs (especially streptomycin and kanamycin).

Infants at greatest risk for hearing loss are those with a family history of hearing loss (43 percent) followed by those admitted to the newborn intensive care unit (24 percent), infants with a low APGAR rating (a well-baby assessment that tests breathing, heartrate, color, muscle tone and motor reactions of newborns) (18 percent) or infants affected by maternal infection (12 percent). See also POSTNATAL AND PARTURIENT CAUSES OF HEARING LOSS; PRENATAL CAUSES OF HEARING LOSS.

Holder, William A 17th-century English rector interested in teaching deaf children to speak. His book *Elements of Speech* detailed the position of all organs related to speech during the production of PHONEMES.

Holder advocated positive reinforcement and systematic speech development in which sounds are taught first, combined into syllables and then formed into words associated with objects.

home sign Sometimes called homemade SIGN LANGUAGE, this refers to the gestures developed by deaf people who are isolated from the deaf community. Home sign is often the first way a deaf child communicates with hearing family members. Home signs are not the same as artificial sign languages, which are created by educators as a representation of a spoken language. See also AMERICAN SIGN LANGUAGE; MINIMAL LANGUAGE SKILLS.

homophones Words that look alike to a person who is SPEECHREADING, causing confusion.

House Ear Institute A private, non-profit, medical research organization specializing in research into the ear—the causes of hearing loss, diagnosis and treatment—and training ear specialists and professionals from allied disciplines.

Founded in 1946 as the Los Angeles Foundation of Otology by patients of Dr. Howard P. House, the institute is supported entirely by private funds and was renamed in 1981 to honor House and his brother, Dr. William P. House, director of research.

Research at the institute includes studies of COCHLEAR IMPLANTS, HEARING AIDS, ear disease and tumors, diagnosis, hearing tests, TINNITUS, and prosthetic devices. In addition, the institute's researchers study normal and diseased tissues removed from patients during surgery. Its labs house the world's largest documented collection of temporal bones for microscopic study.

In 1981 the institute began a cochlear implant program for children, providing rehabilitative therapy and helping parents deal with issues facing deaf children. Parents' organizations sponsored by the institute include Bridging the Gap, Family Camp, Kid Safe and the Young Adult Work Program. See also Appendix II.

Hubbard, Gardiner Greene (1822–1897) This Massachusetts lawyer was passionately interested in educating deaf people, largely because his daughter Mabel (later the wife of ALEXANDER GRAHAM BELL) lost her hearing after a bout of scarlet fever at age four.

When Hubbard was told his daughter would lose her speech and could not attend school for six more years, he realized he would need to educate his daughter himself—or find a teacher who could. Aware of the success achieved by German educators of deaf students, he decided to set up a similar school in Northampton.

Hubbard was instrumental in the establishment of the Clarke Institution for Deaf Mutes, in Northampton, Massachusetts, an oral school for deaf students now called the Clarke School.

With his son-in-law Alexander Graham Bell, Hubbard founded the American Association to Promote the Teaching of Speech to the Deaf, the National Geographic Society and the publication *Science*, the official magazine of the American Asso-

ciation for the Advancement of Science. In addition to his many entrepreneurial ventures, such as bringing gas lights and water to Cambridge, Hubbard led the presidential commission to reorganize the U.S. Postal Service and was a trustee of the Smithsonian Institution.

hypacusis Another word for hard-of-hearing.

hyperacusis An unusually acute sense of hearing.

Hyperacusis Network An international support group established to care for individuals with collapsed tolerance to sound (HYPERACUSIS and RECRUITMENT). The network helps educate the medical community and families about this rare auditory disorder by sharing ways to cope, providing advice on how to secure disability assistance and reporting on current research and/or treatment options. Membership in the network is free. See also Appendix II.

hypoacousia See HYPOACUSIA.

hypoacusia A synonym for hearing loss.

hysterical hearing loss See FUNCTIONAL HEARING LOSS (NONORGANIC).

Hz See HERTZ.

identification audiometry Screening large numbers of people to identify those with hearing problems who need to be given more specific tests on an individual basis. See also AUDIOMETRY.

idiopathic endolymphatic hydrops See MÉNIÈRE'S DISEASE.

immittance tests See AUDIOMETRY.

immune system and hearing loss The immune system is crucial to the defense against infection of both the middle and inner ear. There is evidence that a faulty immune system can induce hearing loss and is responsible for the progression of chronic OTITIS MEDIA and possibly other disorders for which no cause has been found, such as MÉNIÈRE'S DISEASE.

In addition, certain diseases that affect the immune system—such as AIDS—can also result in hearing loss. See AIDS AND HEARING LOSS.

impacted earwax A hard plug of EARWAX firmly filling the ear canal, blocking the passage of sound to the eardrum and interfering with hearing. Symptoms are worsened if water enters the ear, causing the wax to swell.

Normally, earwax (or CERUMEN) is produced by glands in the skin of the outer ear canal and carried outward to the external ear. When it is produced too quickly, it builds up and forms a hard plug.

Large plugs of earwax must be removed by a physician; smaller plugs may be removed at home. A person can remove hard wax with mineral oil drops; soft wax can be removed with hydrogen peroxide drops or a commercial softener. The drops may be applied overnight and then removed by irrigating the ear with warm water from a baby ear syringe.

COTTON SWABS should not be used because of the danger of pushing wax deeper into the ear.

impedance audiometry A test to measure hearing at the level of the COCHLEA and brainstem to determine how well the cochlea and auditory pathways of the medulla are functioning. Impedance refers to the opposition to the flow of energy.

In the test, two tubes are placed into the external ear canal, and sound is sent from a small loudspeaker through one tube. The sound reflected from the eardrum is picked up by the other tube, which leads to a microphone, amplifier and recorder. When a sudden intense sound is applied to the other ear, the stapedius muscle contracts, the impedance is increased and the recorder indicates when more sound is picked up.

This does not, however, measure the actual acoustic impedance of the ear. This is tested by using an acoustic bridge, which allows an OTOLOGIST to listen to a sound as it is reflected from the patient's eardrum. At the same time, a similar sound of the same intensity is reflected in an artificial cavity that is adjusted to equal that of the external canal of the ear.

When the two sounds are matched by changing the acoustic impedance of the cavity, the otologist can then read the impedance of the ear from the scale of the instrument. This test can uncover conductive defects of the MIDDLE EAR (including discontinuity of the ossicular chain and immobility of the malleus or stapes). See also ACOUSTIC IMMITANCE; AUDIOMETRY.

implantable hearing aid Still in experimental stages, this type of hearing aid would be implanted within the ear canal in the hope of overcoming many of the drawbacks of conventional in-the-ear HEARING AIDS. There has been considerable research in the past 10 years into this type of aid. These in-the-ear aids have a tendency toward acoustic feedback and cause discomfort and can also worsen ear infections.

The implantable aid would effectively remove the feedback problem by eliminating acoustic coupling and should provide greater comfort and benefit to hard-of-hearing people. It would also be more acceptable to those who need amplification but cannot (or choose not) to use currently-available hearing aids. See also COCHLEAR IMPLANT.

incus   The middle bone of the three OSSICLES of the middle ear, also known as the ANVIL.

India   It is estimated that out of India's population of more than 700 million, 800,000 are deaf; most of these live in the rural areas. Only about 5 percent of India's deaf children are currently in school. At a deafness rate of 66 per 100,000, India is about midway between Peru's high rate (300) and Australia's low rate (35).

Communication for India's deaf population is complicated by the fact that the country is considered trilingual, with the three languages being Hindi, English and one of the many regional languages. The education a deaf child would receive varies depending on the area in which he or she grows up.

The government is interested in helping provide services for its deaf citizens, but most resources for this purpose are limited.

India's first school for deaf students was opened in 1885; since 1900, 200 more schools have been established—none in the rural areas. Of the 200, only 14 offer secondary school education, and only a few offer vocational training. There is no school for university education for deaf students, although there are a few deaf Indian students studying at universities in the United States.

Education in India is not required, is not free and is based on an oral approach. Although most deaf Indians communicate in sign, its use in schools has been repressed.

INDIAN SIGN LANGUAGE is a highly-structured, grammatical language, and its first dictionary was published in 1980.

Most deaf citizens are unemployed. There is no national captioning service, TELECOMMUNICATIONS FOR THE DEAF (TDDs) are not available and there are almost no interpreters, even in large cities.

Indian Sign Language   Despite India's official languages and more than 200 dialects, Indian Sign Language (ISL) is surprisingly universal in India; there is only one sign language, and more than one million deaf Indians communicate with it.

In general, the signs of the Indian system do not relate to any of the European sign languages, although there are a few signs similar to BRITISH SIGN LANGUAGE and its FINGERSPELLING system.

Because ISL is not used in schools, most deaf speakers use the pure, natural sign language. Initial research in ISL suggests its grammar is complex and is not similar to any languages of India.

induction coil   Another name for a loop device. See also AUDIO LOOP; AUDIO LOOP SYSTEM; LISTENING DEVICE.

induction loop devices   See AUDIO LOOP SYSTEM.

infection, ear   See OTITIS MEDIA.

Ingrassia, Giovanni (1510–1580)   Born in Recalbuto, Sicily, Ingrassia was one of the most well-known Renaissance anatomists, and a contemporary of BARTOLOMEO EUSTACHIO and GABRIELE FALLOPPIO. A professor in Padua, Naples and Palermo, and adviser to the king, he was among the first to describe the tympanic cavity and the OSSICLES and was credited with discovering the STAPES in 1546.

inner ear   An extremely intricate portion of the ear deep within the skull that contains the AUDITORY NERVE and the balance mechanism of the body in a winding maze of passages called the LABYRINTH.

The front of the inner ear, which resembles a snail shell and is concerned with hearing, is called the COCHLEA. The rear part, concerned with balance, is a series of three SEMICIRCULAR CANALS at right angles to each other and connected to a cavity called the VESTIBULE.

These canals contain hair cells continually bathed in fluid, some of which are sensitive to gravity and acceleration and others to position and movements of the head. This sensory information is registered by the cells and conveyed by nerve fibers to the brain.

inner ear diseases and hearing loss Diseases located deep within the auditory structure are difficult to diagnose, especially since it is impossible to visually inspect the COCHLEA. Inner ear diseases involve SENSORINEURAL HEARING LOSSES that are very difficult to pinpoint since they are rarely isolated problems. In fact, the cause of many sensorineural problems, such as MÉNIÈRE'S DISEASE, are often impossible to determine.

Still, the inner ear is susceptible to many of the same problems that affect the middle ear: infection and inflammation, injury and OTOTOXIC DRUGS.

Injuries

Injury to the temporal bone can affect the inner ear and is a common cause of a sensorineural hearing loss since head injuries occur in more than three-quarters of auto accidents. Hitting the front or the back of the head can result in a transverse fracture, causing SENSORINEURAL HEARING LOSS, VERTIGO or TINNITUS. Severe blows to the head can also damage the ORGAN OF CORTI.

Barotrauma (sudden pressure changes in airplanes or deepsea diving resulting in unequal pressure in the ear) can damage the cochlea, membranes of the round or oval windows or REISSNER'S MEMBRANE, all causing a sensorineural hearing loss.

Infection

LABYRINTHITIS (inflammation of the inner ear), carried by bacteria or viruses from the middle ear, brain or bloodstream, can result in a sensorineural hearing loss.

Ototoxic Drugs

The cochlea and VESTIBULAR SYSTEM are susceptible to the effects of a range of ototoxic drugs, especially aminoglycoside antibiotics, which cause a gradual or sudden sensorineural hearing loss. Hearing loss from ototoxic drugs cannot usually be reversed because the drugs damage hair cells, which do not regenerate, and also harm the AUDITORY NERVE.

Ménière's Disease

This disease, which distends the membranous labyrinth, causes sensorineural hearing loss (usually in one ear), sudden attacks of vertigo and tinnitus. Hearing loss usually causes difficulty in hearing low-frequency sounds, progressing to difficulty with high frequency sounds as well. The cause of Ménière's disease is still not known, although a wide range of factors have been suggested.

Aging

As a person ages, the hair cells in the organ of Corti begin to degenerate and the BASILAR MEMBRANE stiffens. Called PRESBYCUSIS, the sensorineural hearing loss of old age is first noticed as a loss of understanding in the higher frequencies in late middle age.

Diseases

Several systemic diseases affect hearing, including certain genetic syndromes. High blood pressure and other vascular disorders can result in a sudden sensorineural loss because of clots in the internal auditory artery or a hemorrhage in the cochlea, destroying hair cells because of decreased blood flow.

Diabetes can cause a sensorineural hearing loss because of degeneration of blood vessels and nerves that supply the ear and internal auditory canal. Kidney disease often causes sensorineural hearing problems in patients who undergo hemodialysis or kidney transplants.

Genetic diseases that result in sensorineural hearing loss include PAGET'S DISEASE and ALPORT'S DISEASE. COGAN'S SYNDROME is an inflammation of the cornea accompanied by vertigo, tinnitus and severe sensorineural hearing loss with unknown cause. See also AERO-OTITIS MEDIA; DIABETES AND HEARING LOSS; GENETICS AND HEARING LOSS.

Institut National des Jeunes Sourds Also called the Paris Institute, this institution was founded by ABBÉ CHARLES-MICHEL DE L'ÉPÉE in the 1700s and is today the oldest permanent school for deaf students in the world.

Begun with a grant from King Louis XVI, the school managed to stay open during the French

Revolution. De l'Epée began the school by teaching two sisters in his home and by the late 1760s had six students; 10 years later there were 30 students, and at the time of de l'Epée's death in 1789, there were more than 60.

After the death of de l'Epée, the school was run by ABBÉ ROCH-AMBROISE CUCURRON SICARD, who convinced the French National Assembly that aid for handicapped students was a natural duty. In response, the assembly nationalized the school in 1791, naming it the National Institution for the Congenitally Deaf (Institut National des Sourds-Muets de Naissance).

The years of the French Revolution were difficult, and Sicard, the school's director, was imprisoned at least twice as a suspected Royalist. He was saved at last by a petition from his deaf students. Sicard directed the spartan program for 32 years until his death in 1822 at the age of 80. At that time, the school had 150 students, all whom used SIGN LANGUAGE (Old French Sign Language).

After the Catholic church was reestablished in France following the Revolution (in 1801), the school began to emphasize religion for its deaf student. See also Appendix II.

intensity   The strength of a sound the brain perceives as loudness; usually measured by the amplitude of its wave. It is also measured in decibels.

internal acoustic meatus   A passage in the temporal bone for the facial and auditory nerves. It is also called the internal auditory meatus or the meatus auditorius internus.

International Catholic Deaf Association   A group promoting ministry to Catholic deaf people and responding to spiritually-related requests worldwide.

In general, Catholics have not had separate congregations for deaf members, although they do provide worship services in which an interpreter or priest signs the spoken portion of the mass. However, there are a few deaf Catholic churches in the United States, including St. Mary Magdalene Church for the Deaf (Denver, Colorado), Mother of Perpetual Help Church for the Deaf (Omaha, Nebraska), St. Francis of Assisi Catholic Church and

Center for the Deaf (Landover Hills, Maryland), St. John's Deaf Center (Warren, Michigan) and the Catholic Deaf Center (New Orleans, Louisiana). See also NATIONAL CATHOLIC OFFICE OF THE DEAF.

International Congress on the Education of the Deaf   For the past century, international meetings have been held to discuss education for deaf students, although early meetings rarely involved deaf educators or deaf persons at all.

For the first 100 years, no group administered these international meetings; a meeting could be called simply whenever a group within a country invited representatives from other countries to meet. But in 1975 in Tokyo, an International Congress Committee made up of the chairs of the three preceding congresses was finally established.

Many different topics were discussed at these meetings, but the prime controversy for almost 100 years was the debate between the ORAL APPROACH and the MANUAL APPROACH. The oral approach was the early favorite, and the second international Congress of Milan 1880 had an enormous effect on the education of deaf students around the world when convention participants decided that speech was "incontestably superior" to sign.

Further, Milan congressional delegates decided they preferred the oral approach over the simultaneous use of signs and speech as well. Milan resolutions cited the long-term benefits of oral education and devised procedures to introduce the oral approach into the schools.

The only votes against these pro-oral approach resolutions were an English delegate and the American delegates led by EDWARD MINER GALLAUDET. The oral-manual controversy continued to rage in nearly all of the congresses up until 1980, when delegates at the Hamburg Congress decided the controversy was pointless and that both the oral and manual approaches could be helpful to deaf persons.

International Games for the Deaf   See WORLD GAMES FOR THE DEAF.

international hand alphabet   See INTERNATIONAL MANUAL ALPHABET.

International Hearing Society (IHS)   A professional association that represents hearing instrument specialists who test hearing and select, fit and dispense hearing instruments. It is a leading consumer advocate and conducts programs on competency qualification, education and training and promotes specialty-level accreditation for its members.

Founded in 1951 by a group of hearing instrument specialists, the society is active in promoting the highest possible standards for its members. Its directory lists members of the hearing health profession approved by the qualifications board of the society. The group also publishes a journal, *Audecibel* and provides consumer information through a toll-free helpline. See also Appendix II.

International Lutheran Deaf Association   Nonprofit organization that promotes Lutheran ministry for deaf people throughout the Lutheran Church-Missouri Synod. The group, which publishes *The Deaf Lutheran,* holds an annual convention.

international manual alphabet   A manual alphabet devised by the WORLD FEDERATION OF THE DEAF and used primarily in Scandinavian countries.

International Organization for the Education of the Hearing Impaired   See ALEXANDER GRAHAM BELL ASSOCIATION FOR THE DEAF.

International Phonetic Association alphabet (IPA)   The most widely used phonetic alphabet, which is used to describe the segmental sound of speech. Most of the symbols in this alphabet are variations of Roman letters and can be used to describe speech in any language or dialect.

A sentence transcribed into a phonetic alphabet would allow a person to correctly speak the transcription, even if in a language that has never been heard.

A phonetic symbol represents a letter as a type of shorthand to describe how that sound is produced. For sounds that also have small differences in how they are pronounced, the alphabet uses basic and secondary symbols called diacritics, which are placed above or below (or before or after) the primary symbols. These diacritical marks indicate differences in sound.

The phonetic symbols used in dictionaries are not generally the IPA but the dictionary's own phonetic symbols, which are defined for readers using key words.

interpreters   See ORAL INTERPRETERS; SIGN LANGUAGE INTERPRETERS.

interpreters and the law   Since the 1960s, federal and state governments have enacted several laws requiring that a certified interpreter be provided for hard-of-hearing people during various court proceedings.

Unfortunately, although each state has some type of law guaranteeing an interpreter for a deaf person, many of the laws are vague, simple or unclear. Some laws state that courts and judges may appoint an interpreter when "necessary," but it is unclear who pays for these services, what the qualifications of the interpreter must be or what "necessary" means. Some states have comprehensive laws stating that interpreters should be appointed at the time of arrest in all civil and criminal cases, for the preparation of depositions, during commitment hearings, before grand juries, for a state exam needed for employment with the state and in juvenile proceedings.

Under state law, it is generally up to the judge to decide the qualifications for interpreters; some states do require consultation with the local or national REGISTRY OF INTERPRETERS FOR THE DEAF.

In criminal proceedings, most states will pay for an interpreter, and some states will pay for these services during civil proceedings as well.

Hard-of-hearing and deaf persons have the right under federal and state law to use the services of interpreters upon their request. When a hard-of-hearing or deaf person states a preference for an oral interpreter, the court must do its best to find one.

The situation is a little more clear in federal courts. When the federal government brings a criminal or civil action against a deaf individual, the law requires that the court appoint a qualified interpreter; in other situations, the federal court can appoint an interpreter if it so chooses. See also COURT INTERPRETER'S ACT; LEGAL RIGHTS.

interpreter services   See ORAL INTERPRETERS; SIGN LANGUAGE INTERPRETERS.

in-the-ear hearing aid   A type of hearing aid that fits completely inside the ear. These types of HEARING AIDS are becoming more popular. They are lightweight devices in a custom EARMOLD and fit inside the ear canal with no external wires or tubes. Most of the device fits into the space in the external ear leading to the ear canal.

The microphone, volume control and battery compartment are located on the outer surface and are visible. Fitted with tone control, these models are generally useful only for mild hearing loss.

intra-aural muscles   The two muscles contained in the middle ear, known separately as the TENSOR TYMPANI and the STAPEDIAL MUSCLE. Their action is reflexive and bilateral and may be initiated either by intense acoustic stimulation or by irritation of the tissues of the external or middle ears.

A number of functions for these muscles have been suggested, but only two are generally accepted: The muscles assist in maintaining the OSSICULAR CHAIN in its proper position, and they act to protect the internal ear from too much stimulation by inhibiting ossicular movement.

Some research data suggest that the intra-aural muscles under moderate levels of tension and at certain frequencies slightly enhance the transmission of sound by the middle ear.

Irish Sign Language   There are three sign systems used in the Republic of Ireland—two based on manual English systems and one indigenous, informal method.

The newest system, called Irish Sign Language, is a manual code for English with one vocabulary for both men and women, unlike the older system with separate styles for men and women. It was introduced in the late 1970s by the Unified Sign Language Committee.

Most signs in the new system are based on the first letter of the word in English and are grouped so that many words of similar meaning will use the same basic sign but with different handshapes. This new sign language is used in some sign language classes taught outside traditional deaf schools and in the manual classes in the oral deaf schools. However, many people in the Irish deaf community prefer the old sign language system.

This older system is also a manual code for English and uses gender-specific vocabularies. Brought over from France in the 1800s, the French signs were modified to express English grammar and also split into "feminine" styles for use with the deaf girls' schools and more "masculine" for the deaf boys' schools. Today, the two vocabularies differ as much as 30 percent, although boys and girls can still understand each other.

Finally, the "informal" sign language, known as Deaf Sign Language, is used by deaf people in informal settings and is less accepted than the first two. It is believed this informal method is derived from the old sign language used in the Irish schools, but it does not parallel English grammar. Like all natural sign languages, however, it does appear to have its own grammatical system.

To a degree, portions of Irish sign systems have been exported to both South Africa and Australia.

Israel   Although there have been no definitive studies of the deaf population in Israel, estimates suggest that the incidence of deafness in Asiatic-African Jewish children and Israel's minority (predominantly Arab) group is about double that of European-American children. This unexpected incidence of hearing problems is probably due to the incidence of intermarriage within these cultures.

By age one, most of the country's deaf children are referred to one of the nationwide nonprofit institutions designed for deaf infants. Two of these centers use Total Communication; three use the oral approach. At these centers, parents are offered a range of services, including sign language classes, special discussions groups and home training. By the age of five or six, most deaf Jewish children are mainstreamed into state-supported kindergartens; about 10 percent attend special kindergartens designed for deaf pupils only. Once a child reaches elementary age, there are several options: a special school for deaf children, integrated classes, mainstreaming or a special school for multidisabled children.

Until 1976, all school programs used the oral approach; today educators use a combined approach (speech and ISRAELI SIGN LANGUAGE). At high school age, a student can choose to attend a vocational high school, integrated classes or mainstreaming.

In addition, the government offers its deaf citizen job placement and training services and private tutoring for deaf children in regular classes.

Israeli Sign Language was developed in the early 1900s and was eventually unified during the late 1950s with the establishment of the Association of the Deaf. In 1977, a signed Hebrew alphabet was created.

In general, Israel's heritage and comparatively concentrated number of deaf citizens has led to a wide network of services and programs for the deaf community.

Israeli Sign Language   About 5,000 deaf Israelis use Israeli Sign Language (ISL), a relatively new language continually infused with new signs from other countries as immigrants come to ISRAEL. In addition, a FINGERSPELLING system for Hebrew was adapted from the American MANUAL ALPHABET and includes 16 handshapes for Hebrew.

Still considered a very new language, ISL appears to be very flexible regarding sign order. The modifying sign follows the sign for the thing it modifies (for example, cat fat) and quantifiers precede the sign for the thing quantified (four horses) or bracket the thing quantified (four horses four). Israeli sign language also has major structural characteristics as in other sign language, such as the simultaneity of signs.

Although deaf schools in Israel have been completely oral since the first school was founded in

1934, teachers today use some ISL signs in their oral classes.

Italian Sign Language   Still widely considered to be simple gestures in ITALY, research has found the sign language of deaf Italians is indeed a complete language with a complex structure and grammar.

The structural features of LIS (Lingua Italiana dei Segni) are different from other languages, and the Italian spoken language influences LIS in the use of speechreading and articulation. FINGERSPELLING is rarely used, although there is an old and a new manual alphabet. The older method, used primarily by older deaf Italians, is a two-handed system employing hands and the face. The new version, used by younger deaf Italians, is a one-handed system using only handshapes.

There is no census information available on the number of people who use ISL, and it is not used in the all-oral school systems.

Italy   The exact number of deaf citizens is not known, but a 1980 survey suggests that there may be at least 70,000 profoundly deaf people in Italy, with the rate of deafness higher in the southern regions of the country. In general, hearing loss occurs in about 8–10 percent of the general population, or about 3.5 million Italians.

Although there is a significant lack of good services and programs for them, deaf Italians do have a strong community among themselves, including a national organization for the deaf, and promote ITALIAN SIGN LANGUAGE, OR LIS (Lingua Italiana dei Segni).

The government provides special services only for preschool through age 14, either in special, mostly residential schools or mainstreamed with hearing children. The ORAL APPROACH is generally the preferred educational mode of communication, and sign language is generally prohibited in class, although it is tolerated elsewhere. In actuality, most deaf students and adults communicate in sign.

Japan Between 320,000 and 7.5 million Japanese have hearing problems, and the programs and services for this population have improved since World War II.

Education is compulsory between ages nine and 15, and in Japan deaf and hard-of-hearing children are treated separately: Deaf children are educated in special schools, and hard-of-hearing children attend special classes or are mainstreamed. Special school populations, however, are decreasing as more and more deaf students are attending regular classes and going to a university. There are 131 deaf institutions in Japan.

Most schools in Japan use the ORAL APPROACH, although more and more schools are introducing CUED SPEECH; students use sign language among themselves. Although JAPANESE SIGN LANGUAGE is not yet considered a language, since it does not match the expressive forms of the Japanese oral language, efforts are being made to make it more systematic.

The Japanese Association of the Deaf and Dumb, with 20,000 members, serves as an advocate for improved services for deaf Japanese. The association offers an annual convention and an annual sports meeting and has local branches in many areas throughout Japan. In addition, the Japanese Society for the Study of Education for the Deaf is a national network of 5,000 teachers in deaf schools. Deaf adults can expect a lower standard of living than hearing Japanese, and less than 32 percent of all Japanese deaf people are employed at all. Still, the outlook has improved since new laws require public agencies and private businesses to hire a certain number of physically disabled people.

Japanese Sign Language More than 95 percent of the 320,000 deaf Japanese are assumed to be able to understand Japanese Sign Language (JSL), called Shuwa (hand talk).

Since all deaf schools are officially oral except for a few that use the simultaneous method (communication combining speech, sign and fingerspelling), JSL does not play a large part in the educational system. In the classes that use the simultaneous method, teachers use Signed Japanese or manually coded Japanese. Their sign language, called simultaneous methodic signs, uses FINGERSPELLING to represent suffixes and postpositions. In general, this language is not accepted by people in the deaf community, who use Pidgin Sign Japanese in communicating with deaf and hearing Japanese. Pidgin Sign Language is also used on TV programs, lectures and so forth.

Still in the early stages of research, JSL is not yet well understood by linguists.

Jena method Developed by Karl Brauckmann in Jena, Germany, the Jena method is a system of teaching SPEECHREADING that focuses attention on the syllable and rhythm patterns in speech.

Jewish Deaf Congress This organization (formerly known as the National Congress of Jewish Deaf) has served as an advocate for religious and cultural ideals and fellowship for Jewish deaf people since it was established in 1956. It serves as a clearinghouse for information about religious, educational and cultural programs for deaf Jews and represents them in projects involving nursing homes, interpreters, legal rights, demographic studies, education, sports and so forth. Publications include *The J.D. Quarterly.* The congress maintains a Hall of Fame honoring well-known deaf Jews and has been active in the campaign against offensive signs and terms for the words

Jews and *Jewish*. The group also participated in founding the World Organization of Jewish Deaf People in Israel in 1977 to serve deaf Jews in Israel and Europe. In the 1960s, the group established an endowment fund to provide for the education of deaf rabbis. The congress holds biennial conventions in major cities. See also Appendix 2.

The Job Accommodation Network (JAN)   This international toll-free consulting service is not a job-placement service, but an information source about job accommodations and the employability of people with hearing problems. JAN also provides information regarding the Americans with Disabilities Act (ADA). It is located at West Virginia University in Morgantown.

Johnston test   A group pure-tone screening test for children in kindergarten through second grade. See also MASSACHUSETTS TEST; SWEEP-CHECK TEST.

journals in the field of deafness   A wide range of professional publications are available for people who work in the field of deafness. Full addresses of publications can be found in Appendix VII in the back of this book.

Journal of Auditory Research

This publication of the C.W. Shilling Auditory Research Center, Inc., was founded in 1961 for audiologists, auditory neurophysiologists, engineers, musicologists, otologists, psychoacousticians, sensory and comparative psychologists, speech scientists and anyone interested in the study of hearing.

It includes experimental papers on a variety of topics, and its board includes otologists, audiologists, psychologists, psychoacousticians and speech scientists. Because the subject matter of the journal is so broad, there is no board of review editors.

Journal of Communication Disorders

This publication discusses a broad spectrum of topics in the field of communication disorders, including pure experimental research and clinical and theoretical issues.

Its audience includes linguists, neurologists, otolaryngologists, psychologists, psychiatrists and speech and hearing specialists. Articles primarily discuss problems related to disorders of communication, including the normal communicative processes, plus the anatomical, physiological, diagnostic, psychodynamic and psychopathological aspects of communication disorders. Most issues also contain a mix of different articles and an international review of publications dealing with communication disorders.

Journal of the American Deafness and Rehabilitation Association

This official publication of the AMERICAN DEAFNESS AND REHABILITATION ASSOCIATION, begun in 1967, is published quarterly. Articles are published on the field of deafness and are reviewed by professionals in medicine-psychiatry, psychology, vocational rehabilitation and education.

Journal of Speech and Hearing Disorders

Published by the AMERICAN SPEECH-LANGUAGE-HEARING ASSOCIATION, this 54-year-old journal is one of six official periodicals of the association. Published quarterly, its circulation includes more than 50,000 practitioners in the field of speech and hearing disorders. The journal accepts articles, reports and letters focusing primarily on clinical issues, including the nature and treatment of disordered speech, hearing and language. The journal does not publish articles on theoretical or experimental research in speech, hearing or language sciences, which are published by the association's *Journal of Speech and Hearing Research*.

The *Journal of Speech and Hearing Disorders* also publishes conference proceedings in its *ASHA Reports* and information on single subjects in monographs. Information on language, speech and hearing services for children (especially in school) are not included in the journal but appear in the association's *Language, Speech and Hearing Services in Schools*.

Journal of Speech and Hearing Research

This publication is one of two journals published by the American Speech-Language-Hearing Association. Designed to appeal to researchers—as opposed to the *Journal of Speech and Hearing Disorders*—the journal is aimed at clinicians in the field of speech and hearing science.

This quarterly journal focuses on studies of the processes and disorders of speech, language and hearing and has more than 50,000 readers.

Journal of the Acoustical Society of America

This 60-year-old monthly publication of the Acoustical Society of America publishes articles in several branches of acoustics, including general linear, nonlinear, physiological, psychological and architectural acoustics; aeroacoustics; atmospheric and underwater sound; ultrasonics, mechanical, shock and random vibration; vibration of plates and shells; noise and its control; acoustic signal processing; speech communication; music and instruments; bioacoustics; acoustical measurements and instrumentation; and acoustical transduction. In addition to research papers in these areas, the journal includes society activities, calendars of meetings of other relevant societies, book reviews of acoustical patents.

Each year, three separate supplements are published by the society; two contain abstracts of all papers presented at the two annual conventions; the third, *References to Contemporary Papers on Acoustics,* is a bibliography of recent articles on acoustics published throughout the world.

Junior National Association of the Deaf   This group, affiliated with the NATIONAL ASSOCIATION OF THE DEAF, tries to develop leadership, scholarship and service among deaf high school students. The organization carries out its mandate by creating opportunities for hands-on experience through participation in various extracurricular activities and a youth leadership camp.

The first Junior NAD national convention was held in 1968 at Gallaudet University, with 120 student delegates from 36 chapters in schools for deaf students. The association also publishes the *Junior NAD Newsletter.* See also Appendix II.

Justinian Code   During the reign of Justinian I from A.D. 527–565, all of Roman law was codified, including the legal rights of deaf citizens (which were basically nonexistent).

Deaf Romans could not marry, and legal guardians were appointed to handle their affairs. The code was more lenient for the adventitious deaf person, allowing those with acquired deafness to handle their own affairs if they could write.

Keller, Helen Adams (1880–1968) This world-famous Alabama woman, blind and deaf from early childhood, became one of the best-known advocates of the education for blind and deaf students and was hailed for her achievement as a writer and lecturer.

She was born June 27, 1880, the daughter of a former officer in the Confederate army. A severe illness at 19 months destroyed both her sight and hearing, and she quickly deteriorated from an energetic, bright child into a spoiled, rebellious youngster who was almost impossible to handle.

Aware that the Perkins Institute for the Blind in Massachusetts had successfully educated a deaf-blind girl 50 years earlier, Helen's parents—on the advice of ALEXANDER GRAHAM BELL—sought help from the institute in educating Helen.

The institute recommended a former graduate, Anne Mansfield Sullivan, then 20 and partially blind herself. Sullivan arrived March 3, 1887, and began trying to teach young Helen names of objects by pressing the manual alphabet into her hand. Eventually, Sullivan managed to break through Helen's dark and silent world when Helen finally connected the feel of the water running over her hand to its manual sign.

A remarkably bright child, Helen's vocabulary increased rapidly, and she went on to be educated at the Horace Mann School for the Deaf in Boston and the Wright-Humason Oral School in New York City, where she learned to read and write in braille. She graduated cum laude in 1904 from Radcliffe, where Sullivan spelled lectures into her hand.

Keller—a close friend of the oralist Bell—was likewise a confirmed oralist who had learned to speak by feeling vibrations in Sullivan's larynx. Although far from perfect, her voice was understood by those who knew her well. Still, aware of the controversy between oral and manual methods of communication, she tried to find a common ground, admitting that no method was perfect and that deaf people need every advantage they can get.

Although her voice required interpretation in public, she became a noted lecturer for 12 years. Eventually, she became affiliated with the American Foundation for the Blind and spent many years traveling and speaking all over the world for this group.

In addition to lectures, Keller was a prolific writer; she wrote speeches, letters, magazine articles and books, including: *The Story of My Life* (1903), *The World I Live In* (1908), *Out of the Dark* (1913), *Midstream* (1929), *Helen Keller in Scotland* (1933), *Helen Keller's Journal* (1938) and *Teacher: Anne Sullivan Macy: A Tribute by the Foster-Child of Her Mind* (1955).

Although known all over the world, Keller lived within a small, protected circle: the ever-present, possessive teacher (Sullivan), Sullivan's husband John Macy and, later, an assistant. In her middle years she intended to marry but decided against it in the face of her mother's reluctance to "lose" her daughter.

A relentlessly kind woman, Keller was a suffragist strongly opposed to racism and war; she joined the Socialist party and ardently supported the Bolshevik Revolution.

Of her blindness and deafness, Keller considered deafness to be the greater loss, and her efforts to help those who were both blind and deaf led to the establishment of the HELEN KELLER NATIONAL CENTER FOR DEAF-BLIND YOUTHS AND ADULTS in Sands Point, New York.

Kendall Demonstration Elementary School
Originating as a school for deaf pupils in the Washington, D.C., area in 1857, the Kendall school became a national demonstration elementary school in 1970 when Congress mandated it provide not only an education to local students but also conduct research into a deaf education for dissemination across the country.

Public Law 91-587 set up the school as a demonstration center and emphasized that it must stress innovative auditory and visual devices, excellent architecture and works of art. Legislation also set up a new high school in 1966 for deaf secondary students located at GALLAUDET UNIVERSITY campus.

Kendall accepts students from birth to age 15 who live in the national capital region (the District of Columbia, northern Virginia and nearby Maryland counties) and have a hearing problem severe enough to warrant placement in a special class. Among its commuter students, 90 percent have a severe to profound hearing loss and the other 10 percent have a severe to moderate loss. About 30 percent have a disability in addition to hearing problems. The school includes a parent-infant program and a pre-school, primary, intermediate and middle school. Because it was designed as a demonstration school, Kendall often serves as a product testing ground and also supports applied and basic research. See also MODEL SECONDARY SCHOOL FOR THE DEAF.

kernicterus A jaundiced area of the newborn brain caused by the destruction of red blood cells. An incompatibility of Rh blood factors between infant and mother causes this destruction.

Untreated, kernicterus can cause central nerve deafness. See also HEARING LOSS; RH FACTOR INCOMPATIBILITY AND DEAFNESS.

kidney failure and hearing loss Kidney disease requiring renal dialysis and transplantation often causes a type of SENSORINEURAL HEARING LOSS. This loss can be caused by a number of factors, including electrolyte imbalance, inadequate dialysis or drug ototoxicity (diuretics or aminoglycosides), which can affect the components of the INNER EAR fluid and alter the normal function of the COCHLEA.

labyrinth, inner ear   This section of the INNER EAR contains the nerve endings of the vestibular nerve (the nerve of equilibrium) and the AUDITORY NERVE (nerve of hearing).

Diseases of the labyrinth may affect both nerves or only the auditory nerve, causing hearing loss, or only the vestibular nerve, disrupting balance and causing VERTIGO. Common inner ear diseases include congenital nerve deafness (a defect of the hearing nerve in the COCHLEA), viral nerve deafness (a hearing impairment caused by a virus, such as mumps, measles or flu), deafness from OTOTOXIC DRUGS, skull fracture, NOISE exposure, LABYRINTHITIS, ACOUSTIC NEUROMA, MENIERE'S DISEASE or PRESBYCUSIS.

labyrinthectomy   Surgical excision of the entire inner ear. This operation has been replaced by selective VESTIBULAR NERVE SECTION, which preserves hearing in those patients with incapacitating VERTIGO.

labyrinthitis   An inflammation of the LABYRINTH (the fluid-filled maze of inner ear chambers that sense balance), labyrinthitis can cause nausea, vomiting, TINNITUS, VERTIGO and deafness. Also called otitis interna, it is almost always caused by either a bacterial or viral infection that enters the inner ear from the middle ear. The main danger is spread of the infection to the meninges (the outer covering of the brain).

Bacterial labyrinthitis can result from MASTOIDITIS or an untreated acute or chronic ear infection, particularly if a CHOLESTEATOMA (infected skin debris) has developed; the bacteria enters the inner ear through the eroded labyrinthine capsule. Infection may also reach the inner ear from a head injury or through the bloodstream from elsewhere in the body. It can also occur from contamination during a STAPES operation or a MASTOIDECTOMY.

Bacterial labyrinthitis requires immediate treatment with antibiotics to treat the infection, which otherwise could lead to meningitis or profound SENSORINEURAL HEARING LOSS, violent vertigo and total deafness.

Viral labyrinthitis is usually transmitted through the bloodstream and attacks the inner ear during illnesses such as measles, mumps, CHICKEN POX, shingles or flu. With this type of sensorineural hearing loss, onset is sudden and results in a severe or profound hearing problem. Viral labyrinthitis will eventually go away on its own, although symptoms can be relieved with antihistamines.

Meningeal labyrinthitis, more common in children, results from the transmittal of an organism to the COCHLEA by way of the internal auditory meatus or the cochlear duct.

Syphilitic labyrinthitis is usually caused by congenital syphilis and results in a sudden, flat sensorineural hearing loss with poor speech discrimination or a sudden increasing fluctuation of sensorineural hearing loss. Acquired syphilitic labyrinthitis is rare. See also VIRUSES AND HEARING LOSS; SYPHILIS.

language   Symbols, words or signs that are composed by strict rules and arranged into sentences also governed by strict rules. All languages have symbols, and all languages have rules about how those symbols are grouped together to form sentences. In spoken languages, symbols are made up of sounds in particular ways; in sign languages, symbols are made up of body movements and positions.

The study of language, called LINGUISTICS, is still a relatively new science and is often controversial, but its basic tenets are universal. All spoken languages have rules about which sounds can be put together in certain ways to form words and sentences; similarly, natural sign languages have rules as well. But in sign language, grammatical rules govern body positions, facial expressions and movements.

Languages can differ at even the smallest levels, in the way in which sounds combine to form words and in the word order used to form sentences.

In English, word order usually follows the subject-verb-direct object format ("I love you"). In other languages, this word order is different; for example, in French, word order is subject-object-verb ("I you love"). Some languages, such as Latin, have no required word order at all but discriminate subjects from objects by word endings.

Because linguistic research into sign languages is still in its infancy, studies are only beginning to provide information on its syntactic rules. The key to understanding the grammatical structure of sign languages is to study the way signers use space.

People, places or objects not in the immediate area will be assigned a spatial location (to the left or right, for example). The signer can indicate the subject and object by moving the verb from one location to another. For example, by first assigning the right location to "Sam" and the left location to "cat," the signer moving the sign "see" from right to left means "Sam sees the cat."

Contrary to the widespread assumption that infant babbling requires normal hearing and an ability to speak aloud, recent research suggests that the brain seems to possess some type of unified capacity for learning both signed and spoken language. Psychologists at McGill University in Montreal studied five infants, two of whom were deaf and whose deaf parents' first language was sign. The three hearing babies had hearing parents who did not use sign language. When researchers videotaped babies at ages 10, 12 and 14 months alone and with their parents, they found that both deaf and hearing babies engaged in their own brand of babbling. Hearing infants initially produced strings of sounds and syllables, emitting their first words by age one. The two deaf babies babbled with their hands, starting out with basic hand shapes for letters and numbers that they saw their parents use. Hand movements and shapes gradually grew more

complex until the first linguistic signs emerged also by age one.

language development   See LANGUAGE.

late-onset deafness   See ADVENTITIOUS DEAFNESS; HEARING LOSS; PRESBYCUSIS.

lateralization   Sound vibrations presented to one side of the head will move through the bones of the skull toward the opposite COCHLEA. Whether the sound reaches the cochlea depends on the decibel level of the sound. All sounds will lateralize, but not all will be heard by the opposite cochlea. See also AUDIOMETRY; HEARING AIDS.

law   See COURT INTERPRETER'S ACT; LEGAL RIGHTS.

legal rights   A number of laws have been enacted since the 1970s guaranteeing legal rights for deaf people. They include:

Rehabilitation Act of 1973

Called the "Bill of Rights" for disabled people, this act was designed to make sure that programs receiving federal funds can be used by all disabled people. The four major sections of the act prohibit discrimination and require accessibility in employment, education, health, welfare and social services.

Section 501:   This section, which applies to federal government hiring practices, requires each executive department and agency to have an affirmative action plan for the hiring, placement and advancement of qualified handicapped people.

Section 502:   This section creates the ARCHITECTURAL AND TRANSPORTATION BARRIERS COMPLIANCE BOARD, which ensures compliance with a 1968 federal law regarding architectural barriers in federally-funded buildings and public transportation systems.

Section 503:   This requires affirmative action for qualified handicapped persons by people who have contracts or subcontracts with the federal government worth more than $2,500 a year or who employ more than 50 people.

Section 504:   This prohibits any form of discrimination against individuals with disabilities in any federally-supported program or activity, including most public and some private schools, nursing homes, museums and airports.

Public Law 94-142

Known now as the Individuals with Disabilities Act, this federal law guarantees public education to handicapped students in the least restrictive environment. It was signed into law on November 29, 1975, by President Gerald Ford.

The law provides states with funds for special education and imposes specific requirements on how such education should be provided—emphasizing special education and related services, protecting the rights of handicapped children and their parents and providing for the assessment of the effectiveness of programs.

The definition of handicapped children includes hard-of-hearing and deaf children, with "deaf" defined as: "a hearing impairment which is so severe that the child is impaired in processing linguistic information through hearing, with or without amplification, which adversely affects education performance." The law defined "hard-of-hearing" as an impairment—either fluctuating or permanent—that affects a child's educational performance.

The act defines "deaf-blind" as a "concomitant hearing and visual impairment" that causes such severe communication and other problems that these children cannot be accommodated in special education programs designed just for deaf or for blind children alone.

The act further provides that each child must have an individualized education program (IEP), a signed, written agreement renewed yearly, that includes a statement about the child's current abilities, annual goals and short-term educational objectives, specific services and the extent of participation in regular educational programs. The IEP is prepared with input from parents, teachers and school administrators.

According to information from the Department of Education, the number of hard-of-hearing students served by this law has steadily decreased over the past 10 years, due to the aging of children deafened in the RUBELLA epidemic of 1963 to 1965. Since the implementation of public laws aimed at assisting handicapped children, the number of hard-of-hearing and deaf students below 21 years of age decreased 19 percent between 1977–78 and 1985–86.

Public Law 97-410

The Telecommunications for the Disabled Act of 1982 addresses the issue of compatibility between hearing aids and telephones.

The law provides that all coin-operated telephones must be hearing-aid compatible; credit card phones must also be compatible unless there is a compatible coin phone nearby. Further, emergency phones (elevator phones, police and fire call boxes) and new public phones in businesses and public buildings must be compatible and an employer must supply a compatible phone on request by a deaf employee.

Hotels and motels must also specify compatibility when installing new phones until 10 percent of the rooms have compatible phones. Further, new phones installed after 1985 in hospitals, convalescent homes, homes for the aged, prisons and other confined areas must be compatible.

Public Law 88-565

Also known as the Vocational Rehabilitation Act, this law provides a number of direct services for deaf people and other disabled Americans. It includes funding and services for continuing education in a university or technical school and funds research and demonstration grants influencing deaf education.

The law led the way for expanded services and organizations for deaf people, including the REGISTRY OF INTERPRETERS FOR THE DEAF, the Professional Rehabilitation Workers with the Adult Deaf (now known as ADARA, the AMERICAN DEAFNESS AND REHABILITATION ASSOCIATION) and the Council of Organizations Serving the Deaf.

Amendments enacted in 1965 (PL 89-333) extended federal support even further to include education as well as rehabilitation and provided for interpreter services in a wide variety of settings.

Public Law 85-905

This important legislation for the deaf community created the Media Services and Captioned Films Branch in the Bureau of Education for the

Handicapped, granting deaf people accessibility to entertainment and educational films. Additional laws (PL 87-715 and 91-230) set up a national advisory committee on deaf education, enlarged the focus of Media Service and Captioned Films and funded a National Center on Educational Media and Materials for the Handicapped to be located at Ohio State University at Columbus.

Public Law 100-533

The National Deafness and Other Communication Disorders Act of 1988 established the NATIONAL INSTITUTE ON DEAFNESS AND OTHER COMMUNICATION DISORDERS within the National Institutes of Health. The law addresses not only hearing disorders but also balance, voice, speech, language, taste and smell.

This law requires the program include investigation into the etiology, pathology, detection, treatment and prevention of all forms of disorders of hearing and other communication processes. It also requires research into diagnostic, treatment, rehabilitation and prevention techniques; prevention and early detection of these disorders; and the environmental agents that influence hearing disorders. Finally, the law establishes a data system to collect, analyze and distribute information from patients, a national information clearinghouse and multipurpose research centers.

Public Law 87-276

In response to a shortage of teachers for deaf students, this law was signed on September 22, 1961, by President John F. Kennedy to provide stipends for undergraduate and graduate study. As a result, the number of approved university teaching training centers doubled.

Public Law 88-136

This legislation set up an advisory committee on deaf education, which began in March 1964 under the leadership of Homer Babbidge. The subsequent "Babbidge Report," which highlighted and analyzed problems in deaf education, was partly responsible for the subsequent creation of the MODEL SECONDARY SCHOOL FOR THE DEAF located on the GALLAUDET UNIVERSITY campus in Washington, D.C.

Vocational Education Act of 1963

This law allowed residential schools for deaf children to qualify for supplementary funding for their vocational departments; amendments in 1968 to this law required that at least 10 percent of the federal funds allocated for vocational education be set aside for handicapped students.

Public Law 89-36

This law, signed on June 8, 1965, by President Lyndon Johnson, established the NATIONAL TECHNICAL INSTITUTE FOR THE DEAF and an advisory committee to administer it. Of 28 competing colleges and universities, the Rochester Institute of Technology in New York was awarded the job.

line 21 The bottom line of a television's vertical blanking system; used in this country for closed captioning.

American television signals are made up of 525 lines, which include both the picture and a black bar, made up of 21 lines, called the vertical blanking interval (these 21 lines roll up or down on the screen when the TV is not adjusted properly).

Digital information encoded on one or more of these 21 lines within the black bar can be transmitted to TV receivers, where they can be decoded and displayed on the TV screen. The 21st line is the bottom line of the vertical blanking system and is used in this country for closed captioning.

Line 21 was first used in 1972, after the National Bureau of Standards and ABC-TV demonstrated that it was possible to place information within this "black bar"; subsequently, the Public Broadcasting Service developed a method that used this 21st line in the black bar for closed captioning. See also CAPTION CENTER; CAPTIONED FILMS FOR THE DEAF; CLOSED CAPTIONS.

linguist A person who uses highly-specialized skills to analyze language and associated cultural patterns in research or applied LINGUISTICS. Current research in the field of deafness includes studies of the history and development of AMERICAN SIGN LANGUAGE, comparative sign languages and language development of deaf children. Applied linguistics is especially useful in schools, where a professional can analyze language patterns of individual students and help the teacher devise strategies to develop new language skills. See also SIGN LANGUAGE.

linguistics The study of language as a system, involving an investigation into its nature, structure, units and modification. Theoretical linguistics tries to establish a theory of the underlying structure of language, isolating the structure of language from actual language production. It does not take into account language acquisition or usage. Applied linguistics tries to use the findings and techniques of the scientific study of language for a range of practical tasks, especially to help improve the teaching of language.

Linguistics of Visual English (L.O.V.E.) One of the five main manually coded English systems, this one was developed by Dennis Wampler. In this system, stress was placed on signing by morpheme (a word that conveys meaning and cannot be broken down into a smaller word). This system, similar to SEE 2 (SEE SIGNING EXACT ENGLISH) and SIGNED ENGLISH, features the use of symbols adapted from William Stokoe's symbols in the *Dictionary of American Sign Language* to show how signs were made, rather than depending on words or pictures to depict signs. This system is not widely used. Because it's considered to be a signing system rather than a language, some people claim that exposure to L.O.V.E. doesn't give children the complete linguistic access needed to internalize whole language.

lipreading See SPEECHREADING.

Little Theatre of the Deaf Working under its parent company, the NATIONAL THEATRE OF THE DEAF, the Little Theatre has presented stories, fables and poetry to young audiences for more than 20 years.

The theater uses body movement, SIGN LANGUAGE and hearing interpreters to bring both classic literature and original works to life. Programs are presented in schools, parks, museums, theaters and libraries throughout the United States and in other places, such as India, the Far East and Scandinavia.

Now composed of two companies of five actors each, the theater offers one-hour performances that include short stories, fables and often an introduction to sign language. The actors form living sculptures during "Your Game," a program using suggestions from the audience to illustrate ensemble performances, such as a washing machine or a videocassette player in fast forward.

The 31-year-old theater, where deaf and hearing actors team to present performances in sign language and spoken words, is the country's oldest, continually producing touring theater. The theater set a global record February 1998 in Antarctica when it became the world's first theater to reach all seven continents.

Lombard test A special test for functional hearing loss in which masking sounds are introduced into the ears while the subject talks. The test is positive if the subject raises the intensity level of his voice in order to hear himself above the masking sound and negative if his voice remains at a fixed level. See also AUDIOMETRY; FUNCTIONAL HEARING LOSS [NONORGANIC].

loop diuretics These powerful drugs are fast-acting chemicals that help remove excess water from the body by increasing the flow of urine; this class of diuretics is named for the part of the kidneys they affect, called Henle's loop. They are especially powerful and fast-acting when given by injection and are helpful in the emergency treatment of heart failure.

Studies suggest that loop diuretics may cause temporary or even permanent hearing loss, TINNITUS and VERTIGO, although symptoms usually disappear between 30 minutes and one day after treatment ends. Loop diuretics include azosemide, bumetadine, ethacrynic acid, furosemide, indapamide, lasix, piretamide and triflocin.

In general, physicians are advised against giving loop diuretics to premature infants or to patients taking aminoglycoside antibiotics. They are also advised against rapid intravenous use of furosemide.

Other diuretics (such as dyazide and the thiazides) have not been found to have ototoxic effects. See also OTOTOXIC DRUGS.

loudness The intensity factor of sound.

L.O.V.E. See LINGUISTICS OF VISUAL ENGLISH.

low birth weight and hearing loss Premature infants with a low birth weight (3.3 lbs or below) are at risk of a SENSORINEURAL HEARING LOSS ranging from mild to severe. Approximately 5 percent of these low-birth-weight infants will have hearing problems.

Full-term babies who have low birth weight are not at risk for hearing loss. See also PRENATAL CAUSES OF HEARING LOSS.

Lutheran religion and deafness The Lutheran church was the second religious group to set up a church specifically for deaf members; Our Saviour Lutheran Church for the Deaf was organized in 1896 in Chicago. It was followed by Emanuel Lutheran Church for the Deaf in Milwaukee, Wisconsin, in 1898.

Soon, there were more than 14 missions to deaf people. These missions supervised programs for deaf people in the United States and provided pastors who were often assigned to more than one city. See also INTERNATIONAL LUTHERAN DEAF ASSOCIATION.

macula A small sensory patch inside both the SACCULE and the UTRICLE (small sacs in the vestibule). Each macula is covered with sensory hair cells and is connected to fibers from the vestibular branch of the eighth cranial (auditory) nerve. These sensory patches are part of the body's delicate balance system.

mainstreaming The process in which a student with hearing problems attends some—or all—classes in a regular school for hearing students. See also EDUCATION OF DEAF CHILDREN.

malignant otitis externa A disorder involving inflammation and damage of the bones and cartilage of the base of the skull, caused by spread of infection from external ear infection (otitis externa). Malignant otitis externa is a relatively uncommon complication of both acute and chronic otitis externa (also known as SWIMMER'S EAR). It occurs in approximately five out of 10,000 people and is more common among diabetics and those whose immune system is compromised from diseases or medications.

The infection, often caused by difficult-to-treat germs such as pseudomonads, spreads from the floor of the ear canal to nearby tissue and into the bones of the base of the skull. The bones may be damaged or destroyed from the resulting infection and inflammation. The infection may further spread and affect the cranial nerves, the brain or other parts of the body.

Symptoms include draining from the ear, yellow or foul-smelling pus, itching of the ear or ear canal, deep ear pain which may worsen with head movement, and persistent hearing loss. The head around and behind the ear may be tender to touch. Neurological examination may show involvement of cranial nerves. A culture of drainage may show bacteria or fungus. A head CT scan, skull X rays, MRI scan of the head or radionuclide scan may show bone infection adjacent to the ear canal.

The goal of treatment is cure of the infection. Treatment is often prolonged, lasting several months, because of the difficulty of treating the involved bacteria and the difficulties reaching an infection that is within bone tissue. Antibiotics that are effective against the involved microorganism are needed for prolonged periods. Antibiotic therapy should be continued until scan or other tests show a marked reduction in the associated inflammation.

Occasionally, surgery is needed to allow drainage and to reduce deterioration of the skull bone. Malignant otitis externa usually responds to prolonged treatment but may recur. Complications include damage to the cranial nerves, skull or brain and the spread of infection to the brain or other parts of the body.

To prevent external ear infection, it is important to treat acute otitis externa completely and not to stop treatment sooner than recommended by your health care provider. The ears should be dried thoroughly after exposure to moisture; the infected person should avoid swimming in polluted water and protect the ear canal with cotton or lamb's wool while applying hair spray or hair dye (if susceptible to otitis externa). After swimming, one or two drops of a mixture of 50 percent alcohol and 50 percent vinegar in each ear will help to dry the ear and prevent infection.

malleus One of the three OSSICLES of the middle ear, also known as the hammer.

manual alphabet See FINGERSPELLING.

manual approach   Method of communication among deaf people using SIGN LANGUAGE and FINGER-SPELLING. Those who believe in the importance of manual communication consider it is a natural mode of communication for deaf people, deaf people should be encouraged to use signs and they should be allowed to sign in school. Opponents of the manual approach generally reject sign language, at least for the purpose of education.

There are intermediate positions between the two ends of the manual-oral spectrum. Some supporters of oral communication agree with the use of FINGERSPELLING in many settings but not in schools; others approve of mouth-hand systems of communication, such as CUED SPEECH.

Many schools in the United States today have tried to reach a compromise between the manual and oral methods by combining the two approaches.

The manual approach was referred to as the "French method" during the 19th century and was the preferred educational method of ABBÉ CHARLES-MICHEL DE L'ÉPÉE of Paris. At the same time, German deaf educator SAMUEL HEINICKE of Leipzig was promoting the oral approach.

L'Épée, as director of the French Royal Institute for the Deaf and Dumb in Paris (now the Institut National des Jeunes Sourds), promoted the use of what he called "methodical signs" for the education of deaf students, becoming the first proponent of sign language usage in schools. Because l'Épée did not believe there was any logical connection between sounds and ideas, it did not matter to him whether a person spoke or signed thoughts—each would be equally useful. All education was taught through his methodical signs, except for proper names for which he used fingerspelling. Still, l'Épée did teach speech and SPEECHREADING as well.

It was at the Paris Institute that THOMAS HOPKINS GALLAUDET learned how to educate deaf children, and it was therefore the French manual method he took back home to the United States. From the beginning of the first permanent school for deaf students in 1817, which Gallaudet founded, until the late 1860s, all instruction in the United States (some 26 separate schools) was based on the manual method.

But in the 1840s, educators began to tour Europe and bring back reports of the oral progress in English and German schools. Eventually, when parents of some deaf children did not want their children to learn signs, they formed a school in 1867 with the assistance of John Clarke, who donated $300,000 to start the first purely oral school in America, the Clarke School of Northampton, Massachusetts.

A more recent refinement of the manual approach is called Total Communication, which implies acceptance, understanding and use of all methods of communication. Proponents of this theory believe people with hearing loss should be exposed to all methods, emphasizing whatever enables them to learn and communicate effectively. See also SIMULTANEOUS COMMUNICATION.

manually coded English   All artificially developed codes that try to represent the English language in sign form are known as manually coded English (MCE). Typically, these systems have been developed primarily for the educational system to help build English language skills by manually incorporating many English language features.

In the past 20 years, a number of these codes have been developed, including SEEING ESSENTIAL ENGLISH (SEE 1), SIGNING EXACT ENGLISH (SEE 2) and SIGNED ENGLISH. All were designed to improve deaf students' English scores.

These codes, also known as manual English, are just that—codes, not languages—that reflect the structure and vocabulary of English. Generally, these systems use AMERICAN SIGN LANGUAGE signs in English word order, along with new signs that have been created to represent English parts of speech normally omitted from ASL. These manually coded systems therefore parallel the word and sentence structure of English.

However, manually coded English can be confusing to those used to American Sign Language. Whereas in English (and MCE) one word can have many meanings, ASL would assign a different sign to each separate meaning of the word. For example, the ASL sign for "run" (meaning a gait) is different from the run in a stocking or running for office.

Preliminary studies suggest these systems may improve students' grammar, but they are cumbersome to use, taking as much as twice as long to sign a word as it would to say it. Because of this, many students and teachers began to drop required signs. In response, Harry Bornstein, the author of Signed English, in 1982 came up with a pared-down version, although he continues to advocate that teachers and parents of young children slow down and sign accurately.

Use of these manual systems outside the classroom is not popular with the majority of deaf people, who view the system as an attempt to interfere with or eliminate ASL. See also SIGN CODES.

Martineau, Harriet (1802–1876) This strong and independent journalist was remarkable for her outspokenness during the Victorian era; she became one of the most famous writers of her time.

Born June 12, 1802, in Norwich, England, to a radical Unitarian family, her severe, painful hearing problem began at the age of 12. Within six years she was severely deafened but was reluctant to use an ear trumpet.

Extremely well-educated for her time, Martineau wrote about economics, education, sociology and philosophy for the leading periodicals of her day, making enemies for her unorthodox views along the way. A believer in mesmerism (hypnotism), her subsequent views on religion (she espoused a form of atheism) brought her even more criticism.

On a visit to the United States, she was appalled at the treatment of women and Indians, and her strong antislavery views made her a controversial speaker.

Despite this, her home in the Lake District was a beacon to other well-known philosophers and writers, including William Wordsworth, Matthew Arnold, Charlotte Brontë, Ralph Waldo Emerson and Nathaniel Hawthorne.

She also wrote widely about deafness and the problems deaf people encountered, ridiculing hearing people for meddling in the affairs of the deaf community and blaming parents and teachers for inadequate education of deaf children.

maskers See TINNITUS MASKER.

masking techniques See TINNITUS MASKER.

Massachusetts test A group PURE-TONE HEARING TEST that can screen 40 students at the same time by presenting pure tones of 500, 4,000 and 6,000 Hz at 20, 25 and 30 dB respectively. See also JOHNSTON TEST; SWEEP-CHECK TEST.

Massieu, Jean (1772–1846) This brilliant, outgoing educator, together with the ABBÉ ROCH-AMBROISE CUCURRON SICARD, helped develop the MANUAL APPROACH of education taught at the famed Paris Institute.

Born in 1772 near Cadillac, France, Massieu was one of six children, all deaf, who communicated among themselves in the family's own system of manual signs. Sent to a school for deaf children in Bordeaux, Massieu met Abbé Roch-Ambroise Sicard, who taught him how to read and write. When Sicard was named head of the Paris Institute, both men moved to Paris in 1790.

As the French Revolution exploded around them, Massieu and Sicard worked to establish education for deaf people. Massieu worked as instructor at the school, together with LAURENT CLERC, and helped teach THOMAS HOPKINS GALLAUDET their manual method of education. Upon Sicard's death in 1822, Massieu was fired for sexual indiscretions and moved to Aveyron, where he became headmaster of a local school for deaf students, retiring in 1839.

mastoid bone Located behind the ear, this prominent portion of the temporal bone is honeycombed with air cells that are connected to a cavity in the upper part of the bone called the mastoid antrum, which is in turn connected to the MIDDLE EAR. OTITIS MEDIA can spread through this bone to cause acute MASTOIDITIS (inflammation of the mastoid bone). See also MASTOIDECTOMY.

mastoidectomy A surgical procedure to remove the mastoid portion of the temporal bone, thereby removing the infected air cells within the bone caused by MASTOIDITIS, OTITIS MEDIA or CHOLESTEATOMA. It may also be used in the repair of a paralyzed facial nerve. It is performed less frequently today because of the widespread use of antibiotics in the treatment of acute OTITIS MEDIA and acute mastoiditis. Most mastoidectomies are performed behind the ear under general anesthesia.

There are several types of mastoidectomy, including antrotomy, cortical, modified radical, radical and a combined approach.

Antrotomy

Now almost obsolete, this operation involves the clearing and draining of the infected bone.

Cortical

Also called a simple or Swartze mastoidectomy, this procedure is used in acute and masked mastoiditis, a severely draining ear and recurrent otitis media. It involves removal of all cells of the mastoid bone.

Modified Radical

This procedure is used for cholesteatoma not involving the MIDDLE EAR but confined to the attic and mastoid, in which part of the bony wall is removed. It is also called a Bondy operation.

Radical

This operation for otitis media and, rarely, cholesteatoma involves removal of the tympanic membrane (EARDRUM), the OSSICLES, the posterior wall of the external canal, the diseased tissue and the mastoid. This converts the mastoid and middle ear into a single, healthy cavity. Unfortunately, a CONDUCTIVE HEARING LOSS of up to 50 dB is usually expected because the middle ear ossicles are removed, although a TYMPANOPLASTY may offset some of the loss. There may also be a partial or complete SENSORINEURAL HEARING LOSS if the footplate of the STAPES is dislodged.

Combined

This treatment for cholesteatoma, also called an intact canal wall mastoidectomy, avoids leaving a mastoid cavity by clearing the mastoid cavity and the middle ear of cholesteatoma while preserving the posterior canal wall. Unfortunately, some of the disease may be overlooked and left behind, which is why some otologic surgeons perform routine follow-up surgeries in several years.

mastoiditis An inflammation of the MASTOID BONE (the bone behind the ear), caused by a spreading infection from the middle ear to the antrum (a cavity in the mastoid bone), and from there to the air cells in the bone.

Mastoiditis causes severe pain, swelling and tenderness behind and inside the ear together with fever, creamy discharge and progressive hearing loss. The real danger is that infection may spread to inside the skull, causing MENINGITIS, a brain abscess or stroke. The infection could also spread outward, damaging the facial nerve and paralyzing the facial muscles.

Mastoiditis has become uncommon since the use of antibiotic drugs for the treatment of ear infections. Antibiotic treatment will clear the infection, although a MASTOIDECTOMY (removal of the infected air cells within the mastoid bone) may be needed if it does not.

McCallum, Heather Whitestone (1973–) Miss America for 1995, Heather Whitestone McCallum is totally deaf in her right ear and profoundly deaf in the other. Born in Dothlan, Alabama, February 24, 1973, she contracted a bacterial infection, *Hemophilus influenzae* at the age of 18 months. She became deaf after taking antibiotics for the infection. But it was unclear whether the infection or the antibiotics were the cause of the problem.

Because her mother did not approve of SIGN LANGUAGE, she enrolled Heather in an oral program that emphasized teaching deaf students to speak. Heather's speech improved dramatically, but it also took her six grueling years to learn how to pronounce her last name correctly. As part of her therapy, she took ballet classes at the age of five, and eventually considered a professional career in ballet. She did not learn sign language until high school; no one else in her family signed.

When Heather was 15, her parents divorced. To pay for Heather's college education, her mother enrolled her in beauty pageants, which culminated in the Miss America pageant in 1995.

Following her reign as America's beauty queen, Heather married John McCallum, with whom she operates Heather Whitestone, Inc., and became a mother of two boys. In recent years, she has received a COCHLEAR IMPLANT in her right ear, but she still depends on the HEARING AID in her left ear. She has written two books, *Listening with My Heart*

(Doubleday, 1997) and *Believing the Promise* (Doubleday, 1999).

She served as a board member of the Helen Keller Foundation for Research and Education from 1995 until 2002. In 2002, she was appointed by President Bush and Secretary Thompson to the Advisory Council for the NATIONAL INSTITUTE OF DEAFNESS AND OTHER COMMUNICATION DISORDERS.

measles   This viral illness causes a rash and fever and can cause hearing problems or deafness from complications of ear infections and ENCEPHALITIS. Measles affects primarily children, but an attack can occur at any age.

Spread by airborne droplets, measles has an incubation period up to 11 days before symptoms appear, and can be transmitted during this period and up to about one week after symptoms occur. Once very common throughout the world, measles today appears much less often in developed countries because of the availability of vaccinations that protect against the disease.

Symptoms begin with a fever, cold symptoms and cough; several days later a red rash begins on the head and neck and spreads downward. Symptoms fade after about three days if no complications develop.

In addition to encephalitis and possible hearing loss, other complications include seizure and coma, sometimes followed by retardation and death. Measles during pregnancy kills the fetus in about one out of five cases.

Treatment includes plenty of fluids and acetaminophen to reduce the fever. Antibiotics will not be helpful against the measles virus, but they may be prescribed to treat a secondary infection.

In the United States, a measles vaccination (usually combined with MUMPS and RUBELLA vaccinations) is given to children over age one and affords protection against the disease in most cases. In recent years, isolated epidemics have required immunizations of infants under age one living in epidemic areas.

meatus   See EXTERNAL AUDITORY CANAL.

membranous labyrinth   A delicate closed system of ducts and sacs filled with a watery fluid called ENDOLYMPH, the membranous labyrinth is suspended in the bony labyrinth of the otic capsule and is part of the body's balance system.

Each of its SEMICIRCULAR CANALS contains a narrow membranous semicircular duct with a rounded expansion (the ampulla) at the end. These ducts open into the tubular sac of the UTRICLE, which is in turn connected to a similar sac called the SACCULE.

Ménière's disease   An inner ear disorder of unknown origin that causes HEARING LOSS, dizziness or VERTIGO, and ringing in the ears. Ménière's disease affects more than 1 million Americans and can be extremely incapacitating; it is related to a problem with the fluid balance system in the inner ear.

First described by the French physician Prosper Ménière in 1861, the disease is characterized by dizziness in which people feel either they or their surroundings, are spinning. This occurs together with hearing loss, nausea and vomiting, tinnitus, and fullness or pressure within the ear. Symptoms may last from a few minutes to eight hours or more, and can be profoundly disturbing. The attacks of vertigo may occur every so often every few weeks.

There are several less common variants of the condition. While most patients with Ménière's disease experience vertigo, hearing loss, and TINNITUS, those with cochlear Ménière's disease have symptoms that include tinnitus *without* vertigo. Another variant—vestibular Ménière's disease—causes vertigo without hearing loss.

Symptoms

Ménière's disease tends to come and go, but the vertigo usually gets progressively worse until it peaks after several years; symptoms will then become less severe until the vertigo finally disappears. By this time, however, the patient is usually severely deaf. Normally, only one ear is affected and the sensorineural hearing loss may get worse and worse over the years, although a few people have experienced hearing loss in both ears. The loss may start with low frequencies and then involve higher frequencies, eventually becoming permanent. Hearing tests can usually reveal loudness recruitment and poor speech discrimination.

Cause

While the exact cause of Ménière's disease is unknown, researchers believe the problem is related to a change in pressure of the fluid in the inner ear. Experts believe that the endolymphatic chamber builds up excess fluid, causing the feeling of pressure, increased tinnitus, and hearing problems. Once the pressure has reached a critical level, the thin membrane separating the endolymphatic and perilymphatic chambers ruptures, mixing the fluids from the two chambers. Because these fluids are chemically different, their mixture short-circuits the inner ear, causing the severe vertigo of the Meniere's attack. Once the pressure has been released, this membrane heals and the fluid chemistries return to normal.

Experts believe that when the ear heals, hearing recovers (although not always completely). However, the fluid pressure buildup can reoccur, causing the symptoms to return. As excess fluid accumulates in the inner ear, delicate nerve endings become damaged.

Treatment

Researchers at the House Ear Institute in California have found a wide range of potential links to the disorder, including allergies, endocrine problems, and trauma. Treating these separate conditions may improve the Ménière's symptoms, but not everyone will get relief this way. Research at the University of Southern California at Los Angeles suggests that allergy-related immune problems may help trigger symptoms of the disease. These researchers found that for many Ménière's patients, allergy shots for airborne allergies or special diets (for food-related allergies) can be very effective in controlling vertigo and tinnitus. This could be because the anatomy of the inner ear makes it a target of histamine and other chemicals released during an allergic reaction. Airbone allergies to dust, mold and pollen, and food allergies (especially wheat) are often associated with Ménière's.

House Ear Institute researchers found that by severely restricting diet, some patients may find their symptoms subside and hearing increases by as much as 20 dB. Unfortunately, diet restrictions are severe, including no wheat, flour, eggs, chocolate, corn or mayonnaise. Some patients at the institute who temporarily disregard the diet restrictions notice an immediate return of symptoms. Ménière's patients who have abnormal insulin levels and/or impaired glucose tolerance should eat six small meals of low-carbohydrate, low-cholesterol food.

Other treatments vary. Some doctors recommend lifestyle changes, including less stress, no cigarettes or alcohol, regular exercise, and a different diet (in addition to the above restrictions, less salt and more low-fat foods).

Strategies to deal with vertigo generally involve ways to minimize stimulation of the balance system by limiting head movements. This allows the eyes, looking at a stationary object, to convince the brain that the body is not rotating. In general, head movements or closing the eyes will make the vertigo worse. Patients should lie or sit as still as possible, while trying to keep eyes fixed on a stationary object some distance away. Movements should be slow and even.

For the relief of nausea and the stress associated with vertigo, one of the following drugs may be prescribed:

- *prochlorperizine (Compazine):* controls nausea, vomiting and anxiety.
- *promethazine (Phenergan):* controls nausea, vomiting, motion sickness.
- *diazepam (Valium):* suppresses anxiety.
- *meclizine (Antivert):* controls nausea, vomiting, motion sickness. Another H1-blocking antihistamine.
- *scopolamine:* controls nausea and vomiting.

While most of these drugs are generally aimed at treating the effects of vertigo in Ménière's disease they may also play a role in controlling the disease by reducing anxiety, since stress is an important factor in triggering Ménière's attacks.

Many physicians prescribe steroids such as prednisone or dexamethasone, which may work by suppressing the immune response (some believe that Ménière's is a form of autoimmune disease). However, glucocorticoids also affect carbohydrate and protein metabolism, lipid metabolism, electrolyte balance, inflammatory responses and immune responses.

Surgical options include placing a tympanostomy tube, a relatively minor albeit controversial procedure that is widely used in children and adults for the relief of middle-ear infections (OTITIS MEDIA). The purpose of the tube is to maintain a tiny hole through the eardrum. Although the medical community has been skeptical that this treatment would have any bearing on Ménière's disease, many doctors are finding that they are very effective with success rates as good as endolymphatic shunt surgery. Studies indicate a high proportion of Ménière's patients get relief from vertigo by this procedure. However, some physicians remain unconvinced.

In addition, there are many surgical (and controversial) procedures involving the endolymphatic sac:

- *Endolymphatic sac decompression:* Drilling away the bone overlying the endolymphatic sac to make a larger "cavity" for the sac to occupy.

- *Endolymph-subarachnoid shunt:* Placing a tube between the endolymphatic sac and the cranium.

- *Endolymph-mastoid shunt:* Placing a tube between the endolymphatic sac and the mastoid cavity of the middle ear to avoid potential problems of opening the cranium in the endolymph-subarachnoid shunt.

However, endolymphatic sac surgery is extremely controversial. Based on a published study, many doctors regard endolymphatic sac surgery as a "placebo" surgery (i.e., the patient gets the same outcome whether or not the sac is actually shunted) and will no longer perform it. Others regard surgery of the sac as a step between nonsurgical therapies and more invasive procedures.

An alternative, less invasive method to alter the vestibular system is by using certain antibiotics that are known to destroy the vestibular hair cells. By destroying these cells, the brain is no longer sent "incorrect" information that the head is rotating. The techniques rely on the fact that for antibiotics such as gentamicin, the sensory cells of the vestibular system are more sensitive to damage than are the cells of the cochlea. This means that at the right dose, vestibular function can be reduced without damaging hearing. The antibiotic is usually injected into the middle ear space through the eardrum, and enters the inner ear through the round and oval windows. This method can be effective, but it is difficult to avoid some damage to hearing. For this reason, many doctors use just enough treatments to ease vertigo without necessarily destroying all vestibular function.

Surgical removal of either a portion or the entire labyrinth can be performed when there is no useful hearing in the affected ear, since collateral damage to the cochlea may produce significant hearing loss.

Vestibular nerve section surgery is a more invasive type of surgery, but it can dramatically cure vertigo. The goal of the surgery is to cut the nerve from the vestibular apparatus while leaving the auditory nerve intact, thereby preserving hearing. During the recovery period, the brain adapts to manage without vestibular input from the operated side, so that normal activity can be resumed.

Ménière's Network, The A national network of patient support groups administered by the EAR FOUNDATION to provide people with the opportunity to share experiences and coping strategies.

meningeal labyrinthitis See LABYRINTHITIS.

meningitis This disease involves an infection and inflammation of the outer coverings of the brain (meninges) and the nerves that lead to it and can cause sudden, profound and irreversible deafness in both ears. Because the deafness is incurable, physicians generally try to prevent or catch meningitis early to head off such complications.

Meningitis can be caused by almost any infectious agent, although bacteria cause the most fatal infections. Symptoms include fever, headache, vomiting, irritability, loss of appetite and a stiff neck.

Most cases of meningitis occur in children under the age of five. Recent studies suggest that about 6 percent of children with bacterial meningitis are left with a SENSORINEURAL HEARING LOSS, although other researchers have reported a higher rate of occurrence.

Occasionally, when deafness occurs during bacterial meningitis, a small amount of hearing remains, and a powerful hearing aid can be of some help but only to amplify sounds, not to recognize speech. TINNITUS is not often present, although there may be a brief experience of VERTIGO. Balance problems can also occur. Mental retardation occurs in about 15 percent of children whose deafness is associated with meningitis.

Meningitis is diagnosed by a spinal tap (insertion of a needle in the lower back to sample spinal fluid). Any bacterial, fungal or tubercular infection must be treated immediately with antibiotics.

Death from bacterial meningitis still occurs frequently, even with prompt antibiotic treatment. On the other hand, viral meningitis does not require any specific treatment, and patients usually recover within five days without lasting symptoms or risk of hearing problems. See also POSTNATAL CAUSES OF HEARING LOSS.

mental health services Finding adequate mental health services for deaf clients has become easier in recent years.

Accurate and appropriate diagnosis and treatment requires a working knowledge of the educational, psychological, social, cultural, linguistic, communication and emotional aspects of deafness—and fluency in SIGN LANGUAGE in particular.

Significantly, it has been demonstrated in the past 10 years that deaf people do respond to and benefit from the various methods of therapy used with hearing clients, as long as treatment is carried out using the preferred communication mode and style of the deaf individual.

There are a number of ways to locate sources of mental health services for deaf and hard-of-hearing people. State and community agencies serving people who are deaf and hard-of-hearing, in addition to community referral centers, often maintain files on service providers working with specific populations in a state. These include:

- State offices/commissions for deaf and hard-of-hearing people
- Community service agencies for deaf and hard of hearing people
- Hearing and speech agencies
- State school(s) for deaf children
- State departments of mental health

Other resources include:

- *Mental Health Services for Deaf People (1992)* A 210-page directory that identifies more than 350 U.S. mental health programs and services for deaf people, including information on services, accreditation, fees, special programs and accessibility. *Mental Health Services for Deaf People: A Resource Directory*, 2000 edition is available for $12.95 per copy plus postage and handling. Copies can be ordered from The Gallaudet Research Institute, ATTN: Dissemination Office, Gallaudet University, 800 Florida Avenue, N.E., Washington, DC 20002 or ordered online at http://gri.gallaudet.edu/Publications/#order.

- *National Directory of Alcohol and Other Drugs Prevention and Treatment Programs Accessible to the Deaf (1995).* This directory identifies programs reporting that they are culturally and linguistically accessible to deaf consumers. Copies are available for $35 plus $5 shipping/handling from Rochester Institute of Technology, Campus Connections Bookstore, 48 Lomb Memorial Drive, Rochester NY 14623-5604.

- *Standards of Care for the Delivery of Mental Health Services to Deaf and Hard-of-Hearing Persons.* The seven chapters of this document present an up-to-date description of the mental health resources and standards of care for deaf and hard-of-hearing persons. Included in the binder are descriptions of the population, referral into the mental health system, methods of access, specialized services, specialized resources and skills. The appendices include a list of state coordinators of mental health services for deaf and hard-of-hearing persons, residential facilities for deaf adults, and residential programs for deaf children and adolescents with emotional/behavioral disturbances. Copies are available for $64.95 plus $4.75 shipping/handling from: National Association of the Deaf Bookstore, 814 Thayer Avenue, Silver Spring MD 20910.

mental illness Research has shown that the rates of psychological disorders and mental illness are about the same for both the deaf and hearing populations. However, the lack of access to quality mental health services for deaf patients often precludes preventive mental health care.

In addition, hearing mental health professionals tend to diagnose psychological disorders and mental illness in deaf patients where none exist because they are unfamiliar with the educational, psychological, social, cultural, linguistic and communication aspects of deafness and are unable to use sign language to communicate.

To the inexperienced mental health professional, deaf people may appear to be psychologically disturbed or mentally ill when in fact they are not, according to Barbara A. Brauer, Ph.D., psychologist and research scientist at the Mental Health Research Program at GALLAUDET RESEARCH INSTITUTE. Because AMERICAN SIGN LANGUAGE and English have very different structures, styles and syntax, the English comprehension and writing levels of deaf people may appear pathological when in fact they are normal. Standardized tests are also culturally biased, as the tests are given in the context of the hearing experience, which may in many respects be different from the deaf experience. Consequently, the results often yield erroneous information about psychologically healthy deaf individuals.

For this reason, a number of psychological and personality tests have been translated by Dr. Brauer into American Sign Language on videotape as part of Gallaudet University's Mental Health Research Program. According to Dr. Brauer, preliminary findings suggest normal profiles for most deaf individuals tested.

Mercer, William (1765–1839)   Little is known about the early life of this deaf American painter, other than that he was born deaf in Fredericksburg, Virginia, in 1765, the first of five children. At the age of 18, he was sent to be apprenticed to Charles Willson Peale, a well-known Philadelphia artist. For three years, Mercer boarded with the Peale family and studied painting under the master artist.

Mercer's artworks include *The Battle of Princeton,* and a half portrait of his grandmother, Mrs. John Gordeon (both of which are owned by the Historical Society of Pennsylvania), and an oval miniature of a Virginian official (owned by the Virginia Historical Society of Richmond).

Although Mercer returned to Fredericksburg in 1786, where he continued to work as a painter, no other pictures by him are known to have survived.

message relay service   A generic term for a one-way service in which an operator relays a message from a hearing person without a TELECOMMUNICATIONS DEVICE FOR THE DEAF (TDD) to a deaf person who has a TDD, or vice-versa. This is distinguished from a RELAY SERVICE, in which both hearing and deaf parties are on the line at the same time with an operator acting as a go-between.

methods of instruction   There are currently four primary methods of instruction for deaf students used in the United States—the oral, auditory, Rochester, and simultaneous methods—as well as a more recent method—total communication.

Oral Approach

Also called the oral-aural method, children learning under this system are taught through SPEECHREADING (lipreading) and amplification of sound; they express themselves by speaking. Gestures and signs are prohibited.

Auditory Method

This system concentrates on helping children develop listening skills by relying primarily on hearing. Early reading, writing and speechreading (lipreading) are discouraged. This system is generally used for people with moderate hearing loss, but it is sometimes used with profoundly deaf students as well.

Rochester Method

Rarely used in this country today, this system combines the oral approach with FINGERSPELLING. Children receive input through speechreading, amplification and fingerspelling, with great emphasis placed on reading and writing.

Simultaneous Method

This features a combination of the oral approach plus signs and fingerspelling. Children are taught through speechreading, amplification, signs and fingerspelling.

Total Communication

In addition to the above four methods, Total Communication has received widespread attention in the past several years. According to the Conference of Executives of American Schools for the Deaf, Total Communication is a philosophy incorporating aural, manual and oral modes of communication to ensure effective communication with and among deaf people.

Mexican Sign Language   Known as LSM (Lenguaje de Señas Mexicanas), this SIGN LANGUAGE is used throughout Mexico by many of its more than 1.3 million deaf citizens.

As is typical for sign language, LSM does not parallel Spanish grammar. Sign meaning can be altered by varying speed, size and duration of the sign, and placement of signs depends on context. As in written Spanish, a sign for "question" appears at the beginning of the sentence.

There are no manual codes that follow Spanish-language structure, such as the manual codes for English in the United States.

Education is still widely oral in Mexico, although deaf educators are working to include LSM in the schools.

Mexico   With more than 1.3 million deaf and hard-of-hearing citizens there has been growth in the number of services provided for deaf people in Mexico, although there is still much more to be done in the field of education for deaf students and in the training of deaf teachers. According to a 1940 census, the prevalence rate of deafness in Mexico was 39 per 100,000; the count rose to 46 per 100,000 in the 1974 census. Still, this represents a fairly low rate compared to those of other developed nations that report data on deafness, which range from 35 per 100,000 to 300 per 100,000.

Mexico does not have any national organizations or regional groups for deaf people, although there are two deaf sports associations.

Although education for deaf Mexicans began in the late 1860s, few new schools were established until the middle of the 20th century as the educational philosophy changed from the MANUAL to ORAL approach. In 1951 the first institute for deaf people in Latin America was established, called the Mexican Institute of Speech and Hearing (IMAL). The institute, primarily oral, offers courses for teachers, audiologists, speech pathologists, technicians and deaf people, conducts research and provides social services.

microphone hearing aid   See HEARING AIDS.

middle ear   The small cavity between the EARDRUM and the INNER EAR that houses the three bones of the middle ear (OSSICLES). The middle ear transmits the vibration of a sound from the air outside to the fluid in the inner ear by the chain of these three tiny bones, which link the eardrum to an OVAL WINDOW in the wall on the opposite side of the middle ear cavity.

The first of the three bones, called the malleus or hammer, is joined to the inside of the eardrum. The second, called the incus or anvil, is joined to the malleus and has another delicate joint to the third bone, called the stapes or stirrup. The base of the stapes fills the oval window, which leads to the inner ear.

Although the eardrum cuts off the middle ear from the outside, it is not completely airtight. A ventilation channel, called the EUSTACHIAN TUBE, runs forward and down into the back of the nose. Although the eustachian tube is normally closed, it opens during yawning and swallowing.

middle ear cavity   See TYMPANUM.

middle ear diseases and hearing loss   There are a number of conditions that occur in the MIDDLE EAR and result in a CONDUCTIVE HEARING LOSS. These include injuries, inflammation, tumors and diseases of the OTIC CAPSULE.

Injuries
Injuries to the middle ear that produce conductive hearing loss can include an imbalance in air pressure (such as found in a descending plane), head injury and foreign objects.

A ruptured eardrum and SEROUS OTITIS MEDIA can develop in the wake of barotrauma (when the EUSTACHIAN TUBE can't equalize the pressure during an airplane landing or deepsea dive). Severe blows to the head, auto accidents or even a slap directly on the ear can fracture the temporal bone, fracturing or dislocating the OSSICLES (usually separating the incus and stapes) and causing a conductive hearing loss.

Inflammation

One of the most common causes of hearing loss in children is caused by inflammation of the middle ear. In acute and chronic suppurative otitis media, ear infection caused by bacterial or viral infection of the nasopharynx, most often by streptococcus pneumonia, staphylococcus aureus and hemolytic streptococcus, can spread to the middle ear.

In acute infections, the patient has a fever and headache with possible rupture of the eardrum and draining of fluid.

Complications include MASTOIDITIS (infection of the MASTOID BONE with pus in the air cells) which requires surgery, LABYRINTHITIS, or MENINGITIS. If the acute suppurative ear infection is not properly treated, frequent repeated ear infections can result in a resistant form of mastoiditis and in a permanently ruptured eardrum, discharge and a mild to moderate conductive hearing loss.

Another type of chronic middle ear infection features a lesion made up of skin debris called a CHOLESTEATOMA and can either be congenital or acquired. The rare congenital variety of cholesteatoma can appear in any part of the temporal bone. An acquired cholesteatoma may appear as skin migrates from the external ear canal into the middle ear through a small hole in the eardrum; as the lesion grows, it damages the middle ear structure and can cause a conductive hearing loss. Serious complications can be associated with an invasive cholesteatoma, including labyrinthitis, meningitis, brain abscess or facial nerve paralysis.

Glue ear (also called nonsuppurative otitis media or serous otitis media) is the most common cause of hearing loss in children and may be a result of an ear infection treated with antibiotics but with poor drainage of ear fluids. In adults, it may be caused by a dysfunctioning eustachian tube due to barotrauma or head colds; the resulting negative air pressure in the middle ear pulls the eardrum back, forcing fluid out of the middle ear. Glue ear can lead to the formation of a cholesteatoma.

Chronic middle ear infection can also scar the eardrum and cause it to collapse (ADHESIVE OTITIS MEDIA), adhering to the ossicles and causing hearing loss. Such chronic infection can also cause new bone to form in the middle ear lining.

OTOSCLEROSIS is a disorder involving the overgrowth of bone that immobilizes the stapes (the innermost bone of the middle ear) and prevents sound vibrations from passing to the INNER EAR, resulting in conductive deafness. Generally, both ears are eventually affected. The disease begins in early adulthood, is more common among women and affects about one in every 200 people. Hearing loss progresses slowly over a period of 10 to 15 years, often accompanied by TINNITUS and sometimes by VERTIGO.

Tumors

Tumors of the middle ear are fairly rare. Primary malignant tumors that may involve the middle ear space include adenoid cystic carcinoma, adenocarcinoma, rhabdomyosarcoma, and squamous cell carcinoma.

Squamous cell cancer usually appears in middle age and spreads rapidly, resulting in a conductive hearing loss until the tumor invades the labyrinth. In later stages, pain is intense and may result in blood-stained discharge.

Glomus tumor is a usually benign slow-growing mass that occurs more often in women and causes a conductive hearing loss and tinnitus, followed eventually by a SENSORINEURAL HEARING LOSS, dizziness and nerve palsy. Surgical removal is usually required. See also AERO-OTITIS MEDIA; TUMORS OF THE MIDDLE EAR; TYMPANOSCLEROSIS.

middle ear effusion   See SEROUS OTITIS MEDIA.

mild to moderate hearing loss   Generally considered to be a 30 decibel to 55 dB loss.

minimal language skills   A controversial term meaning a diminished communication repertoire of some individuals with hearing loss. This term replaced the negative "low verbal" description used before the 1970s, which was incorrectly used to label people who were proficient in AMERICAN SIGN LANGUAGE but not in spoken English.

Minimal language skills does *not* mean a person has problems with spoken language (especially English), has problems speech-reading or is illiterate.

A person who is not competent in sign language *or* in spoken language may be said incorrectly to have minimal language skills.

Miss Deaf America   A national competition designed for young deaf women between the ages of 18 and 28 who have already won their state competitions, it takes place during the biennial convention of the NATIONAL ASSOCIATION OF THE DEAF. Miss Deaf America serves as a role model for young deaf people and increases awareness of deafness among the general public through her appearances around the country. The pageant's goal is to encourage and foster future leaders and is one of several youth programs of the National Association of the Deaf.

The MDAP began as a vision of the late Douglas J. Burke, who in 1966 established a National Cultural Program within the NAD for the purpose of finding the hidden talents of deaf people in the visual arts. As a way of discovering deaf actresses at an early age, Burke created the Miss Deaf America Talent Pageant as a part of the National Cultural Program.

The first pageant took place in Miami Beach during the 1972 NAD Convention, with just five contestants; in 1976, the word *talent* was removed, and it simply became known as the Miss Deaf America Pageant, following closely the structure of the Miss America Pageant. Women are judged across a broad spectrum of categories including community service, academics, current events and deaf culture.

mixed hearing loss   A combination of conductive and sensorineural loss that occurs in the outer or middle plus the inner ear. Conductive deafness is often treatable, depending on cause; sensorineural deafness is seldom treatable. See also CONDUCTIVE HEARING LOSS; SENSORINEURAL HEARING LOSS.

Model Secondary School for the Deaf (MSSD)   Established by an act of Congress on October 15, 1966, the MSSD was designed to provide an outstanding example of a secondary school program for students with hearing problems and to stimulate the development of similar programs around the country.

Congress stipulated that the school should serve as a regional high school to prepare deaf students for college or a vocational career and should upgrade education for deaf students, using the newest research in testing, methodology and curriculum development.

In the beginning, admission requirements mandated that students be at least 14 years of age and have a third-grade reading level, a hearing loss of 70 decibels or more in the better ear and no other major problems. (These criteria were loosened following the passage of PL 94-142, the Education for All Handicapped Children Act.)

Students between 14 and 21 attending MSSD come primarily from Maryland, Delaware, Pennsylvania, Virginia, West Virginia and Washington, D.C., although students from other states are admitted if there is space. In that case, preference is given to students who have no access to a full-service high school.

Today, the school—located on 17 acres in the northwest corner of GALLAUDET UNIVERSITY—includes residence halls, health facilities, dining rooms, an infirmary and playing fields and serves about 400 deaf students a year. If offers students a continually-updated curriculum of more than 180 courses, including foreign language, art and theater arts. About 75 percent of the students live on campus; the rest commute from nearby Washington. Approximately 70 percent of MSSD students continue their education after graduation.

The school also offers a wide variety of interest clubs, a yearbook and service organizations, such as the Junior National Association of the Deaf.

The school provides curriculum development, workshops, seminars and internships for professionals and graduate students. School staff publish *Perspectives,* a professional journal for teachers, and *The World Around You,* a national high school student publication.

Input is received from the Parent Advisory Council and a National Advisory Council, which helps maintain goals and direction. See also KENDALL DEMONSTRATION SCHOOL.

modiolus   The central column of the COCHLEA in which the spiral ganglion of the eighth cranial nerve is located.

monaural   Pertaining to one ear.

monaural hearing aid   A single-ear hearing aid available in various styles, including the body, ear level, in-the-ear or eyeglass types. See also HEARING AIDS.

Mondini's dysplasia   A developmental problem of the inner ear characterized by malformations of the cochlear and semicircular canals that may cause severe SENSORINEURAL HEARING LOSS, PERILYMPH FISTULAS or recurrent meningitis. In a Mondini malformation, only one-and-a-half turns of the normal two-and-one-half turns of the cochlea is completed. The defect occurs during the seventh week of gestation after development of the basal turn (high frequency hearing is usually preserved). The vestibule and semicircular canals may or may not be normal. A problem with development between the fourth and fifth week gestation will lead to a common cavity between the cochlea and vestibule. The semicircular canals may or may not be normal, and hearing loss is usually profound. The diagnosis is confirmed by a high-resolution CT scan of the temporal bone.

For patients without symptoms, most otologists recommend a waiting period before treating the condition. Patients with symptoms may require surgical exploration and packing of the ear. Research suggests that a multichannel COCHLEAR IMPLANT may be of some benefit to those who have lost hearing due to Mondini dysplasia; at worst, the condition is not a contraindication for cochlear implantation.

mouth-hand systems   Mouth-hand systems are not a language but an aid to the visual transmission of spoken languages using handshapes close to the mouth to differentiate PHONEMES that look the same when spoken. (Phonemes are a family of closely related speech sounds regarded as a single sound; for example, the "r" in "bring," "red" and "car.") Used as aids for speechreading and speech training, there are two major forms of mouth-hand systems: CUED SPEECH and Danish.

Cued Speech

Cued Speech was developed in 1966 as a speechreading support system which (in English) uses eight hand configurations and four hand placements near the mouth to supplement visible speech. Each "cue" (hand placement or configuration) identifies a special group of two to four speech sounds. The combination of cues and mouth movements makes all the essential speech sounds appear different from each other so that the spoken message is clarified.

The hand configurations and locations are called "cues," not cued speech, which is the combination of the cues with speech (the cues are not readable alone).

Each hand configuration identifies a group of consonants; each hand location identifies a group of vowels. Further, cued speech can be used to indicate approximate voice pitch for each syllable uttered, which is important in tonal languages (such as Thai, Cantonese, Mandarin and Igbo).

For example, in Cantonese, the syllable "ma" can mean "mother," "scold," "horse" or "right?" depending on the pitch. Tone cueing is also helpful in speech therapy. In order to cue a tone, a person changes the inclination of the cueing hand to indicate changes in pitch.

Cued speech has been adapted to many languages, and audiocassette lessons designed for self-instruction by hearing persons are available. The system is generally the same in all languages.

Proponents believe cued speech makes spoken language visually clear and solves the communication problem at home and that it helps children learn a spoken language more easily. It is also an easily-learned system, taking only about 12 to 20 hours to master.

Initial research does suggest that cued speech helps make the spoken language clear, but the long-term effectiveness of the language is not known. Cued speech is not widely used by adults in the deaf community.

Danish

The mouth-hand system was invented in 1900 in Denmark by Georg Forchhammer, head of a deaf oral school, who believed that visual communication was necessary. Married to a deaf woman, he realized it would be helpful to improve SPEECHREADING capability by making similar-sounding words clear.

In the Danish system, there are 14 different hand positions, each making clear a sound that is hard to speechread. Hand positions are designed to symbolize the sound, and the most-often used sounds are the easiest to make.

Easy to use, the system is the most common visual aid in Denmark by hard-of-hearing people who don't know sign language. On the other hand, this system tends to slow down communication and is tiring to read or produce over a period of time.

Among the Danish deaf population, the mouth-hand system is used as a way to improve speech training and has also become a part of SIGN LANGUAGE in much the same way that the MANUAL ALPHABET is used in conjunction with other sign languages. In Denmark, the system is used to spell out names and words with no equivalent in Danish sign language.

This system can be used with any language, with additional shapes used for sounds that are not made in Danish. These hand positions have been developed for use in English, French, German, Swedish and Norwegian. See also Appendix XIV.

mucous otitis media A middle ear infection caused by thick sticky fluid in the middle ear, instead of the thin watery fluid in SEROUS OTITIS MEDIA. The fluid that collects in the middle ear causes hearing loss, which may vary between a mild high-tone loss to a considerable loss for all tones. In the presence of thick mucus, the hearing loss is most severe and may mimic the type of hearing loss seen as a result of OTOSCLEROSIS.

Hearing is restored when the thick fluid is removed by puncturing the eardrum. If the fluid is not removed, the CONDUCTIVE HEARING LOSS will persist, and the condition may lead to the formation of adhesions in the middle ear that firmly fix the ossicular chain with fibrous tissue bands. See also OSSICLES.

multisensory teaching approach This method, one of two philosophies used in teaching speech to deaf and hard-of-hearing children, calls for the use of all sensory channels—hearing, sight, feel—as opposed to the AUDITORY-ORAL METHOD, which teaches the child to rely solely on the auditory system, however flawed.

The proponents of the multisensory method believe that the hard-of-hearing or deaf child has an auditory system that is inadequate for the development of good speech and that this calls for the use of other senses, including sight and touch. See also SPEECH TRAINING.

mumps Mumps is the most common cause of severe one-sided deafness, which is usually sudden in onset and happens without ear pain or discomfort.

The deafness often goes unnoticed for many days—or years—after onset; often a patient will claim that he only recently noticed deafness in one ear. Close examination and history will reveal, however, that the deafness has been present since an attack of mumps in childhood.

Deafness due to mumps usually causes complete loss of hearing in one ear by irreparably destroying the INNER EAR without affecting the balance mechanism. If any hearing does remain in the affected ear, the deafness does not become progressive.

Mumps is an acute viral illness that usually occurs in childhood and produces swelling and inflammation of the salivary glands on one or both sides of the face. After an incubation period of two to three weeks, symptoms of pain and swelling appear. Fever, headache and difficulty swallowing may develop, but temperature and swelling soon pass.

In people past puberty, there may occasionally be swelling of the testicles in men or swelling of the breasts and ovaries in women. One attack of mumps confers lifelong immunity.

There is no specific treatment for mumps other than painkillers and plenty of fluids. In the United States, most children at age 15 months are given a combination measles, mumps and rubella vaccination to protect against these diseases. The vaccination is given earlier in areas experiencing a measles epidemic. See also VIRUSES AND HEARING LOSS.

mutism The inability to speak due to deafness.

myringoplasty See TYMPANOPLASTY.

myringotomy A surgical procedure used to open the eardrum to drain the middle ear cavity. It is usually performed in children to treat persistent SEROUS OTITIS MEDIA (a sticky secretion in the middle ear cavity causing hearing loss). This hearing loss may become permanent if the condition isn't treated. Before antibiotics, a myringotomy was used to treat acute OTITIS MEDIA by releasing the pus, relieving pressure on the eardrum.

While the patient is under general anesthesia, the otolaryngologist makes a small incision in the eardrum, removing most of the fluid by suction. At the same time, a small tube may be inserted in the hole to allow any remaining fluid to drain into the outer ear. The patient can leave the hospital the next day, and the tube usually falls out several months later as the hole in the eardrum closes. A second operation may be needed to insert another tube if the condition does not clear up.

Some experts advocate the use of allergic management or decongestive therapy, which eventually allows the effusion to clear. Unfortunately, the hearing loss that occurs while the effusion exists may cause developmental problems in children. Some research suggests that long-term treatment with antibiotics may help clear some cases of effusion.

NABTS   See NORTH AMERICAN BASIC TELETEXT SPECIFICATION.

NAD Law Center   Formerly known as the NAD Legal Defense Fund, this organization has protected the legal rights of deaf and hard-of-hearing people through the courts since 1976. Law center attorneys also work closely with deaf and hard-of-hearing individuals, parents, lawyers, employers and service providers to ensure broad national compliance with laws that have a direct impact on the deaf community. The goal of the NAD Law Center is to assure that deaf and hard-of-hearing individuals receive equal opportunity under the law.

In spite of laws that provide important civil rights to effective communication, deaf people experience discrimination because of their deafness, sometimes in life-threatening situations such as hospital emergency rooms and police stations, and sometimes on a continuing basis in classrooms and on the job. The law center vigorously enforces federal and state laws and by seeking to establish powerful legal principles of equality and access.

The NAD Law Center is also a national resource of expertise and information on law and deafness.

Important state and federal laws protect the rights of people with disabilities, but passing a law is not always enough. Often a law must be enforced through court action. Law center attorneys represent individuals and organizations in carefully selected cases. Through litigation, the law center has expanded the boundaries of federal disability law and clarified how these laws apply to the unique needs of deaf and hard-of-hearing people.

The NAD Law Center reviews hundreds of cases involving problems with employment, education, social services, access to commercial and nonprofit services, technology, court and police procedures. The center attorneys advise deaf people with legal problems involving deafness and provide technical assistance to lawyers who represent deaf clients. Because the law center staff is small, it cannot represent every person who asks for help, but selects cases with the best mixture of legal and factual issues to be successful. It identifies cases that will have the widest possible impact and that will be the most helpful to the overall interests of the deaf community.

The law center was established as a litigation-oriented disability law firm, staffed with attorneys who were knowledgeable about deafness, American Sign Language, and issues of importance to deaf and hard-of-hearing people. Today more attorneys are willing to take on the kinds of cases the NAD Law Center has always specialized in. The NAD works closely with attorneys in private practice, through formal and informal cocounseling arrangements, and as a clearinghouse for advice and assistance on legal precedents, strategy and techniques. Attorneys around the country consult with the NAD about disability law and deafness. Law center attorneys provide information, leadership, strategic advice, research and assistance to private attorneys in a wide variety of cases. The law center represents all deaf and hard-of-hearing people, regardless of whether or not they are members of the NAD, regardless of type of communication method or degree of deafness, regardless of geographical location and regardless of age, sex, race, religion or national origin.

The NAD Law Center is a national resource for general legal information and technical assistance about disability and discrimination law, and provides legal information to thousands of individuals and organizations with questions about disability law. See also Appendix II.

name sign   A sign used in the deaf community that serves as the first, middle and last name of a person.

Since most deaf children do not have deaf parents, most deaf offspring of hearing parents receive a name sign from their deaf peers or teachers once they begin school. Name signs can change in different groups of people or when a person's status changes, such as after marriage.

Name signs may be descriptive, in which they describe a person's physical characteristics; research has discovered that many of these emphasize negative physical characteristics, such as being overweight or having a scar. Arbitrary name signs (usually given by deaf parents) all have alphabetically-based handshapes affiliated with the first, middle or last name.

FINGERSPELLING is also sometimes used to spell out an abbreviated form of the name.

narcotics and deafness   Deafness from overuse of narcotics has been rarely reported. However, recent studies show that overuse of a combination of the narcotic pain reliever hydocodone and acetaminophen (a product called Vicodin) can lead to total deafness. Typically, hydrocodone and acetaminophen in combination are often used to alleviate pain. This rapid and progressive hearing loss has been treated successfully with COCHLEAR IMPLANT.

nasopharynx examination   In order to diagnose auditory disorders, it is important to examine the nasopharynx (the passage connecting the nasal cavity behind the nose to the top of the throat behind the soft palate). Part of the respiratory tract, the nasopharynx forms the upper section of the pharynx and contains the openings to the eustachian tubes.

A nasopharynx examination is important because infections can obstruct the eustachian tube, causing abnormalities in the middle ear. Examining the nasopharynx can uncover problems such as SEROUS OTITIS MEDIA (production of sticky fluid in the middle ear), retraction of the eardrum, chronic and acute OTITIS MEDIA (ear infection), infections of the nasopharynx, sinusitis (inflammation of the membrane lining the sinuses), allergy, adenoid enlargement and adenoiditis (inflammation of the adenoids).

The nasopharynx can be examined by looking through the mouth with a mirror placed behind the free edge of the soft palate, or a right-angle telescope can be used through the mouth to look around the soft palate into the nasopharynx. Other ways to examine the nasopharynx include using a nasopharyngoscope (a thin right-angle telescope passed through the nose) or a flexible fiber-optic endoscope to look through the nose or the mouth. Feeling with the finger can also be helpful and is usually performed under general anesthesia. Imaging techniques may also be used, especially in determining the size of adenoid tissue in children.

National Association for Hearing and Speech Action   This organization was founded in 1910 in New York City to advocate and provide information for deaf and hard-of-hearing people and is the consumer affiliate of the AMERICAN SPEECH-LANGUAGE-HEARING ASSOCIATION.

The group operates a toll-free speech and hearing helpline (800-638-TALK) and has produced brochures and television public service announcements promoting healthy hearing.

The association was first called the American Association for the Hard of Hearing and was designed for people interested in teaching SPEECH-READING to hard-of-hearing people. During the 1920s, the association moved to Washington, D.C., and led an aggressive campaign to prevent hearing problems and establish screening programs in schools.

In 1966 the association was renamed the National Association of Hearing and Speech Agencies and emphasized community organization and professional service, education, diagnosis and research.

Its final name change occurred in 1972. Today, its members are involved in promoting the interests of people with speech and hearing problems and emphasizing consumer advocacy, prevention and social action.

National Association of the Deaf (NAD) NAD is a consumer advocate organization concerned about and involved with everything affecting opportunities for the more than 28 million deaf and hard-of-hearing people in the United States.

With 51 affiliated state associations, NAD changed its orientation in 1960 from a group of individuals to a federation of state associations. The first association founded by deaf people, it was started in 1880 by a group of deaf leaders concerned that deaf people were not included in the decision-making processes affecting their own lives.

In 1964, the group abandoned its policy of allowing only deaf people to become members, but today fewer than 100 of its more than 22,000 members can hear. Most of these 100 are professionals who work with deaf clients.

Today, NAD serves as a clearinghouse of information on deafness and is an advocate for the employment of deaf people. The organization promotes the use of AMERICAN SIGN LANGUAGE and supports the philosophy of TOTAL COMMUNICATION—the right of all deaf people to select and use any form of communication, including SIGN LANGUAGE, gestures, writing, reading, FINGERSPELLING, SPEECHREADING and listening with amplification.

Over the years, NAD has received a number of federal grants to conduct the first national census of deaf Americans, to set up a communication skills program and to establish the REGISTRY OF INTERPRETERS FOR THE DEAF, among others.

NAD—together with its affiliate state association in Massachusetts—operates D.E.A.F., INC., a rehabilitation facility serving the deaf population in New England, and administers a survey research organization, the Deaf Community Analysts. The organization also subsidizes the NAD LEGAL DEFENSE FUND, the International Association of Parents of the Deaf and the JUNIOR NATIONAL ASSOCIATION OF THE DEAF and holds an annual leadership camp for deaf youth.

The association also administers the Captioned Media Program (CMP) with funding from the U.S. Department of Education. CMP evaluates and selects materials for open-captioning and distributes open-captioned materials on a free-loan basis to individuals, schools, agencies and other groups across the country. The CMP offers outreach, technical assistance and research to captioning agencies, video producers, and distributors. It handles thousands of inquiries each year from the general public requesting information about the NAD, its programs and services, the deaf community and deaf culture, heritage and language. It promotes deaf awareness and other topics related to issues impacting the lives of deaf and hard-of-hearing people.

Finally, the NAD publishes a national monthly tabloid, *The Broadcaster,* featuring columns, articles, a special sports section and advertisements of special interest to the deaf community. Its quarterly magazine, *The Deaf American,* carries full-length feature articles on topics of interest to the deaf community. NAD also publishes and sells books on deafness and sells assistive devices for deaf people.

Its home office, Halex House, is located in Silver Spring, MD, where it offers for sale more than 200 books on various aspects of deafness. The NAD is a member of the WORLD FEDERATION OF THE DEAF. See also MISS DEAF AMERICA; Appendix II.

National Black Association for Speech-Language and Hearing A nonprofit organization dedicated to sharing information about communication impairments and differences among black people; professional development of SPEECH-LANGUAGE PATHOLOGISTS, AUDIOLOGISTS and students; and advocacy of quality service delivery to the black community. See also Appendix II.

National Black Deaf Advocates, Inc. This organization promotes leadership, deaf awareness and active participation in the political, educational, religious and economic processes that affect the lives of deaf black citizens.

National Board for Certification in Hearing Instrument Sciences Founded in 1981, the NBC-HIS is a voluntary non-profit organization designed to establish a standardized testing and certification program to measure the competency of hearing instrument specialists. The designation BC-HIS stands for board certified in hearing instrument sciences and is given to hearing instrument specialists who have passed the rigorous national competency exam and are certified by the National Board for Certification in Hearing Instrument Sciences. See also Appendix II.

National Captioning Institute (NCI)   This non-profit corporation was founded in 1979 to develop a national closed-captioned television service for the entertainment industry in order to provide deaf and hard-of-hearing people with the words accompanying current news, drama, comedy and special events.

CLOSED CAPTIONS—hidden subtitles that appear on certain programs when a signal triggers a TeleCaption decoding device—enable even profoundly deaf people to understand television programs and movies. The decoders are available nationally through major mail order catalogs and in more than 900 stores.

After the first several demonstrations of closed captioned television in the early 1970s, the then-called U.S. Office of Education (now the Department of Education) supplied seed money to develop the captioning technology. In 1976, the Federal Communications Commission reserved LINE 21 in the vertical blanking interval of the TV signal for the closed caption signal; in 1978 the television networks agreed to participate in the service, provided it was run by a nonprofit group. Consequently, the next year, the Education Department awarded a $6.9 million grant to help establish NCI.

The first closed captioning programs aired on March 16, 1980—*Once Upon a Classic* and *Masterpiece Theatre* (PBS), *The Wonderful World of Disney* (NBC) and *The ABC Sunday Night Movie* (ABC). Over the past 20 years, NCI has grown into the largest captioning company in the world with almost 200 employees. With a highly skilled captioning staff and state-of-the-art facilities, NCI provides the highest-quality captioning services for broadcast and cable television, home video and DVD, and government and corporate video programming. NCI also provides subtitling and language translation services in more than 40 languages and dialects.

As part of NCI's commitment to television access, NCI now offers video service for people who are blind or have low vision. Headquartered in Vienna, Virginia, the company also has offices in Burbank, Dallas, and New York City.

Private support of the service has increased since 1982, when all federal funding of the program ceased. In addition, the NCI Caption Club was formed in 1983 to accept contributions toward expanding the number of closed captioned programs.

Although originally designed for a hard-of-hearing audience, NCI has expanded its market to include people learning English as a second language and people learning to read—especially students with learning disabilities. Similarly, the Annenberg/CPB Project and NCI joined together to produce closed captioning for eight educational telecourses in 1984 that can be taken for college credit.

NCI had been the sole developer, manufacturer and distributor of the consumer device that once was needed to view captioned television, the TELE-CAPTION DECODER. Since 1991, NCI supplied TV manufacturers with an integrated circuit chip that provided built-in decoding capacity for televisions. All TVs now include the chip.

Publications of NCI include its free newsletter, *CAPTION,* and a marketing memo sent to commercial advertisers and corporations. See also Appendix II.

National Catholic Office for the Deaf   This group organizes workshops and provides information and teaching materials for the religious education of hard-of-hearing people. It also coordinates preparation programs for pastoral workers. See also INTERNATIONAL CATHOLIC DEAF ASSOCIATION; Appendix II.

National Center for Law and Deafness   The first national center designed to meet the legal needs of the deaf population, which had been located at GALLAUDET UNIVERSITY in Washington, D.C. The center, which was abolished by Gallaudet in 1997, had been designed to provide a variety of legal services and programs for the deaf community.

The center provided free assistance to Gallaudet University students and low-income hard-of-hearing people in the Washington, D.C., area. The clinic primarily handled common legal problems (wills, immigration, consumer issues, landlord-tenant disagreements and so forth).

During the school year, law student interns—supervised by staff attorneys—worked at the center, gaining valuable experience in meeting the legal and communication needs of deaf people. The law schools at both George Washington University and Catholic University offered courses in conjunction with the law center.

The center's attorneys tried to eliminate discrimination caused by the communication barriers between deaf and hearing people in education, employment, health care, legal services and governmental programs. Efforts included technical assistance with federal and state statutes and regulations dealing with interpreter services, civil rights of deaf people and the right to good mental and physical health care. Center attorneys also provided information to a variety of groups, including other lawyers, employers, schools and the federal government, on issues that affected deaf people.

Importantly, the center concentrated on the areas of television and telephone access for deaf people and was instrumental in petitioning the FCC to require all TV stations to present emergency information in visual form; it also helped the Public Broadcasting Service reserve LINE 21 to be used for closed captioning.

Interpreters were available for interviews at the center, and all staffers had been trained in sign language. Many of the center's tasks have been taken over by the NAD LEGAL DEFENSE FUND, which maintains an office at the National Association of the Deaf in Silver Spring, Maryland. The defense fund represents deaf and hard-of-hearing people with discrimination problems and helps provide education and legal aid.

National Congress of Jewish Deaf (NCJD)   See JEWISH DEAF CONGRESS.

National Cued Speech Association   The membership organization that provides advocacy, information and support on the use of CUED SPEECH. Members include both families and professionals in the field of deafness. The association's board of directors are geographically diverse and each regional director provides services for people in his or her area. Publications of the association include the *Cued Speech Journal* and newsletters *On Cue* and *On Cue News Flash.* See also CORNETT, R. ORIN; Appendix II.

National Deaf Education Center   Located on the campus of GALLAUDET UNIVERSITY, the Laurent Clerc National Deaf Education Center shares the concerns of parents and professionals about the achievement of deaf and hard-of-hearing students in different learning environments across the country. The Clerc Center has been mandated by Congress to develop, evaluate and disseminate innovative curricula, instructional techniques and strategies, and materials. The aim of the Clerc Center is to improve the quality of education for deaf and hard-of-hearing children and youth from birth through age 21. The KENDALL DEMONSTRATION ELEMENTARY SCHOOL and the SECONDARY SCHOOL FOR THE DEAF, which are part of the Clerc Center, focus their development and evaluation activities in three priority areas: literacy, family involvement, and transition to postsecondary education and employment. In addition to operating the demonstration schools, the Clerc Center also works collaboratively with schools and programs across the country to meet critical needs.

National Directory and Resource Guide   A national directory of residential numbers of TTY users in each state, together with fax and e-mail information, a business section of listings by states in such categories as *auxiliary* (hearing and speech services), *health* (including mental health), *human resources* (including social services) and *interest groups* (including associations and organizations).

Copies are available for $20 for nonmembers, $10 for members, plus $4 shipping/handling from: Telecommunications for the Deaf, Inc. (TDI), 8716 Colesville Road, #300, Silver Spring, MD 20910.

National Fraternal Society of the Deaf   This group was founded in 1901 by a group of young deaf adults interested in forming a fraternal society solely for deaf people and in providing low-cost insurance protection denied to deaf individuals at that time. (Insurance was denied because at the beginning of the 20th century, insurers thought that deaf people didn't live very long and were prone to accidents.)

The society was incorporated as a mutual benefit organization by the state of Illinois in 1901, and by 1984 there were 106 divisions with assets totalling $9 million. Although it began strictly as a men's fraternal organization, by 1937 it was able to form social auxiliaries; in 1951 women were granted regular insurance membership.

Today, the society provides low-cost insurance to deaf and hard-of-hearing people, granting membership with the purchase of a life insurance policy. The society also insures deaf children, hearing children and grandchildren of deaf members and hearing adults involved in the field of deafness. The society holds conventions every four years and publishes a bimonthly newsletter, *The Frat.*

In addition to providing insurance, the society each year awards more than 50 savings bonds to outstanding deaf or hard-of-hearing graduates of deaf schools and 10 university scholarships to deaf students. The NFS gives annual All-American awards to outstanding deaf football and basketball players and an annual Athlete of the Year award to a deserving deaf athlete. The society also maintains a library. See also Appendix II.

National Index on Deafness, Speech and Hearing

See DEAFNESS SPEECH AND HEARING PUBLICATIONS, INC.

National Information Center for Children and Youth with Disabilities

This group collects and shares information helpful to handicapped youths, sponsors workshops and publishes newsletters. The group publishes information for the public and professionals to help deaf youths become participating members of the home and community. See also Appendix II.

National Institute for Hearing Instruments Studies (NIHIS)

The educational division of the National Hearing Aid Society, NIHIS accredits educational programs in the hearing instrument sciences as offered by approved providers or the institute. See also Appendix II.

National Institute on Deafness and Other Communication Disorders

One of the institutes of the National Institutes of Health that was established in 1988 to conduct and support research and training on disorders of hearing and other communication processes. These disorders include diseases affecting hearing, balance, voice, speech, language, taste and smell.

The institute, which was established by the National Deafness and Other Communication Disorders Act of 1988 (Public Law 100-533), requires a wide range of research and development programs, including investigations in the etiology, pathology, detection, treatment and prevention of all forms of hearing disorders and evaluations of diagnosis, treatment, rehabilitation and prevention techniques. Emphasis is also placed in early detection of disorders in infants and the elderly and on exploring environmental causes of deafness.

National Rehabilitation Information Center

A rehabilitation information service and research library that provides reference, research and referral services, conducts custom database searches, publishes a quarterly newsletter *NARIC Quarterly,* and disseminates rehabilitation-related information. The center offers a database called REHABDATA, a computerized listing of rehabilitation literature. See also Appendix II.

National Technical Institute for the Deaf (NTID)

The world's largest technological college for deaf students; established in 1965 in Rochester, New York. It is a federally-funded institution, one of eight colleges of the Rochester Institute of Technology (RIT).

The institute's 1,151 deaf and hard-of-hearing students may select from courses in 34 programs in business, computer science, engineering technology, photography and printing. The institute is one of nine colleges of RIT, sharing campus facilities, library, bookstore and athletic areas. Students may also pursue a bachelor's or master's degree in other colleges at RIT, including the Colleges of Applied Science and Technology, Business, Engineering, Fine and Applied Arts, Graphic Arts and Photography and Liberal Arts. Nearly 20 percent of RIT's deaf students are enrolled in another college of RIT.

Instructors at NTID use SIGN LANGUAGE, speech and FINGERSPELLING, and students may use whatever communication mode they prefer. Although instructors in other RIT courses don't use sign language, professional interpreters and trained notetakers are available. Deaf students may also obtain interpreters for student activities, counseling, theater, sports, religious services and cultural events.

The school was established in 1965 with the National Technical Institute for the Deaf Act (PL 89–36), which created the school and provided that the institute must be established within a school that already existed. The law defined NTID as a postsecondary educational and residential institution with a range of basic responsibilities. The Rochester Institute of Technology was selected as the host school by a national advisory board from among 20 applicants.

Applicants to NTID must be U.S. citizens with an overall achievement level of eighth grade with good grades and have a hearing loss of 70 dB or greater without a hearing aid in the better ear.

In addition to educating deaf students, NTID cooperates with other institutions in deafness research and offers a range of programs to improve the quality of deaf education in the United States. In addition, RIT and the University of Rochester cosponsor a graduate program that qualifies secondary school educators to work with deaf people.

A placement program is offered for NTID graduates, 95 percent of whom find jobs upon graduation. NTID also staffs the National Center on Employment of the Deaf, which assists both employers and deaf people seeking jobs. See also Appendix II.

National Temporal Bone Hearing and Balance Pathology Resource Registry

A registry formerly called the National Temporal Bone Bank (NTBB) program, which was established in 1960 with the support of the National Institutes of Health and the Deafness Research Foundation (DRF).

The principal purpose of the NTBB was to solicit temporal bone donors for four regional centers. In 1992 the National Temporal Bone Hearing and Balance Pathology Resource Registry was established by the NATIONAL INSTITUTE ON DEAFNESS AND OTHER COMMUNICATION DISORDERS (NIDCD), to assume the responsibilities of the previous NTBB and, most important, to add to the objectives the creation of a more effective temporal bone network.

Of the 28 known human temporal bone collections in the United States, 15 are still active in the collection and study of specimens. All of the 15 active laboratories and 11 inactive temporal bone laboratories have collaborated with the registry. See also Appendix II.

National Theatre of the Deaf (NTD)

A professional ensemble of deaf and hearing actors, this theater company uses mime, body language and SIGN LANGUAGE augmented by reverse interpretation of the signs for hearing audiences. Founded in 1970, the company has given more than 8,000 performances of classical repertory as well as original works in 31 countries.

The company's professional actors put on a new play each fall and go on tour to the major theaters of the world; it is the only theatrical company to have performed in all 50 states. The NTD has appeared on many TV specials and on *Sesame Street* and received a Tony Award in 1977 for theatrical excellence. In 1984, the group represented the United States at the Los Angeles Olympics Arts Festival, and in 1986 it became the first Western theater company to tour the People's Republic of China.

Most of the actors are deaf, and the cast takes English scripts and translates them into a theatrical form of sign language, which may also include new signs created to express a dramatic point. Two hearing actors also translate orally for the primarily-hearing audiences who come to the shows.

In addition to formal performances, the company supports the LITTLE THEATRE OF THE DEAF for young audiences and presents numerous workshops and lecture-demonstrations. The company also supports a professional theater school during the summer to teach deaf individuals basic and advanced theater skills at the company's headquarters in Chester, Connecticut.

The National Theatre of the Deaf is located at the Hazel E. Stark Center, a converted mill and residence housing offices, rehearsal space, classrooms and theater shops. Funding for the theater comes from grants, gifts, performances and the Media Services and Captioned Films section of the Bureau of Education. See also PROFESSIONAL SCHOOL FOR DEAF THEATRE PERSONNEL.

Navarrete, Juan Fernández de (1526–1579)
Also known as "El Mudo" (the mute), Juan Fernández de Navarrete was born in Spain and became deaf at age three from unknown causes. As a child, he began to draw as a way of communicating and received his first art lessons in his hometown of Logrono. Eventually he was sent to study art in Italy upon his teacher's recommendation.

He toured the primary cities of Italy, studying art as he went, until King Philip II of Spain summoned him to Madrid, where he became the most important of the group of Spanish and Italian painters commissioned to work in the famed monastery and royal palace of the Escorial.

A member of the Madrid school, El Mudo painted during a time of transition in the Spanish art world. He was the first to abandon the mannerist movement, which had begun in the 16th century, and was the bridge to the naturalists of the 17th century. Almost all of his paintings are religious in nature; those that remain at the cloister of the Escorial hang in the gallery of the upper cloister.

El Mudo died on March 28, 1579, in Toledo, Spain, before completing his commission to paint the pictures for 30 altars in the Basilica of the Escorial.

neonatal hearing screening programs   See AUDIOMETRY.

nerve deafness   See SENSORINEURAL HEARING LOSS.

Netherlands   About 3.4 percent of this population of 14.4 million is hard-of-hearing, and about 28,000 to 931,761 of these are deaf, representing a fairly low rate of deafness.

There are 44 deaf institutions, including preschool, elementary and vocational training, with varied programs offering day and residential, oral and TOTAL COMMUNICATION approaches. Few students are mainstreamed or are educated beyond high school.

The oral approach has been the basis of social interchange in the Netherlands from preschool to adult aftercare programs, but more and more experts are beginning to acknowledge the value of the manual.

Adult deaf people communicate with a blended form of Signed Dutch, DUTCH SIGN LANGUAGE and lip movements.

neural prosthesis   See COCHLEAR IMPLANT.

neurogenic communication disorder   The inability to exchange information with others because of hearing, speech and/or language problems caused by impairment of the nervous system (brain or nerves).

newborn screening programs   Because prompt diagnosis of hearing problems could help offset lapses in language development, the American Academy of Pediatrics now recommends that all newborns be checked for HEARING LOSS. Hearing impairment in infants can cause delays in speech, language and cognitive development, according to the academy experts. Often, hearing loss is not diagnosed in children until they are two or three years old and not speaking properly.

Yet if hearing problems are detected early enough, babies can be fitted with HEARING AIDS or watch others using SIGN LANGUAGE. Children learn language by exposure to language; without exposure either to spoken or sign language, it's hard for these children to catch up.

Hearing loss is more frequent than other disorders that are now assessed at birth: hearing loss occurs in four out of every 1,000 births; yet screening is only required in 10 states. Meanwhile, babies are routinely checked for the metabolic disorder of phenylketonuria (PKU), which occurs in only one out of every 16,000 births.

Screening for hearing is noninvasive and painless and usually includes either the vibration of the small hair cells in the COCHLEA when exposed to sound or the use of ear cuplets and sensors on the baby's head to measure brain response to sound.

In the past, only babies in certain high-risk categories were tested at birth for hearing problems. These high-risk categories included lack of oxygen at birth, bacterial MENINGITIS, infections at birth, exposure to rubella or herpes, defects of the head or neck (such as cleft palate or malformation of the ear itself), severe jaundice requiring transfusion, family history of childhood hearing loss, and low birth weight. Among these high-risk infants, chances of having a congenital hearing problem is between one out of 20 to one out of 50. See also AUDITORY BRAINSTEM RESPONSE TEST; HIGH RISK QUESTIONNAIRE.

New Zealand This tiny country of only three million people includes a scattered deaf population of 7,700 deaf and hard-of-hearing people.

The first state oral school for deaf students in the world was opened in 1880 by Gerrit Van Asch, whose work was praised by ALEXANDER GRAHAM BELL. Beginning in the 1940s, a host of changes were introduced: free hearing aids, formal teacher training, nursery school and guidance programs for parents and students.

Since 1960, educators for deaf students in New Zealand have tried to develop new, expanded services, serving classes for deaf children in ordinary elementary and high schools with special teachers and for students mainstreamed in regular classes. They have also developed two state residential schools. Further, the schools for deaf students are affiliated with polytechnic colleges and community colleges; they also send deaf students to regular universities.

As in many European countries, New Zealand for many years favored the oral approach; today, it has modified this approach to include TOTAL COMMUNICATION with a standardized SIGN LANGUAGE system (the Australian or Victorian) and two-handed FINGERSPELLING.

Because of the country's small size, no one school limits itself to one communication mode but consults with parents in deciding which method to use with each individual child.

Although many deaf people in New Zealand are not hired in positions that fully utilize their abilities, the increased availability of further education has raised the standard of living for deaf people.

Because the school system relied on oral instruction for many years, no formal sign language system was developed. Most deaf New Zealanders do communicate with signs they originated, but no fingerspelling is used. With the introduction of TOTAL COMMUNICATION, two-handed fingerspelling and a wide range of signs has been introduced.

nicotine and hearing loss Nicotine, a known vasoconstrictor, inhibits the flow of blood throughout the body by narrowing blood vessels, including those to the ear.

Nicotine can cause TINNITUS in addition to hearing loss. Also, research suggests that smokers have a higher failure rate following MYRINGOPLASTY (reconstruction of the eardrum), one of the least dangerous and simplest operations of the ear. See also SMOKING AND HEARING LOSS.

Nigeria The exact number of deaf people in Nigeria is difficult to ascertain since there has been no census of this population, but it is estimated that there are about 70,000 deaf citizens out of a population of 80 million. About 7,000 of these are believed to be between six and 18 years of age.

Too often in this country, deafness in children is unnoticed or ignored by illiterate parents; many infants are born at home, and physicians may rarely see these children. In addition, the society looks negatively at deaf children and their parents, and therefore many are hidden away. Because most cases of deafness occur after birth and during adolescence or adulthood, many deaf Nigerians can learn to speak fairly well.

Today, there are 20 schools for deaf students in addition to special classes in regular schools, and about 50 deaf Nigerian students study in the United States each year. Most schools use the American MANUAL ALPHABET and SIGN LANGUAGE.

noise One of the most prevalent—and preventable—causes of deafness in the United States, exposure to excessive noise levels accounts for 10 million of the 28 million Americans with HEARING LOSS.

Hearing occurs when sound enters the outer ear, striking the eardrum; vibrations move deep inside the inner ear where they pass over 30,000 microscopic hair-like cells, which convert vibrations into the electrical signals the brain can interpret.

Damage to hearing from excess noise occurs primarily in the COCHLEA, overloading the tiny, irreplaceable "hair cells," and possibly resulting in a sensory hearing loss. In addition, excess noise can reduce enzymes and energy sources in the cochlear fluids and change the structure of the cochlear mechanism, which provides most of the nourishment to the hair cells.

As exposure to noise continues, stress on the hair cells increases, the tiny hairs on top of the cells become fused together, the hair cells disintegrate, and finally the nerve fibers to the hair cells disappear. At this point, since hair cells do not regenerate, damage is permanent.

In the case of acoustic trauma—a sudden, sharp, very loud noise—the entire mechanical INNER EAR system vibrates so violently that its attachments are disrupted, membranes in the cochlea may rupture, and hair cells are torn from the BASILAR MEMBRANE. The rupture of the cochlea membranes results in a mixing of ear fluids that poisons any hair cells that were not destroyed in the initial blast.

Most sounds (other than acoustic trauma) that can produce lasting damage are high-intensity noises that occur over a long period of time—eight hours a day for more than ten years, for example. Such noise-induced hearing loss is quite common, for example, among rock musicians and disc jockeys.

While it's generally true that the younger a person is, the better the hearing, almost all adults in this country notice some decrease in hearing ability by age 30; by age 65 at least one out of six Americans has a severe hearing loss.

Recent research has uncovered an astonishing loss of hearing acuity among students: 15 percent of school-age children and 61 percent of college freshmen tested all showed hearing problems. Conversely, studies have found that natives in the African jungle—exposed to no excess noise at all—show almost no decrease in hearing acuity as they age. But the biggest increase in hearing loss is among "baby boomers" in their 40s and 50s. From 1971 to 1990, hearing problems in this group jumped 26 percent, almost all due to increased noise levels.

New research has found that pregnant women who work in noisy environments may be at risk for damage to the hearing of their unborn children. In the past, sound was thought to be muffled by the mother's abdominal tissues and fluids in the uterus. However, in a recent study of unborn lambs, chronic loud noises and short, loud bursts of noise (such as the sound of a weapon firing)

RANGE OF SOUNDS AUDIBLE TO HUMANS

Typical Decibel	Example
0	Lowest sound audible to the human ear.
30	Quiet library, soft whisper.
40	Living room, quiet office, bedroom away from traffic.
50	Light traffic at a distance, refrigerator, gentle breeze.
60	Air conditioner at 20 feet, conversation, sewing machine.
70	Busy traffic, office tabulator, noisy restaurant. At this decibel level, noise may begin to affect hearing if exposure is constant.

The Hazardous Zone

80	Subway, heavy city traffic, alarm clock at two feet, factory noise. These noises are dangerous if exposure to them lasts for more than eight hours.
90	Truck traffic, noisy home appliances, shop tools, lawn mower. As loudness increases, the "safe" time exposure decreases; damage can occur in less than eight hours.
100	Chain saw, stereo headphones, pneumatic drill. Even two hours of exposure can be dangerous at this decibel level; with each 5 dB increase the safe time is cut *in half*.
120	Rock band concert in front of speakers, sandblasting, thunderclap. The danger is immediate; exposure at 120 dB can injure ears.
140	Gunshot blast, jet plane. *Any* length of exposure time is dangerous; noise at this level may cause actual pain in the ear.
180	Rocket launching pad. Without ear protection, noise at this level causes irreversible damage; hearing loss is inevitable.

Source: American Academy of Otolaryngology; © 1983.

triggered hearing loss while the lamb was in the womb. Not only did the lambs' hearing become less sensitive after chronic loud noise exposure, but after birth, the tiny hairs that pick up sounds in the lambs' inner ears were often deformed. Because developing lambs are about the same size as humans, the animals are good models for human pregnancy.

For this reason, experts are now suggesting that pregnant women avoid loud noise if possible, such as rock concerts, jet skiing, snowmobiling and mowing the yard. If a woman has to speak loudly to be understood, the noise level is potentially dangerous to both the adult and the unborn child.

However, data are not yet solid enough to recommend that employers bar pregnant women from jobs with high noise exposure. Although a few human studies have shown mild hearing loss among children of women who work in noisy places, the studies aren't conclusive because hearing was not measured right at birth.

Studies have indicated that hearing loss in the workplace begins once noise exceeds 80 dB, although there is not a significant effect until noise reaches 90 dB. Although studies indicate that continual exposure to 90 dB noise will result in a hearing loss of about 15 dB, it does not mean that everyone who works in this environment at 90 dB will have the same loss; some workers' ears will remain healthy while others might incur a hearing loss of over 30 dB. This is because hearing loss is also related to noise environment outside of work, which can vary a great deal.

It is also possible that noise-induced hearing loss can be made much worse by certain OTOTOXIC DRUGS that, if taken in the presence of excess noise, could harm an ear it would otherwise leave unaffected. So far, efforts to link noise damage with smoking, diet, posture and social drugs have failed.

At this time, the only way to protect the ears against damage from noise in excess of 80 dB for eight hours a day is to wear protective ear devices, such as earplugs or earmuffs. See also EAR PROTECTORS; NOISE CONTROL LAWS; OCCUPATIONAL HEARING LOSS.

noise blocker   Also called an automatic signal processor, these are innovative devices operating on the theory that most noise occurs at low pitch; consequently, they are designed to pick up the low pitch sounds and automatically reduce their noise level.

However, if the wearer's speech discrimination is poor, the noise blockers may not help, particularly if the noise is coming from large groups of people talking.

noise control laws   Legislation aimed at controlling noise in public, first enacted in 1968 by the U.S. Congress as part of its amendment to the Federal Aviation Act. One year later, Congress included hearing-conservation rules for plants with federal contracts as part of the Walsh-Healy Act.

Unusual in its inclusion of safety provisions for private enterprise, the regulations paved the way for the Occupational Safety and Health Act of 1970 that brought together a host of safety regulations in industry. Included in the act was section 1910.95, which applied the noise regulations of the Walsh-Healy Act to all workers in all industries.

The law required industry to define areas in their plants where noise exceeded an equivalent of 90 dBA for an eight-hour workday; each time noise level increases 5 dBA, the allowable exposure time is cut in half.

If possible, noise in areas of excessive noise should be lowered; if workers' hearing can't be protected by limiting the exposure or the level of the noise, then the law requires they be protected by provision either of protective hearing devices or annual hearing tests to identify people experiencing progressive hearing loss.

The 1970 legislation was followed two years later by the Noise Control Act, which gave the Environmental Protection Agency power over federal regulatory action in noise control. However, the labor department maintained control over the Occupational Safety and Health Administration, and the Federal Aviation Agency retained authority over aircraft noise regulatory action.

noise exposure and hearing loss   See NOISE.

nonhuman signing   Manual communication taught to nonhumans (typically apes) in an attempt to teach these animals language.

The earliest attempts to teach apes to communicate focused on speech rather than SIGN LANGUAGE. Although years of research occasionally produced an ape that could utter one or two words, forcing the apes to produce vocal human speech was doomed from the start because of the different vocal apparatus between the species.

The first successful attempt at teaching apes communication came in 1966, when two researchers, R. Allen and B. T. Gardner, taught their 10-month old chimpanzee, Washoe, AMERICAN SIGN LANGUAGE (ASL). They began Washoe's training by raising her in the social environment of their own family, living with humans by day and in a separate house trailer at night. In addition, Washoe could play in the back yard with a sandbox, gym and a large tree.

Since chimps lack the ability to produce speech and because in the wild they use gestures to communicate, the Gardners chose to teach Washoe ASL because it was a gestural and human language.

In Washoe's first four years, she acquired more than 130 signs, using them spontaneously and in correct context. She carried on everyday conversations, initiated conversation and commented to and questioned her human companions. She could ask about friends who were not there and generalized her signs to a variety of uses. For example, she would sign "dog" not just for a real dog but for photos of dogs and sounds of barking dogs.

Further study with Washoe looked at the capacity of chimps to use cross-modal transfer between auditory words and visual signs. Researchers also compared individual differences between chimps, generic and specific use of signs, comprehension, use of prepositional phrases and the conceptual use of signs.

Still, the Gardners' research with Washoe was criticized in the late 1970s by people who argued that the conclusions of the Gardners and others were false because the evidence was ambiguous, suggesting that the Gardners wanted to believe Washoe could sign and were therefore biased, and that scientists inadvertently cued the chimp. Critics also charged that the form and structure of the ape's signs showed no resemblance to ASL.

In 1978, researchers tried to design a study to answer critics, stopping all signs around the chimp except for seven signs: who, what, want, which, where, sign and name. Researchers believed if Washoe's infants acquired sign language, it was because they had learned it from her.

After Washoe's first infant died, a 10-month-old male was given to her to adopt. Eight days later, little Loulis used his first sign: "person." At 15 months, he started using two-sign combinations, and five years later, he used 54 different signs—all learned from Washoe and signing chimp friends.

Loulis was therefore the first chimp to acquire human language from another chimp.

In 1980, three new chimps were raised in their early years at the Gardners' house, intended for testing in cross-chimp communication. To control the use of human signing, the chimps were videotaped and observed on monitors from a separate room in 20-minute segments three times a day for 15 days, thereby restricting access to their human caretakers.

In the 15 hours taped, 617 chimp conversations were recorded. Together with research from another study examining many more conversations, scientists found that almost 90 percent of these chimp "conversations" centered around play, reassurance and social interactions. Only 5 percent had to do with food.

nonmanual behaviors   The features of AMERICAN SIGN LANGUAGE that are not portrayed with the hands. These include facial expression, head and body movement and posture.

nonorganic hearing loss   See FUNCTIONAL HEARING LOSS (NONORGANIC).

nonsuppurative otitis media   See SEROUS OTITIS MEDIA.

nonverbal communication   Nonverbal communication includes tone of voice and noises, shrugs, body position, facial expressions and gestures to enrich and modify speech. Hearing people generally assume this nonverbal communication is inferior to speech, because it is less variable and not a systematic form of language.

SIGN LANGUAGE, however, is *not* a form of nonverbal communication. Deaf people use nonverbal communication in much the same way hearing people do. The reason why sign languages have often been misclassified as nonverbal systems of communication is probably because their form is visual-gestural, which is also the most common form of nonverbal communication among hearing people.

North American Basic Teletext Specification
Also known as NABTS, this is the teletext system
that provides CLOSED CAPTIONS similar to those
offered by the LINE 21 type of closed captioning.

Teletext systems use several lines of the vertical
blanking interval to send closed captions to TV sets
equipped with a teletext decoder (different from
the TELECAPTION DECODER needed for decoding line
21 captioning).

The only television network that offers both
teletext and line 21 closed captions is CBS-TV. See
also CAPTION CENTER; NATIONAL CAPTIONING INSTITUTE.

Northampton vowel and consonant charts A
printed system to help deaf children learn to speak,
read and write syntactically correct sentences.

Devised in 1884, the system uses alphabet symbols to describe English pronunciation and was first
used for teaching how sounds and words were
related in reading. It is now more commonly used
to help develop speech.

Norwegian Sign Language There are three
major sign dialects of Norwegian Sign Language
(NSL), spoken by about 4,000 deaf Norwegians,
which originate with the three schools for the deaf.

In these schools, teachers use a manual code
for Norwegian called Signed Norwegian, together
with speech in addition to signs. As is typical
around the world, Norwegian students use SIGN
LANGUAGE when speaking among themselves outside of school.

In addition to NSL, the INTERNATIONAL MANUAL
ALPHABET developed by the WORLD FEDERATION OF THE
DEAF and considered to be the best system for deaf-
blind people, has been used since 1970.

Since the 1970s, there has been a growing
demand for the use of NSL in education by the deaf
community.

Unlike AMERICAN SIGN LANGUAGE, NSL vocabulary
uses almost no fingerspelled signs. It does, however, emphasize the use of lip movements of spoken words.

occupational hearing loss   A number of industrial environments produce enough noise to impair hearing. In part, this occurs because although noise above 90 decibels can harm hearing, a person can work in the presence of noise up to 120 dB before it begins to be painful.

At the end of a day in the presence of 90 dB noise, there might be slight ringing or muffling of noises, but after an evening or weekend away from the noise, these symptoms would be gone. A person tested after working all day in the presence of 120 dB noise might show a slight loss of hearing, but after a few days away from the job, a retest would show hearing has returned to normal. This is called a temporary THRESHOLD shift.

After several months of this type of exposure, the hearing loss becomes permanent. A worker probably would not notice work-induced hearing loss because the deficits show up first among the high frequencies, which interferes very little with the understanding of speech. Not until the loss worsens and begins to affect the middle frequencies would a hearing loss be noticed. By that time, the loss could be permanent. A person does not become "used" to working around noise; if after some months or years the noise seems less noticeable, it is only because a hearing loss has already occurred.

Jobs that put workers at risk for hearing loss include boilermaking, weaving, aircraft maintenance, blacksmithing, chipping, riveting, blasting, machine manufacturing, metalworking and loud rock music production. Also at risk are people employed in any job involving large presses, high-pressure steam, large wood saws and heavy hammering (such as iron and steel working).

People involved in work around noisy machinery should understand that if it is necessary to raise the voice to be heard by someone less than two feet away, protective devices should be worn. A person working in an environment this noisy should have a hearing test once a year and always wear EAR PROTECTORS or find other employment. See also NOISE; OCCUPATIONAL HEALTH AND SAFETY ACT.

Occupational Safety and Health Act   An essential requirement of this act is that any industry in which employees are exposed daily to continuous NOISE levels greater than 90 decibels for an eight-hour working day over many years must either reduce the noise or protect the hearing of exposed workers.

The 90 dBA level specified is the level at which conservation of hearing should begin. Occupations that pose a risk to hearing include boilermaking, weaving, aircraft maintenance, blacksmithing, chipping, riveting, blasting, machine manufacturing and metal-working, as well as any job using large presses, high-pressure steam, large wood saws or heavy hammering (such as in iron and steel works). Persons involved in the production of loud rock music are also at risk of a permanent hearing loss. See also OCCUPATIONAL HEARING LOSS.

on-the-body hearing aids   See BODY HEARING AID.

open captions   Ordinary subtitles that appear on films (such as foreign films with English subtitles) and that are available for everyone to see. These are the opposite of CLOSED CAPTIONS, which are visible only to people with special decoding devices.

open-set speech recognition   Understanding speech without visual clues (speechreading).

oral approach A communication method that stresses the use of speech among deaf and hard-of-hearing people together with SPEECHREADING and auditory training as a way of merging with the hearing world.

The roots of the oral approach may be traced to the 1500s, when a Spanish monk named PEDRO PONCE DE LEÓN taught the deaf children of nobility at his monastery. Using his own methods, he taught the children to use language, speech and speech-reading. His methods were handed on to other Spanish teachers of deaf children at the end of the 16th century, including Manuel Ramirez de Carrion. At about the same time, JUAN PABLO BONET published what was the first book describing oral teaching methods for deaf students.

Gradually, the oral method movement spread throughout Europe and found a special home in Germany in the 18th century, where SAMUEL HEINICKE became its leading proponent. Heinicke, a devout oral proponent, opened the first German school for deaf students in 1778. At the same time in England, the Braidwood family headed by THOMAS BRAIDWOOD was opening oralist schools for deaf children using its own secret methods of instruction.

In 1819 American educator THOMAS HOPKINS GALLAUDET came to the Braidwoods to learn the oralist tradition. When the Braidwoods refused to reveal their methods to Gallaudet, he went on to France to learn the manual method, which he subsequently brought back to the United States.

The MANUAL APPROACH was the sole method of instruction for deaf students up until the mid-1800s, when the Clarke School opened in Northampton, Massachusetts. From then on, aided by the European success of oralist education, the tide began to change in the United States, and from 1880 to 1930 oralism replaced the manual approach as the primary method of instruction. After World War I, about 75 percent of American deaf pupils were taught almost entirely by the oral method.

As time went on, however, schools began combining their methods; elementary students were taught orally, with signs used in some classes in high school. But studies in the 1960s and 1970s found that the educational achievement of deaf children educated orally fell short of their hearing peers and that students taught in sign from the beginning generally functioned at a higher level.

The 200-year debate over the oral and manual methods centers on the place in society in which a deaf person should fit. Those who supported the oral approach in this country were generally opposed to the segregation of deaf people and did not approve of special camps, churches or social organizations. Critics of the oral approach, on the other hand, believed in maintaining deaf culture and in making accommodations in communication and social organizations.

Oral supporters (whose chief champion was ALEXANDER GRAHAM BELL) promote the use of hearing aids, speechreading and speech as the right of all deaf children and do not favor the use of sign language in schools. In fact, for many years, sign language was forbidden in oral schools. This objection to sign is primarily because proponents of the oral method believe it is too difficult to learn two languages at once (speech and sign). However, not all object to sign language as a means of communication *outside* the school.

There are also differences of opinions among oral method supporters over auditory, multisensory or CUED SPEECH teaching methods. The first method uses auditory training and specialized training that does not emphasize speechreading.

The multisensory teaching method is more traditional, encouraging students to use speechreading, body language or tactile methods to communicate. Some multisensory programs also permit the use of FINGERSPELLING.

Cued Speech supporters believe in the Cued Speech system, which supplements what a person hears with a hearing aid, a combined form of speechreading and hand cues. See also SIMULTANEOUS COMMUNICATION; TOTAL COMMUNICATION.

Oral Deaf Adults Section (ODAS) A service organization, this group was formed in 1964 as part of the ALEXANDER GRAHAM BELL ASSOCIATION FOR THE DEAF. Its members choose to communicate through spoken language and SPEECHREADING and have joined together to encourage the oral-aural approach in educating deaf children. Supporters of the oral approach believe students can learn to communicate effectively using speech, speechreading and auditory training.

The section was founded by H. LATHAM BREUNIG and ROBERT H. WEITBRECHT, the developer of teletypewriters (TTYs) for deaf people. It publishes a membership directory and a newsletter for members, offers educational scholarships and plans outings for families with deaf children.

The group maintains its own member speakers' bureau in order to portray these deaf adults as role models for younger deaf people.

oral interpreters Persons skilled in the specialized interpreting ability of translating the meaning of spoken words by silently mouthing a speaker's words for a deaf person who prefers the oral approach. Oral interpreters use no sign language and are skilled in substituting words for those that are difficult to speechread. However, oral interpreters are used by only a very few deaf people.

Oral interpreters are also available to repeat to a hearing audience a spoken message from a deaf person whose speech may not be clear. They use a variety of skills and techniques to convey the message and emotions of the speaker; these are most helpful when the person with a hearing loss does not use sign language.

An oral interpreter may not be the best interpreter for a person who uses listening skills and SPEECHREADING since it is difficult to watch an oral interpreter while listening to the speaker. Because of the delay between the sound of the speaker's voice and lip movements of the oral interpreter, the oral interpreter is always several words behind the speaker.

Oral interpreters are certified by the REGISTRY OF INTERPRETERS FOR THE DEAF, the only national professional organization in the United States that certifies both oral and SIGN LANGUAGE interpreters. The registry lists interpreters in various specialties, including legal, medical and educational interpreting. In 1979, the registry established a separate certification process for oral interpreters similar to the one for sign language interpreters. Three oral interpreting certifications are awarded by the registry: Two for different levels of accuracy by hearing candidates and one for candidates with hearing problems.

Oral interpreters are listed with local and state chapters of the Registry of Interpreters for the Deaf, local speech and hearing centers, the Office of Vocational Rehabilitation, the ALEXANDER GRAHAM BELL ASSOCIATION FOR THE DEAF, a school or college with support services for hard-of-hearing students and programs and agencies serving hard-of-hearing people.

A hard-of-hearing person does not have to pay for oral interpreters under several conditions. For example, Section 504 of the Rehabilitation Act of 1973 requires that interpreting services for hard-of-hearing people must be provided free for all meetings, classes and other group activities sponsored by an agency that receives federal funds and has 15 or more employees. In an educational setting, the Education for All Handicapped Children Act of 1975 (PL 94–142) requires that the services of an interpreter must be written into a student's individual educational plan. Such an interpreter service would then be paid for by the child's school. At the same time, hard-of-hearing or deaf parents must also be given an interpreter for parent/teacher conferences and meetings. In addition, federal law requires the federal court to appoint a qualified interpreter in criminal or civil actions against a hard-of-hearing person, and the court must provide an oral interpreter if so requested. Most states also pay for an interpreter in criminal proceedings; several pay for an interpreter in civil cases as well. See also INTERPRETERS AND THE LAW; LEGAL RIGHTS.

organ of Corti The organ of Corti is contained in the COCHLEA and is the most important part of the hearing process.

The organ is covered with many fine hairs arranged like the strings of a harp, with the shorter, thinner hairs picking up high sounds and the longer, thicker hairs picking up low sounds. When a sound wave makes the eardrum vibrate, the vibrations are carried across the middle ear by the hammer, the anvil and the stirrup, which pass the vibrations through the oval window to the fluid in the tubes of the inner ear.

This makes the hairs of the organ of Corti vibrate; the more hairs that vibrate, the louder the sound. The AUDITORY NERVE picks up the message from these hairs and sends it to the brain, where the sound is processed.

osseous labyrinth   See LABYRINTH, INNER EAR.

ossicles   The three small bones of the MIDDLE EAR (the malleus or hammer, the incus or anvil and the stapes or stirrup) that help carry sound and speech from the eardrum to the inner ear. See also OSSICULAR CHAIN.

ossicular chain   Attached to the eardrum is a chain of three small bones called the ossicular chain. Located in the pea-sized middle ear cavity, the ossicles are the smallest bones in the human body and are full size when a child is born.

The individual bones are smaller than a grain of rice: the bone attached to the eardrum is the malleus (hammer); the second bone is the incus (anvil); and the third is the stapes (stirrup). As sound waves move the eardrum, it moves the ossicles. The three bones actually serve as a type of level that transfers the energy of the sound waves from the outer ear through the MIDDLE EAR into the INNER EAR.

ossicular interruption   A separation of the three tiny ossicles that carry sound vibrations from the eardrum membrane to the fluid inside the inner ear. It is caused by an infection or by a blow to the head.

The separation usually occurs at the weakest point of the OSSICULAR CHAIN, where the anvil (incus) joins the stirrup (stapes). A partial separation causes mild hearing impairment; a more complete separation results in a severe hearing loss.

Ossicular interruption can be diagnosed by hearing tests that indicate the hearing nerve in the inner ear is normal but sound is not being conducted from the eardrum to the inner ear.

Treatment of ossicular interruption is one of the most successful operations to restore hearing— performed by an otolaryngologist, it involves repositioning the ossicles so they can again conduct sound. See also OSSICULOPLASTY.

ossiculoplasty   Surgical repair of the middle-ear OSSICLES to treat hearing loss, usually caused by chronic OTITIS MEDIA or CHOLESTEATOMA or a temporal bone fracture. Ossiculoplasty may be combined with MYRINGOPLASTY or MASTOIDECTOMY. See also OSSICULAR INTERRUPTION; TYMPANOPLASTY.

osteitis deformans   See PAGET'S DISEASE.

osteogenesis imperfecta   A bone disorder causing the entire skeleton to have brittle bones with many fractures. About half of these patients have a syndrome called van der Hoeve's syndrome, in which there is a CONDUCTIVE HEARING LOSS and a blue tinge to the whites of the eyes. It is believed that this syndrome is caused by a disease similar to OTOSCLEROSIS, which causes the STAPES (stirrup) footplate to adhere to surrounding bone. The conductive hearing loss occurs because of fractures in the stapes.

osteoma   An osteoma of the ear canal is a bony knob close to the eardrum, occurring particularly in people who swim frequently in cold water. Unless the growth blocks the ear canal and therefore interferes with hearing, it does not need to be removed.

otic capsule   The bony case enclosing the inner ear. Part of the otic capsule forms the inner wall of the middle ear.

otitis externa   See SWIMMER'S EAR.

otitis media   An infection of the MIDDLE EAR (the cavity between the eardrum and the INNER EAR) that can produce pus or fluid and cause hearing loss. The inflammation can occur as the result of an infection extending up the eustachian tube, the passage that connects the back of the nose to the middle ear. This tube may become blocked by the infection or by enlarged adenoids (often associated with infections of the nose and throat). Fluid produced by the inflammation can't drain off through the tube and instead collects in the middle ear.

Acute otitis media causes sudden, severe earache, deafness, TINNITUS (ringing or buzzing in the ear), sense of fullness in the ear and fever. Occasionally, the eardrum can burst, which causes a discharge of pus and relief of pain; a physician will sometimes incise the eardrum (MYRINGOTOMY) to relieve pressure. Chronic otitis media is usually caused by repeated attacks of acute otitis media, with pus seeping from a perforation in the eardrum together with some degree of deafness. Complications include otitis externa (inflammation of the outer ear), damage to the bones in the middle ear (sometimes causing total deafness) or a CHOLESTEATOMA (a matted ball of skin debris which can erode bone and cause further damage to the ear). Rarely, infection can spread *inward* from an infected ear and cause a brain abscess.

Otitis media can be detected by examining the ear with an instrument called an OTOSCOPE. A sample of discharge may be taken to identify the organism responsible for the infection.

Acute otitis media usually clears up completely with treatment with antibiotic drugs, although there may occasionally be continual production of a sticky fluid in the middle ear known as persistent middle ear infection. Deafness can occur, but usually disappears with treatment. Otitis media is treated with antibiotics (usually penicillins) and analgesics for pain. A physician may also remove pus and skin debris and prescribe antibiotic ear drops, if necessary. Ephedrine nose drops can help establish drainage of the ear in children.

Children, probably because of the shortness of their eustachian tubes, are particularly prone to otitis media. About one in six infants under age one suffers from this problem, and some children have recurrent attacks through age 10. Chronic otitis media is much less common because most cases of acute ear infection clear up after treatment. See also EAR INFECTION VACCINE.

otoacoustic emissions (OAE) test The otoacoustic emissions test is a new, quick method of hearing testing that can be given to the youngest children—it can even be used for screening in the newborn nursery. It's based on the fact that the ear not only hears noise, but also makes noise. By measuring the very faint noises made by the ear, the test estimates how well the ear hears. An ear that does not hear will not make the expected noises. These noises are much too faint to be heard by our ears, but there are machines that can measure them. See also CHILDREN AND DEAFNESS.

OtoLAM A laser technique for treating infants and young children with ear infections by creating a tiny hole in the eardrum to drain fluid and immediately ease pain. The hole stays open for several weeks and provides ventilation of the middle ear without the need for a surgical procedure under general anesthesia to insert tubes. Special ear drops make the procedure painless, and there is no bleeding, postoperative grogginess or any of the side effects usually associated with general anesthesia. Parents stay with their child during the office procedure, which takes less than five minutes once the ear drops have taken effect.

Normally, the holes close up on their own in three to four weeks, but the time the hole remains open can be varied depending on the child's specific condition. Three to four weeks of middle ear ventilation prevents fluid from building up again in the middle ear and provides enough time, in most cases, for the underlying infection to clear. In addition to promoting healing, this reduces the likelihood of recurrence.

OtoLAM won't replace tubes (especially for children with chronic infections), but it may soon be another widely used effective treatment for ear infections. Studies have not yet found whether OtoLAM is better than tubes. Although the procedure was approved by the FDA in 1996 for treating ear infections, the technology is expensive, and doctors intending to use it will need extensive training.

The procedure can be performed on an appropriate child at the first sign of ear infection, limiting repeated courses of antibiotics. It can also prevent an acute episode from progressing to a chronic condition, reducing the risk of hearing loss and other cognitive learning disabilities.

Candidates for OtoLAM include ear infection patients who have not responded to typical antibiotic treatment or a tympanostomy, as well as those for whom the risk of general anesthesia and conventional MYRINGOTOMY surgery is too high. Clinical studies show OtoLAM to be safe and effective for infants and young children with ear infections.

otolaryngologist Also called otorhinolaryngologists, or ear, nose and throat (ENT) physicians, an otolaryngologist is a medical/surgical specialist who treats ear, nose and throat problems ranging from common conditions (such as ear infections and minor hearing loss) to more complex problems like MÉNIÈRE'S DISEASE and OTOSCLEROSIS. Otolaryngologists are also sometimes referred to as head-and-neck surgeons.

In addition, otolaryngologists are expert in the diagnosis and testing of different types of hearing loss. This specialist can advise whether a hearing aid will help, and if so, what kind would be suitable.

To qualify for the American Board of Otolaryngology certification examination, a physician must complete five or more years of post-M.D. specialty training in otolaryngology.

otolaryngology   A specialty medical field concerned with treatment and surgery of the ear, nose and throat and related structures of the head and neck.

It includes cosmetic facial reconstruction, surgery of benign and malignant tumors of the head and neck, management of patients with loss of hearing and balance, endoscopic examination of air and food passages and treatment of allergic, sinus, laryngeal, thyroid and esophageal disorders. See also OTOLARYNGOLOGIST.

otologist   A physician specialist primarily interested in diagnosing ear diseases, specifying causes of hearing loss and treating physical defects of the auditory mechanism. Otology is one division of the ear, nose and throat field (OTOLARYNGOLOGY) of medicine. An otologist may work together with an audiologist (a specialist in hearing tests).

An otologist/neurotologist is a physician who specializes in the treatment of the ear. Besides completing medical school, general surgery training, and OTOLARYNGOLOGY training, an otologist/neurotologist has also completed fellowship training in diagnosing and treating diseases of the ear and skull base. Patients often are referred by other otolaryngologists because the case is difficult and complicated and has not responded to conventional therapy. See also OTOLARYNGOLOGIST.

otology   The branch of medicine concerned with the ear. As in many other fields of medicine, the roots of the practice of otology began well before recorded history, although actual surgery on the ear did not begin before the 18th century.

Some of the first descriptions of early otology are found in the *Ebers Papyrus,* written about 1600 B.C., in which Egyptian priests specialized in ear treatments. These treatments might include injections into the ear of olive oil, red lead, bat's wings, ant eggs or goat's urine. By the fifth century, Pythagoras was exploring the physics of sound; he constructed a musical scale by listening to different pitches that occurred when a blacksmith struck his anvil with different hammers.

It was in the 19th century that modern otology began, with the surgical advances of Sir Astley Cooper in London who cut into the eardrum to ease certain cases of deafness. Parisian surgeon Gaspard Itard explored the diseases of the ear while MARIE-JEAN-PIERRE FLOURENS discussed the action of the SEMICIRCULAR CANALS and realized that the acoustic nerve has branches for hearing and for balance. By 1860, Prosper Ménière reported the case of a girl with VERTIGO, nausea and TINNITUS during a fatal illness, and in 1851 ALFONSO CORTI, an Italian anatomist, published his studies about the organ that now bears his name.

otorhinolaryngology   The full name of the surgical specialty focusing on diseases of the ear, nose and throat. See also OTOLARYNGOLOGY.

otorrhea   The medical term for a discharge from the ear. This is usually fluid resulting from an ear infection, although it can include blood or cerebrospinal fluid following a skull fracture. A physician should evaluate any case of otorrhea.

otosclerosis   Also called otospongiosis, a disorder that occurs when an overgrowth of spongy bone immobilizes the stapes (the innermost bone of the middle ear), preventing sound vibrations from passing to the inner ear and resulting in CONDUCTIVE HEARING LOSS. In most cases, both ears are usually affected. It is caused by the absorption of bone followed by the production of new, loose "spongy" bone. Eventually, this soft bone will harden and eventually become as dense as surrounding bone.

While the problem can occur anywhere on the temporal bone, it usually begins in front of the oval windows, gradually spreading to the oval window and then the footplate of the stapes. Eventually, this will imbed the stapes to the surrounding tissue, restricting stapedal movement. In addition, otosclerosis can affect the cochlea, causing a sensorineural hearing loss.

The disease, which begins in early adulthood (between age 20 and 30) and is more common among women, affects about one in every 200 people and often occurs during pregnancy. People with otosclerosis tend to talk softly and hear muffled sound more clearly when there is background noise. Hearing loss progresses slowly over a period of 10 to 15 years, often accompanied by TINNITUS and sometimes by VERTIGO. Eventually, there may be some SENSORINEURAL HEARING LOSS caused by damage spreading to the inner ear, which makes high tones hard to hear.

Hearing tests can uncover otosclerosis showing a conductive hearing loss greater in lower frequencies. There is no medication or local treatment to the ear itself that will improve hearing in people with otosclerosis. In some cases, medication may prevent further nerve hearing loss. A medication known as Florical (sodium fluoride and calcium carbonate) is sometimes prescribed to prevent further nerve hearing loss. This medication slows down and can eventually stop the growth of otosclerosis. Ideally, it should be taken twice a day for two years; after two years, the hearing level, the degree of tinnitus and the severity of imbalance should be reevaluated. If these conditions have stabilized, the Florical may be discontinued or the dosage reduced. Florical should be avoided during pregnancy.

STAPEDECTOMY is recommended for patients with otosclerosis who are good candidates for surgery. This operation is performed under local or general anesthesia with the use of laser and microscopic techniques. The procedure usually requires an outpatient or short hospital stay. Convalescence at home for about a week or so is recommended. Nearly 90 percent of these operations are successful in improving the conductive hearing loss.

otoscope   An instrument used for examining the ear that includes magnifying lenses, a light and a funnel-shaped tip that is inserted into the ear canal. The instrument can be used to inspect the outer ear canal and the eardrum, and to detect certain diseases of the MIDDLE EAR. See also OTOSCOPY.

otoscopy   Visual inspection of the ear with an OTOSCOPE to detect ear disease. Using an otoscope equipped with a bulb, magnifying lens and speculum (a device designed to open a body orifice for examination), the client's ear pinnacle is pulled slightly upward and backward and the speculum is inserted into the outer ear canal.

Pneumatic otoscopy adds a bulb syringe attachment to alternate pressure, allowing a more accurate assessment of the position and mobility of the tympanic membrane.

otospongiosis   Another name for OTOSCLEROSIS.

ototoxic drugs   Certain drugs and chemicals can affect hearing and balance through functional impairment of the inner ear. The actual incidence of drugs and resultant deafness has been hard to establish because of the problems and complexity in studying the ear.

The negative effects of some ototoxic drugs are increased when taken in combination with other drugs or for long periods of time. Often, TINNITUS (ringing in the ears) is the first symptom, although some damage can occur before any symptoms appear.

A number of factors place some people at higher risk when taking ototoxic drugs, including age, earlier ear infections, SENSORINEURAL HEARING LOSS, impaired kidney or liver function, extreme drug sensitivity, simultaneous use of LOOP DIURETICS or drugs that are toxic to kidneys.

Ototoxic drugs are particularly damaging to the developing fetus, especially during the sixth or seventh week of pregnancy. Chloroquine, streptomycin, aspirin and thalidomide are most strongly associated with ototoxic effects during pregnancy.

Substances that may temporarily reduce hearing ability or increase tinnitus include alcohol, carbon monoxide, caffeine, oral contraceptives and tobacco.

FAMILIES OF DRUGS WITH DOCUMENTED OTOTOXIC EFFECTS

1. *Aminoglycoside antibiotics*

Reaction to these drugs is most severe when therapy is extended beyond 10 days. Any patient treated for longer than this period should undergo cochlear and vestibular testing before, during and after therapy. They include:

- kanamycin
- gentamicin
- tobramycin
- amikacin
- ribostamycin
- netilmicin
- dihydrostreptomycin

streptomycin   Onset of hearing loss can occur within five days of treatment.

neomycin   Hearing loss may continue after drug is stopped. It is the most cochleartoxic of all drugs. Warning symptoms: tinnitus or balance impairment (not always present).

2. *Other antibiotics*

erythromycin   All known cases of ototoxicity with this drug have been reversed, usually within 24 hours after treatment has been stopped. Only large doses (more than 4 grams) per day are ototoxic.

viomycin   Can cause permanent hearing impairment.

3. *Diuretics*

Diuretics should be avoided in premature infants and in those receiving aminoglycoside antibiotics. Hearing loss, vertigo and tinnitus is usually reversible, with recovery between 30 minutes to 24 hours: however, permanent hearing loss is possible.

- furosemide (Lasix)   rapid intravenous administration increases chances of ototoxicity.
- ethacrynic acid (Edecrin)
- lasix
- bumetadine (Bumex)
- piretamide
- azosemide
- triflocin
- indapamide
- torsemide (demadex)
- acetazolamide mannitol

Other drugs that have been suspected to cause ototoxicity but are as yet unproven include antipyrine, atropine, chlordiazepoxide, cisplatin, fenoprofen, hexadimethrine bromide, ibuprofen, morphine, naproxen, nitrogen mustard, phenylbutazone and sulindac.

ototoxicity   Having a poisonous effect on the ear and its hearing mechanisms. High doses of certain drugs can damage the COCHLEA and the SEMICIRCULAR CANALS in the inner ear. See also OTOTOXIC DRUGS.

outer ear   The portion of the ear that contains the external ear (the pinna, or auricle). The pinna leads into the ear canal (or meatus), which is about one inch long in adults and closed at its inner end by the eardrum. The part of the ear canal nearest the outside is made of cartilage and covered with skin

FAMILIES OF DRUGS WITH DOCUMENTED OTOTOXIC EFFECTS

4. *Salicylates*

High doses of salicylates cause tinnitus and bilateral hearing loss to 40 dB. Amount of hearing loss depends on blood concentration of drug. Both tinnitus and hearing loss are reversed 24–72 hours after the drug is stopped. Aspirin is a salicylate.

5. *Quinine derivatives*

Less than 2 grams per day may cause transient tinnitus, hearing loss, vertigo, headache, nausea or vision problems. There have been cases of permanent hearing loss and tinnitus but usually only when high doses were continued after symptoms appeared.

Quinine derivatives include:
• quinine
• chloroquine
• quinidine
• hydroxychloroquine
• tonic water

6. *Anticancer drugs*
• cisplatin
• bleomycin
• vincristine
• nitrogen mustard
• vinblastine

that produces earwax which together with hair, traps dust and small particles. See also EXTERNAL AUDITORY CANAL.

oval window A tiny opening in the bony wall of the COCHLEA. It is actually an entrance to the INNER EAR.

overtone Any partial tone included in a complex tone except the lowest tone.

Paget-Gorman sign system (PGSS) A SIGN LANGUAGE system designed by Sir Richard Paget and further developed by Lady Grace Paget and Dr. Pierre Gorman of Great Britain.

It developed in almost total isolation from the language of the deaf community; the sign vocabulary of PGSS is not related to BRITISH SIGN LANGUAGE and is not intelligible to British deaf people. Children learning PGSS have nothing linguistically in common with deaf adults.

Paget's disease Also called osteitis deformans, this common genetic disease often occurs in middle age and affects the normal process of bone formation, weakening and deforming bones of the skull, pelvis, collarbone and long bones of the leg.

Changes in the skull can cause inner ear damage, resulting in TINNITUS, VERTIGO and a SENSORINEURAL HEARING LOSS. The disorder can also distort the face, cause pain and paralysis because of pressure on the spinal cord and cause severe arthritis of the hips.

Many people do not require treatment, but others find pain relief and normal bone formation occurs with analgesic drugs or, in severe cases, calcitonin. Surgery may be required to repair deformities.

painful hearing Painful hearing is produced by moderate or loud sounds that may be a single symptom or part of a range of problems, such as those found in MÉNIÈRE'S DISEASE.

Painful hearing may occur in cases of inflammation of the eardrum, when the additional stress of loud sound can hurt. Even with a normal, healthy ear, if the sound is loud enough (generally above 140 dB) it can cause pain, although there are wide differences among individuals as to the extent of pain experienced.

A sudden loud sound, such as an explosion, is much more painful than sound at the same level reached in successive small steps.

paracusia willisiana The ability to hear speech better in a noisy environment. Named for Dr. Thomas Willis, the English physician who described it in 1672, paracusia willisiana occurs in people with all forms of CONDUCTIVE HEARING LOSS.

Normally, a person in a noisy environment will raise his voice about 40 decibels louder in order to be heard above the background sounds. The person with a conductive hearing loss at frequencies that match the background noise won't be able to hear it but will be able to hear the speaker's voice well at an intensity level 40 decibels higher. With a pure conductive disorder, the sense organ is normal, and the speech at this louder decibel level will be completely understandable. On the other hand, a person with normal hearing hears not only the speaker's louder voice, but the entire range of background noise as well. Finally, a person with SENSORINEURAL HEARING LOSS has more trouble hearing in noise because of the masking effect.

PB words A phonetically balanced list of words for articulation hearing tests that feature speech sounds in approximately the same relative frequency of occurrence as normal speech. See also AUDIOMETRY.

Pendred's syndrome An inherited condition that causes deafness (usually at birth) and development of goiter (enlarged thyroid) in childhood, and the most common of syndromic hereditary HEARING LOSS. People with the syndrome have different degrees of hearing loss, but it is severe for more than half of them. The syndrome is probably the most common form of deafness that appears with another condition (in this case, goiter).

In 1996, two research groups that had studied large, inbred families with Pendred's syndrome reported that they had mapped the responsible gene to chromosome 7. Scientists now know that the syndrome is caused by mutations in the PDS gene (also known as DFNB4), which encodes a protein called pendrin. The gene encoding pendrin is active in the adult thyroid gland and also may be active in the developing fetal cochlea, which may explain the deafness associated with Pendred's syndrome. Scientists suspect that this protein plays a direct role in the development of the inner ear; the cochlea is like a spiral staircase, and in people with Pendred's, it does not have the right number of turns.

However, investigators also found that certain mutations in the pendrin gene can cause deafness without thyroid problems. Not all individuals develop goiters, which may mean that mutations in the pendrin gene account for many more cases of deafness than researchers had previously suspected. It has been estimated that between 4 and 8 percent of deaf children have Pendred's.

percent of hearing loss   The percent of HEARING LOSS used for medical and legal purposes can be estimated by approximating the number of damaged hair cells within the COCHLEA. Because it is impossible to count the damaged cells among the 15,000 in the ear, a percent of loss is made by using the AUDIOGRAM.

The amount of hearing loss is based on threshold levels at 500, 1000 and 2000 Hz. Hearing sensitivity better than 26 dB is not considered a loss; hearing worse than 93 dB is a total loss. Therefore, the percentage (0 to 100) of hearing loss covers a range of 67 dB. Each decibel above 26 dB is rated as a 1.5 percent loss. To calculate percentage of hearing loss, an audiologist averages the thresholds at 500, 1000 and 2000 Hz and subtracts 26 dB from this average. The remainder is multiplied by 1.5.

Although percentage is used to describe hearing loss, it does not give a clear picture of the actual hearing deficit. For example, a 40 percent hearing loss does not specify whether the loss is within the high, low or middle frequencies for speech recep-

tion. But this is important to know since *where* the damage occurs in a frequency range determines the ability to hear speech.

A group of people, all with a 40 percent hearing loss, will not each have the same ability to understand speech—one person's loss may be in the low frequencies, one in the high, another in the middle, with uncounted degrees in between.

Pereira, Jacobo Rodriguez (1715–1780)   This 18th-century Portuguese teacher is known as the first teacher of deaf students in France. Born in Berlanga, Portugal, Pereira moved to Bordeaux, where he demonstrated his techniques before the Parisian Academy of Science.

Advocating a low student-teacher ratio, Pereira accepted payment for his work depending on how quickly his pupils progressed. He used a one-handed manual alphabet that represented phonic qualities, not letters—the position of the fingers indicated the position of the speech organ used in making that sound. Similar to CUED SPEECH, this alphabet was used as a pronunciation aid.

perichondritis   An unusual infection of the cartilage of the outer ear, this disorder is caused by an organism and can be contracted while swimming in polluted water or by an injury.

This microorganism, *Pseudomonas aeruginosa*, creates a greenish brown musty discharge from the outer ear canal. Perichondritis can be suspected when the outer ear is tender, red and thicker than normal. Prompt treatment will prevent a permanent deformity of the outer ear.

perilymph   The fluid, almost identical to spinal fluid, that is contained in the canals of the COCHLEA. See also PERILYMPH FISTULA.

perilymph fistula   An abnormal opening between the air-filled middle ear and the fluid-filled inner ear. In most instances it is a tear or defect in one or both of the small, thin membranes between the middle and inner ears (the oval and round windows) or between in the bone of the ear (the otic capsule). This opening can occur spontaneously or after some type of damage to the eardrum.

The changes in air pressure that occur in the middle ear (for example, when a person's ears pop in an airplane) normally don't affect the inner ear, but when a fistula exists, changes in middle ear pressure will directly affect the inner ear, stimulating the balance and/or hearing structures and causing symptoms including dizziness, vertigo, imbalance, nausea and vomiting. Patients typically report an unsteadiness that increases with activity and is relieved by rest. Some people experience ringing or fullness in the ears, and many notice a hearing loss. Other people with fistulas find that their symptoms get worse with coughing, sneezing or blowing their noses, as well as with exertion and activity. Even speaking or playing a musical instrument can cause dizziness (this is called the Tullio's phenomenon).

A direct blow to the ear is the most common cause of fistulas, but they may also develop after ear surgery or following rapid or profound changes in pressure (BAROTRAUMA) during scuba diving or an airplane descent. Rarely, forceful coughing or sneezing may cause a fistula. Fistulas may be present from birth (usually in association with deafness) or may result from CHOLESTEATOMAS. Rarely, they occur spontaneously. Fistulas may occur in one or both ears, but bilateral fistulas are rare.

A fistula can be diagnosed with a sensitive recording of eye movements while pressurizing each ear; an ELECTROCOCHLEOGRAPHY TEST may also be of help. Hearing tests and an ELECTRONYSTAGMOGRAPHY are nearly always necessary to establish the location of the problem and to exclude other potential causes of symptoms. Magnetic resonance imaging (MRI) or a temporal bone CT scan are usually helpful to exclude additional possibilities. Unfortunately, in some cases, only direct inspection of the inner ear will confirm or rule out the diagnosis of perilymph fistula.

Patients with blocked eustachian tubes (due to a cold or allergy) may find relief with decongestants, allergy medication and ventilating tubes. Tranquilizers such as Valium or Ativan help some individuals; Antivert and Phenergan are also medications that some find helpful. In many cases, a fistula will heal itself if the patient's activity is restricted. In such cases, strict bed rest is recommended for one week or more to give the fistula a chance to close.

During this time, the patient should minimize pressure changes in the ear so that scar tissue will seal the leak. Earplugs are sometimes helpful for those who develop dizziness related to loud noise or rapid fluctuation in air pressure. Patients with severe symptoms that don't respond to bed rest or those with a progressive hearing loss may require surgical repair of the fistula.

Surgery may be recommended to close the leak if the body doesn't repair the damage on its own. The surgery is usually performed under local anesthetic. Through the ear canal, the otologist explores the middle ear, inspecting the area around the stapes bone and the round window (the two most common sites where a leak can occur). The otologist looks for any signs of clear fluid coming from these areas. If there is evidence of leakage, the surgeon will patch the areas with soft tissue obtained from a small incision behind the ear. The risks of any further hearing loss are minimal, but the success rates are variable. About 50 percent of the explorations are negative. If the leak is around the round window, the success rates approach 90 percent. However, the success rates around the stapes footplate are considerably less, at 20 to 30 percent.

perinatal causes of hearing loss   Several conditions during and after the birth process may result in hearing loss in infants. These include loss of oxygen, low birth weight, excess bilirubin and infection.

During Birth

About 6 percent of newborns experience a SENSORINEURAL HEARING LOSS ranging from mild to severe if deprived of oxygen at birth. In premature infants, about 5 percent will experience some type of mild to severe sensorineural hearing loss.

Extremely high levels of bilirubin (bile pigment) can cause a condition called KERNICTERUS, which damages the cochlear nuclei in the brain, causing hearing loss. In addition, several kinds of bacteria and viruses in the birth canal can transmit an ear infection (acute OTITIS MEDIA) to the newborn, which can cause hearing loss. These infections are usually caused by *Streptococcus pneumoniae* or *Hemophilus influenzae*.

At least 20 percent of babies born with hearing problems acquired them during the birth process. Causes can include maternal high blood pressure, prematurity, lack of oxygen (ANOXIA) or jaundice. In other cases of birth-induced deafness, the cause is unknown.

After Birth

One of the most common causes of acquired sensorineural deafness in a newborn after birth is bacterial MENINGITIS. Meningitis is a disease involving an infection and inflammation of the coverings of the brain and the nerves that lead to it.

Bacterial meningitis in infants is usually caused by *Escherichia coli (E. coli)* bacteria, and can result in a hearing loss ranging from mild to profound. About half the infants who contract this disease will have a profound hearing loss, which is usually permanent.

Often, the COCHLEA is damaged when bacteria from the covering of the brain enter the cochlea from the cochlear nerve. Prognosis for children who contract bacterial meningitis is poor; about half of those who live will have severe problems, including hearing loss, retardation and seizures.

Sometimes, children with meningitis get an ear infection with a conductive deafness; this can be cured with antibiotics.

peripheral auditory system   All of the anatomic structures from the pinna or auricle (actual ear visible on the outside of the head) to the end of the auditory nerve in the brain. Generally, the system is divided into three parts: the outer, middle and inner ear structures.

Any problem with the conduction of sound in the OUTER EAR (such as excess wax) or the MIDDLE EAR (such as fluid) that blocks the transmission of sound to the INNER EAR can result in a CONDUCTIVE HEARING LOSS.

If there is a problem with the sensory cells in the COCHLEA located in the inner ear, however, both the ability to hear and understand the sound will be affected; this is called a sensory hearing loss.

If a hearing problem is caused by a condition affecting the hearing nerve to the brain (also called the auditory nerve), the resulting hearing problem is called a neural loss. Since it is common for both

a sensory and a neural loss to occur at the same time—or it may be impossible to tell the difference between them—such a loss is often called a SENSORINEURAL LOSS. A mixed hearing loss results from conditions affecting both the conductive and sensorineural structures.

pharyngotympanic tube   See EUSTACHIAN TUBE.

Philippines   About 100,000 to 4.2 million people of this republic have hearing problems.

For many years, there was only one school for deaf students—the Philippine School for the Deaf, but by 1982 there were more than 17 educational programs.

Communication modes vary from school to school and often change as administrators come and go. Deaf students may continue their education past high school, either with short-term vocational courses or college.

The schools may vary in their communication styles, but many graduates of deaf schools communicate as adults in sign language; those who have not gone to school use natural signs.

phonemes   The essential and smallest elements of a finite number of speech sounds. They are the code signals that give meaning to speech. Phonemes are really abstractions, a bit like an averaging of the types of sounds that actually occur in speech.

For example, the phoneme "t" in the words "cat" and "tea" sounds very much the same yet is produced very differently. In "cat," the "t" sound is really just a stop made with only a very slight explosion of breath. The same "t" sound in the word "tea" is exploded with an audible breath. There are many different variations of pronouncing the phoneme "t," which are called its ALLOPHONES.

phonetics   The study of the smallest units of language. See also LINGUISTICS.

phonology   The study of how the smallest units of language (PHONEMES) can be combined to form words or signs. See also LINGUISTICS.

phonophobia   An extreme sense of discomfort caused by sounds above the threshold of hearing.

Pidgin Sign English (PSE)   A sign language system most often used by hearing people learning to communicate with deaf people. Also called Sign English, it combines the English word order and simplified grammatical structure with the vocabulary and nonmanual features of AMERICAN SIGN LANGUAGE. Signs for definite and indefinite articles are omitted, and only one sign is used for the verb "to be," unlike the MANUALLY CODED ENGLISH systems.

Another name for PSE is "Siglish." See also SIGN LANGUAGE; SIGN LANGUAGE CONTINUUM; SIMULTANEOUS COMMUNICATION.

pinna   The part of the outer ear that we can see; also called auricle. The pinna helps gather sound waves and funnels them into the ear canal to the eardrum. In humans, the pinna has no useful muscle and so remains relatively immobile.

pitch   The perception of sound frequency, measured in terms of the number of cycles per second at which a sound wave vibrates. Pitch can vary with the intensity, duration or complexity of the sound vibration.

In music, "perfect" pitch (also called absolute pitch) is the very rare ability to identify the position of a tone within an octave (in other words, the ability to identify a note, A through G, without using a reference pitch). Perfect relative pitch is the ability to identify a note with the aid of a reference pitch. Perfect relative pitch is more common and is a skill that can be learned.

Plater, Felix (1536–1614)   A 17th-century Swiss physician who published a detailed study of the bones of the ear, including the way in which sound is transmitted through the bones of the head.

In his book, Plater described both sensorineural and conductive deafness. He understood that the root of deafness was found sometimes in the brain and sometimes in the cavity of the ears. He found that if the cause of deafness is found in the brain, there is no cure. Plater is also known for his

descriptions of the presence of TINNITUS in many of his deaf patients.

polymography   The process of taking X rays of the inner ear.

Ponce de León, Pedro (?–1584)   This 16th-century Benedictine monk is considered to be the father of education for deaf people and is thought to have been the first person to invent a method to teach deaf students.

Ponce de León was born in the province of León in northern Spain and entered a local monastery in 1526. Taking as his first pupil a man who had been denied admittance to the Benedictine order because he could neither hear nor speak, Ponce de León taught him to speak so he could make his confession. This student, Gaspard Burgos, went on to write several books of his own.

When transferred to a monastery in the mountains of north-central Spain, he met the two deaf sons of the wealthy marquis of Berlanga, Juan Fernández de Velasco. The marquis' family was known for hereditary deafness, probably caused by intermarriage. Becoming close to Francisco and Pedro Velasco, aged nine and 12 respectively, Ponce de León taught them both to speak. Pedro also learned how to write, speak and read books in Latin, Italian and Spanish before his death at age 30. Ponce de León also taught about 12 other deaf people to speak, including the marquis' deaf daughters Bernardina and Catalina.

He next established a school at the Ona monastery for teaching wealthy deaf students to talk, beginning his teaching with writing and progressing to speech. Historians believe he taught speech to his students by tracing letters and indicating pronunciation with his lips. Historians also suspect that the manual alphabet he used was probably the same one published by the Franciscan monk Melchor Yebra in 1593. This alphabet is almost identical to the one used by 16th-century deaf teachers JUAN PABLO BONET and Manuel Ramírez de Carrión, who also taught deaf members of the Velasco family.

Ponce de León is also assumed to have used signs in the education of his deaf pupils, since the

Benedictines took strict vows of silence and had developed their own signs as a result.

In addition, he is said to have written a book, *Instruction for the Mute Deaf,* which was probably lost during the social upheavals common in Spanish monasteries at that time. Although books and documents from the monastery of Ona were sent to the National Archives in Spain, Ponce de León's book has never been found.

postlingual deafness   Deafness occurring after language has been acquired. See also ADVENTITIOUS DEAFNESS.

prelingual deafness   Deafness occurring before language skills have been acquired.

premature birth and hearing loss   See POSTNATAL AND PERINATAL CAUSES OF HEARING LOSS.

prenatal causes of hearing loss   Loss of hearing from prenatal causes occurs in between 7 percent and 20 percent of deaf and hard-of-hearing people. All of these prenatal causes are preventable.

There are three major threats to the hearing mechanism of a woman's unborn baby: viral diseases, OTOTOXIC DRUGS and the condition of the woman's uterus during pregnancy.

The largest number of cases of prenatal deafness are a result of viral diseases contracted by the mother, including TOXOPLASMOSIS, RUBELLA, CYTOMEGALOVIRUS (CMV) and HERPES SIMPLEX.

A mother who contracts rubella during the first three months of her pregnancy may have a child who is born with some degree of hearing loss. This risk is less likely today because a vaccination is available for those women who have never had rubella but who would like to become pregnant. In fact, following the rubella epidemic of the 1960s, many states require rubella testing for women when applying for a marriage license.

Other viral diseases contracted by the mother may also cause a hearing loss in the fetus, including MUMPS and influenza (particularly during the first three months). An active herpes simplex type II lesion in the genital area during a vaginal delivery can also infect the infant, causing hearing loss.

Ototoxic drugs taken by the mother during pregnancy are known to cause hearing problems in the sensorineural structures of the developing fetus, especially the developing cochlea. These drugs include the aminoglycosides, thalidomide and alcohol.

- *Aminoglycosides:* The incidence of prenatal deafness due to the aminoglycosides (kanamycin, neomycin, gentamicin, tobramycin and amikacin) is extremely low. These drugs have been reported to cause hearing loss in infants only when mothers who took them had kidney problems and received diuretics (ethacrynic acid and furosemide) in addition to an aminoglycoside. It has been suggested that there may be a genetic susceptibility to hearing problems associated with aminoglycosides.

- *Streptomycin:* When the antibiotic streptomycin is given to a pregnant mother at any time, it can cause a sensorineural hearing loss ranging from mild to high-frequency to severe bilateral.

- *Thalidomide:* Although the drug thalidomide taken during the first trimester of pregnancy caused a large number of malformations of the ear in Europe during the 1960s, the drug was never released in the United States.

- *Alcohol:* It has also been reported that FETAL ALCOHOL SYNDROME may cause hearing loss in up to 64 percent of infants born to alcoholic mothers.

Infections in the mother transmitted to the infant in the blood before birth can cause pneumonia or MENINGITIS; other infections in the amniotic fluid can be swallowed by the fetus and then pumped up the eustachian tube into the middle ear, where they can create an ear infection. SYPHILIS transmitted from mother to child during pregnancy may also result in a hearing loss in the child, either during the first two years of life or at puberty.

Incompatible Rh blood factors also pose a threat to the hearing mechanism of the unborn child. When a mother with Rh negative blood has a child with Rh-positive blood, cells from the baby sensitize her and she will develop antibodies to Rh-positive blood. While this will not harm the first baby, subsequent pregnancies risk damaging the baby when the mother's antibodies attack the red blood cells of the Rh-positive fetus.

However, problems for the newborn due to Rh sensitization are becoming rare since the development of Rh (D) immune globulin (anti-D serum). When injected into the mother 72 hours before delivery, it prevents 99 percent of the incidences of sensitization.

A range of other conditions in the mother during pregnancy may be connected with prenatal hearing loss. These include maternal diabetes, hypothyroidism, toxemia and malnutrition. See also NEWBORN SCREENING PROGRAMS; PERINATAL CAUSES OF HEARING LOSS; RH-FACTOR INCOMPATIBILITY AND DEAFNESS.

presbycusis   More than 10 million Americans suffer from presbycusis, a type of SENSORINEURAL HEARING LOSS that comes with age. It is one of the most common chronic problems among older people.

After about age 50, most people slowly begin to lose some ability to hear. A person with presbycusis hears sounds less clearly and tones (especially higher ones) less audibly. People with presbycusis often have trouble understanding speech, particularly in the presence of background noise.

But presbycusis is not just caused by physiological aging; it may simply be a result of wax build-up in the ear or of damage to the inner ear from infection, disease, injury or a loud noise. In fact, some experts believe excessive noise accounts for more hearing loss than all other factors combined.

Medications—most commonly aspirin, antibiotics and hypertension drugs—can also cause hearing problems in the elderly.

Studies at the HOUSE EAR INSTITUTE and elsewhere have shown that as a person ages, there is a loss of nerve cells in the base of the COCHLEA where high-frequency sounds are perceived. But researchers don't know whether the degeneration of cells in the cochlear nucleus is primarily due to aging or whether it is due to a decrease in the specific frequencies supplying those cells from the cochlea.

Each person experiences the development of presbycusis differently. Generally, it involves a slow decline in hearing ability. First a person loses the ability to hear high-pitched sounds, followed by a loss of hearing in the middle frequencies and finally the lowest. Because normal speech covers all these frequencies, the ability to understand conversation may vary according to the extent of presbycusis.

A person who notices hearing loss should immediately see either an OTOLOGIST (specialist in diseases of the ear), an OTOLARYNGOLOGIST (specialist in diseases of the ear, nose and throat) or an AUDIOLOGIST (professional who often works with a physician to assess hearing loss and provide auditory training). Unfortunately, most people with presbycusis wait an average of five years before doing anything about it.

Although HEARING AIDS can help most people, not everyone will benefit from them (people who cannot discriminate different speech sounds, for example). For those who can, an aid should not be prescribed or fitted before an examination and hearing test are given. See also AGING AND HEARING LOSS.

Professional Rehabilitation Workers with the Adult Deaf   The former name of the AMERICAN DEAFNESS AND REHABILITATION ASSOCIATION.

Professional School for Deaf Theater Personnel   America's only professional theater school for deaf students has offered deaf actors a concentrated four-week session in basic and advanced theater since 1967.

The faculty includes professional stage actors, academic instructors and company members of the NATIONAL THEATRE OF THE DEAF. Courses include acting, directing, playwriting, dance, costume design, fencing, storytelling, set design and Japanese dance and theater. Deaf and hearing teachers instruct both deaf students and hearing students involved in deaf culture who are proficient in sign.

The program is accredited by Connecticut College and is supported by the U.S. Department of Education's special education program. Full scholarships for 20 deaf Americans are granted each year. The application process each year ends April 15 for the session beginning in June.

profound hearing loss   Generally considered to be a loss greater than 90 decibels.

psychogenic hearing loss See FUNCTIONAL LOSS (NONORGANIC).

Public Law 94-142 See LEGAL RIGHTS.

Public Law 97-410 See LEGAL RIGHTS.

Public Law 100-533 See LEGAL RIGHTS.

Puerto Rican Sign Language There are at least four varieties of Puerto Rican Sign Language (PRSL) used today on the small Caribbean commonwealth island. It is similar to AMERICAN SIGN LANGUAGE and is believed to have developed from the introduction of ASL in the early 1900s. American Sign Language was brought to Puerto Rico in 1907 by nuns who founded a deaf school; in the 1950s a Spanish teaching order of nuns introduced the oral approach and forbade SIGN LANGUAGE.

Puerto Rican Sign Language is different from ASL in that it does not use FINGERSPELLING and has many signs that are different or do not appear in ASL. Its structural characteristics, as in other sign languages, include the use of space to show relationship between objects or ideas, classifiers and size- and shape-specifiers and the use of compound signs to describe new ideas.

In addition, Signed Spanish, which uses signs in Spanish word order, is used by deaf persons in communicating with Spanish-speaking hearing people.

Signed English is used by deaf Puerto Ricans who were educated in mainland United States. Of the two, Signed Spanish is more commonly used in Puerto Rico to communicate with hearing people, especially for interpreting and watching television.

pure tone audiogram The graph of a person's ability to hear pure tones. See also AUDIOGRAM; AUDIOMETRY.

pure tone average (PTA) The average level of THRESHOLDS elicited for each ear for frequencies believed by some to be essential to understanding speech—500, 1000 and 2000 hertz. The PTA is used to determine the level at which to start presenting words to find a person's speech reception threshold. See also AUDIOMETRY.

pure tone sweep-check test The most reliable method of screening large numbers for hearing loss by testing for auditory response to different frequencies presented at a constant level. It is generally possible to screen one person every two or three minutes. See also AUDIOMETRY; JOHNSTON TEST; MASSACHUSETTS TEST.

pure tone hearing test A hearing test presenting pure tone sounds through a speaker or earphones. See also AUDIOMETRY.

quinine derivatives and hearing loss Drugs derived from quinine in doses of about two grams per day may cause a combination of TINNITUS, decreased hearing, VERTIGO, headache, nausea or blurred vision. Symptoms can quickly disappear when the drugs are discontinued, although permanent hearing loss and tinnitus have been reported after high doses were continued after symptoms began.

Quinine derivatives include quinine, chloroquine, quinidine and hydroxychloroquine. See also OTOTOXIC DRUGS.

Quota International, Inc. A service group that helps individuals with hearing and speech problems. The group publishes *The Quotarian,* offers fellowships and conducts an annual Outstanding Deaf Woman of the Year program. See also Appendix II.

Rainbow Alliance of the Deaf   A national organization serving the deaf gay and lesbian community, this group has 24 chapters throughout the United States and two in Canada. See also Appendix II.

receiver   The part of a HEARING AID that carries amplified sound and speech to the earmold. See also HEARING AIDS.

receptive aphasia   See AUDITORY AGNOSIA.

receptive skill   The ability to understand what is being communicated in both FINGERSPELLING and SIGN LANGUAGE.

recruitment   An abnormal, rapid increase in loudness as the strength of the acoustic signal is increased. A person with normal hearing would notice a gradual increase in loudness as the level of sound is increased; someone with a cochlear impairment would find that loudness increases more rapidly as the signal becomes more intense. Conversely, a person with a dysfunctional AUDITORY NERVE would notice loudness decruitment—as the signal level intensifies, loudness growth decreases or even declines.

Audiologists therefore find recruitment tests very useful in deciding whether a hearing problem originates in the COCHLEA or the auditory nerve.

In order to test for recruitment, audiologists use a loudness balance test—either the ALTERNATE BINAURAL LOUDNESS BALANCE TEST (ABLB) or the monaural bi-frequency loudness balance test (MLB). The ABLB is used to compare loudness growth in both ears for patients with hearing loss on one side. In the test, the client must judge the loudness of a tone at a specific frequency in both the good and poor ear.

If a patient has lost hearing in both ears, the MLB can determine recruitment, especially in high-frequency hearing loss, by presenting two different frequency tones in one ear. The reference tone is set for a frequency the person can hear normally; the variable tone is set at a frequency the person cannot hear, and the examiner notes at what frequency the variable tone is judged to be equal in loudness to the reference tone.

In an excessive case of recruitment, the range of useful hearing between the THRESHOLD and the level at which loudness becomes uncomfortable may be very narrow. Hearing aids would therefore be of limited value for such a problem.

Refsum disease, infantile   This rare disorder is characterized by the reduction or absence of cell structures that get rid of toxic substances in the body, and by the buildup of phytanic acid in blood and tissue. Infantile Refsum disease (IRD) should not be confused with classical REFSUM'S DISEASE; the two are different conditions. However, IRD is closely related to Zellweger's syndrome and neonatal adrenoleukodystrophy. IRD is one of a group of genetic diseases called leukodystrophies that affects the growth of the fatty covering of nerves in the brain.

In addition to hearing loss, symptoms may include eye problems such as retinitis pigmentosa (a potentially blinding eye disease) and nystagmus (rapid, jerky eye movements), decrease in muscle tone, failure to thrive, developmental delays, poor muscle coordination, enlarged liver, low cholesterol levels and abnormalities of the face.

The disorder begins in infancy. There is no cure, although a few physicians around the world are studying the effectiveness of DHA (docosahexaenoic acid) or AA (arachidonic acid). Otherwise, treatment is supportive. The prognosis for patients is poor; death usually occurs in the person's 20s.

Refsum's disease This rare disorder of fat metabolism is inherited as a recessive trait and can cause HEARING LOSS and retinitis pigmentosa, among other symptoms. Also known as heredopathia atactica polyneuritiformis, it is characterized by a high level in blood and tissue of a fatty acid called phytanic acid, a substance derived from phytol (a component of chlorophyll). Humans absorb phytol from milk and the fat of cows and sheep, and most people can break down the phytol and phytanic acid. Those with Refsum's disease can't break it down, and so as they eat food containing phytanic acid the amount in their body gradually rises. While small amounts of phytanic acid are harmless, it becomes toxic as the level rises. In Refsum's patients, it causes three groups of problems:

Congenital: A few abnormalities, such as short fingers and toes, are present at birth in a small group of patients, and rarely cause problems.
Progressive: Deafness, retinitis pigmentosa and inability to smell begin slowly in childhood, and very slowly progress as the person ages. Some evidence suggests that if phytanic acid is controlled, blindness won't progress.
Sudden-onset: Weak, unsteady gait can suddenly appear in a Refsum's patient, but if treated it can improve just as quickly. Caused by nerve damage, the unsteadiness will not improve only if it has gone untreated for a long time.

Refsum's disease was first described in 1946 by Professor Refsum in Oslo, Norway, who noticed two Norwegian families with an unusual combination of impaired vision and weak gait. It was not until 1963 that the high phytanic acid level in the blood was discovered. The condition may affect men and women equally, appearing at any time from childhood to middle age, but symptoms usually appear by age 20.

In 1997 the gene for Refsum's disease was identified on chromosome 10. The protein product of the gene (PAHX) is an enzyme that is needed to metabolize phytanic acid. Refsum's disease patients have problems with PAHX.

The main treatment involves dietary changes. First, patients should try to maintain the same weight, since fat stores are used for energy during weight loss, which would release phytanic acid. Patients should avoid eating food containing animal fat from plant-eating animals, including milk products and fat from mutton and beef. This lowers the blood level of phytanic acid. Plasmapheresis (removal and reinfusion of blood plasma) may be necessary. Once hearing and vision problems appear, however, treatment can't usually repair the damage. See also REFSUM'S DISEASE, INFANTILE.

Registry of Interpreters for the Deaf (RID) The largest national organization of interpreters in the United States. The registry maintains a national list of people skilled in the use of AMERICAN SIGN LANGUAGE and other sign systems.

The RID provides information on interpreting and evaluation and certification of interpreters for deaf people. When it was first established in Muncie, Indiana in 1964, the organization was designed simply as a way to register certified interpreters. But in the early 1970s, the registry began to expand its interests: It set up both the first national certification system and the first performance evaluation for interpreters in the world. At the same time, interpreter associations were founded at the local and state level to advocate legislative reform in the area of interpreter laws.

Today, RID members—most certified interpreters—work to further the profession of interpretation of American Sign Language and English. Its national office produces the bimonthly newsletter *Views* and serves as a clearinghouse of information about interpretation. See also COURT INTERPRETERS ACT; INTERPRETERS AND THE LAW; ORAL INTERPRETERS; SIGN LANGUAGE INTERPRETERS; Appendix II.

Rehabilitation Act of 1973 See LEGAL RIGHTS.

Reissner's membrane The thinnest membrane in the COCHLEA with the thickness of just two cells, this separates the perilymph and endolymph fluids.

relay service   A generic term for a service in which an operator relays a conversation between a hearing person without a TDD and a hard-of-hearing or speech-impaired person who has a TDD. It is also called a "dual party relay service."

The operator serves as a bridge between the two callers and uses two phones, one connected to a TDD. The caller phones the relay service; while the caller waits, a relay service operator places a call to the other party. When both parties are on the line at the same time, the operator speaks the deaf person's typed message and types the hearing person's spoken message. This term distinguishes relayed calls from a message relay service, in which a message is relayed in one direction only and not while both parties are on the line.

Most of the early relay services were staffed completely by volunteers, but as the number of TDD users rose, so did the demand for statewide relay services. Some states have already established statewide dual party message relay services, which are funded by tax revenue or a surcharge on telephone lines. In other states, the relay service is considered part of the telephone companies normal operating expenses.

The NATIONAL CENTER FOR LAW AND THE DEAF at Gallaudet University in Washington, D.C., provides information on the funding and administration of mandated state and federal dual party message relay systems. The TELE-CONSUMER HOTLINE in Washington, D.C., provides a "TDD Relay Center Comparison Chart" offering comparative information about areas served, membership requirements, fees and service limitations. See also MESSAGE RELAY SERVICE; TELECOMMUNICATIONS DEVICE FOR THE DEAF.

residential schools   See EDUCATION OF DEAF CHILDREN.

residual hearing measurement   See AUDIOMETRY.

retracted eardrum   When the pressure inside the middle ear is lower than the pressure on the outside in the external canal, the EARDRUM is gradually pushed inward by the extra pressure from the outside. Sometimes the eardrum can be pressed so far into the middle ear that it touches the cochlea itself, almost completely obliterating the middle ear.

This retraction occurs during a head cold, an allergy attack or an infection in the back of the nose and throat, any of which force the eustachian tube closed so that no air can get into the middle ear. In such a situation, the air normally present in the middle ear becomes locked in, and some of it is absorbed by the lining of the middle ear, reducing the pressure in the middle ear.

This can reduce the efficiency of both the eardrum and the OSSICULAR CHAIN in transmitting sound to the inner ear, although the amount of retraction is no indication of the amount of hearing loss. The amount of hearing loss is determined instead by the site and type of damage in the ossicular chain, and this cannot be determined by appearance alone.

retrocochlear lesion   A type of lesion located on the AUDITORY NERVE (not the cochlea) that causes SENSORINEURAL HEARING LOSS.

reverse interpreting   See SIGN-TO-VOICE INTERPRETING.

Rh factor incompatibility and deafness   Red blood cells carry the Rh (Rhesus) factor, an antigen present in about 85 percent of the population (Rh-positive) and absent in about 15 percent (Rh-negative). Having Rh-negative blood causes no harm unless Rh-positive blood enters the bloodstream of an Rh-negative person.

When an Rh-negative mother has an Rh-positive child, the mixture of these blood factors can cause the mother to develop antibodies against the Rh-positive blood of the child. Because it takes some time for these antibodies to develop, the first child is rarely affected by them. However, in a second pregnancy, the antibodies in the mother's blood will pass through the placenta, damaging the child's blood cells. This destruction of blood cells can cause many problems, including erythroblastosis (a disorder causing severe jaundice) and athetoid cerebral palsy; a fair number of these children also have congenital hearing loss.

Children who become deaf through Rh incompatibility have a series of similar characteristics: a nonprogressive hearing loss, the same in both ears and usually worse in the high frequencies; reduced bone conduction; hearing loss present at birth; and a frequent speech difficulty, particularly in pronouncing the letter *s*.

Rh-negative mothers are now easily identified in this country, and treatment is available to prevent or modify the damage. As a result, few children born in developed countries have this form of deafness.

Rinne test   This common test compares a patient's ability to hear a tuning fork by air and bone conduction. The vibrating fork is first placed about an inch from the ear (air conduction), and the patient is asked how loud it is. Then the base of the fork is quickly pressed against the mastoid bone (bone conduction). The patient is then asked in which position the fork sounds louder. (See also AUDIOMETRY.)

People with normal hearing can hear the sound better and longer through air conduction—almost twice as long as sound through bone. This test result is called a "positive Rinne."

Although people with a sensorineural hearing loss can also hear better with air conduction, they can't hear the sound as loud or as long as people with normal hearing.

Patients with a conductive hearing loss will show a "negative Rinne"—hearing better by bone conduction, since the bone-conducted sound bypasses the conductive block and is then accurately perceived by the healthy cochlea.

Rochester Method   See FINGERSPELLING.

Ronsard, Pierre de (1524–1585)   This "Prince of Poets" was one of the outstanding writers during the French Renaissance and was responsible for a renewed interest in poetry. He was deafened at age 15, a loss that diverted his interests from a diplomatic career toward literary pursuits. Today he is considered to be one of the leading poets in the history of French literature.

He was born on September 11, 1524, in Possoniere castle, the son of a noble family, and embarked at a young age on a career as a diplomat in the royal household. Unfortunately, in 1540 an ear infection and high fever resulted in a severe hear-

ing loss that eliminated further advancement as a diplomat.

Much to his father's displeasure, Ronsard turned to a career in literature. Although he took preliminary steps toward the priesthood, his heart was never in it. After the death of his father, life as a literary figure became easier, and he began to study poetry and literature more seriously.

In 1547, Ronsard joined with Joachim du Bellay, who was also deaf, in forming a group of aspiring poets. He was also frequently at the royal court, eventually earning a job administering kneeling cushions and holy water for the king.

Ronsard published his first collection of poems in 1560 and was at this time an important spokesman at court and defender of the Catholic faith. Still, he was best known for his love poetry, although it is not known to what extent he pursued these relationships in actuality.

round window   An elastic membrane opening between the MIDDLE EAR and INNER EAR. Within the internal ear, the VESTIBULE and COCHLEA are filled with virtually incompressible fluid. The STAPES (stirrup) can move toward the vestibule because of the pressure relief points provided by the round window and the oval window.

rubella   This viral illness (also known as German measles) causes hearing problems in about half of all infants born to mothers who contract the disease while they are pregnant. When infection occurs during the first trimester, 68 percent of babies will be born deaf; when infection occurred during the second trimester, 40 percent of babies will be deaf. There is significantly less risk to babies whose mothers contract rubella during the third trimester, although deafness is still a possibility.

Even if the mother is exposed to the disease at any time during her pregnancy but does not develop symptoms, her baby can still become deaf. For this reason, any female of childbearing age who is unsure whether she has been immunized should have her immune status checked. Vaccination is performed only if there is no chance that a woman is pregnant since there is a risk that the vaccine itself can cause rubella in the fetus.

Typically, hearing loss as a result of prenatal rubella produces a SENSORINEURAL HEARING LOSS and can be progressive during the childhood years. Less commonly, prenatal rubella infection can result in a conductive hearing disorder.

During the rubella epidemic of 1963–65, the disease caused 8,000 cases of prenatal deafness in the United States and was responsible for 20 percent of all cases of deafness during that time.

The introduction of a successful rubella vaccine has slashed the number of prenatal cases of deafness due to rubella to only 5 percent. See also PRENATAL CAUSES OF HEARING LOSS.

saccule   One of the structures of the INNER EAR, this is a small sac located in the VESTIBULE, which encapsulates a single sensory patch called a MACULA. The macula, which resembles the letter *j*, lies against the inner wall of the vestibule directly over the bone.

The UTRICLE and the saccule together with their maculae are also called otolith organs and gravity receptors (since they respond to gravitational forces). These receptors—particularly the utricle—are important in the balance reflexes and in maintaining the contractions of the muscles that keep the body standing upright.

The role the saccule plays is less well understood, although it is believed it may respond to vibration and backwards-forwards positions of the head.

Of the two, the utricle seems to be the dominant receptor.

SAI   See SOCIAL ADEQUACY INDEX.

SAL   See SENSORINEURAL ACUITY LEVEL.

scala media   This tube-like structure lies upon the BASILAR MEMBRANE and follows the turns of the COCHLEA. Inside the entire length of the scala media is the extremely sensitive mechanism of hearing called the ORGAN OF CORTI, which contains about 15,000 minute hair cells responsible for sending impulses on to the brain.

scala tympani   A spiral fluid channel containing PERILYMPH; located in the cochlea below the basilar membrane.

scala vestibuli   A spiral fluid channel containing PERILYMPH; located in the cochlea above the basilar membrane.

scarlet fever   Also known as scarletina, this is an acute infectious disease caused by the streptococcus bacterium. It can lead to complications such as sinus infections, followed by abscesses of the ear and MASTOIDITIS.

Symptoms of the disease begin from two to seven days after exposure, starting with fever, sore throat, headache and (in children) vomiting. A rash appears about two or three days later on the neck, armpits, groin and chest. The throat is red with red spots on the palate and the tongue is coated and inflamed. The rash and fever can last for more than a week, sometimes followed by skin peeling.

Scarlet fever, which today is fairly uncommon in the United States, is treated with penicillin, bed rest and plenty of fluids. It is believed that the reduced threat of the disease is due to a change in the virulence of the bacteria and has nothing to do with the development of drugs to treat the condition.

Schenck, Johannes (1530–1598)   A 16th-century physician who explored the etiology of deafness. Schenck was able to describe the idea of hereditary deafness by exploring the case of a family with several children with congenital deafness. He also discussed how a person might lose the ability to hear following an injury.

Schwabach test   This test compares the patient's ability to hear a tuning fork by BONE CONDUCTION through the MASTOID BONES with a normal hearing person's ability to hear the fork in the same position. (Generally, the listener with normal hearing is the OTOLOGIST.)

In this test, the examiner holds the vibrating tuning fork on the patient's mastoid bone, who then tells the examiner when the fork's tone ceases. The examiner then places the fork on his own bone and notes the time elapsed until the vibration is no longer heard.

If the patient hears the tone longer than the examiner (Schwabach-shortened), the hearing loss is probably conductive. If the patient hears the tone for a shorter time than the examiner (Schwabach-prolonged), than a sensorineural loss is indicated. See also AUDIOMETRY.

Scotland There are an estimated 4,000 deaf adults in Scotland, with another 2,000 students receiving help for some form of hearing loss.

The history of deaf education in Scotland is long, beginning in 1769 with the establishment of a school operated by THOMAS BRAIDWOOD in Edinburgh. As in the United States, deaf education in Scotland has gone through constant evolution, beginning with an emphasis on residential schools and now centering on MAINSTREAMING. Similarly, philosophies of communication have included the ORAL and MANUAL approaches and TOTAL COMMUNICATION.

Today, most deaf children attend regular schools, and about 25 percent go to special units or schools. The scattered deaf population in the country, together with its isolated location, has made services sometimes difficult to provide for this population.

Since the 1970s, pressure has grown to provide more schools closer to home, with a resulting growth in local clinics and programs for deaf people. But the quality and type of programs still varies considerably from town to town.

secondary tympanic membrane A membranous flap at the base of the COCHLEA that closes the SCALA TYMPANI at the ROUND WINDOW.

secretory otitis media See SEROUS OTITIS MEDIA.

SEE 1 See SEEING ESSENTIAL ENGLISH.

SEE 2 See SIGNING EXACT ENGLISH.

S.E.E. Center for the Advancement of Deaf Children The S.E.E. (SIGNING EXACT ENGLISH) Center is a nonprofit organization dedicated to improving the communication and English literacy skills of hard-of-hearing children and hearing language-delayed students.

Signing Exact English (SEE 2) is a manual communication system first published in 1972; the center was established in 1984 in response to requests for workshops, materials and information for implementing S.E.E. 2 in homes and schools across the country.

The center provides information, materials and referral services for new parents emphasizing the importance of early communication stimulation for preschool children utilizing the S.E.E. 2 approach. It also provides information for training and evaluating sign language instructors and educational interpreters in the use of S.E.E. 2.

Further, the group offers videotapes and helps educators, audiologists, psychologists and speech therapists implementing S.E.E. 2 as part of a total communication program and provides support for research assessing the impact of S.E.E. 2.

Seeing Essential English (SEE 1) One of at least five separate codes for English, SEE 1 takes much of its sign vocabulary from AMERICAN SIGN LANGUAGE.

SEE 1, published in 1971, was the first MANUALLY CODED ENGLISH system. David Anthony, the congenitally deaf son of deaf parents born in England, originally began SEE 1 as a graduate degree project in 1962 at GALLAUDET UNIVERSITY.

The system features the sound-spelling-meaning principle: that is, each criterion is used to determine a sign for a particular word. A single sign is used when two of these three are the same. Therefore, "I have a right to vote," "It's on the right" and "You're right" would be signed the same ("right" in this case sounds and is written the same way but has different meanings), but the word "write" would use a different sign since it sounds the same but has a different spelling and meaning.

Seeing Essential English has specific signs for morphemes, suffixes and prefixes.

Self Help for Hard of Hearing People, Inc. (SHHH) A volunteer educational organization devoted to the interests of people who cannot hear. The group's activities include social activities, education, advocacy and consumer activism.

The group publishes *Shhh,* the only bimonthly journal in the United States written specifically for hard-of-hearing people and offering information on hearing loss, assistive technology, coping techniques and personal experiences for more than 200,000 readers.

The organization also offers referral and advisory services and operates an information and resource center. See also Appendix II.

semantics   The interpretation of the meaning of words, signs and sentences. See also LANGUAGE.

semicircular canals   Also called the LABYRINTH, this very important organ inside the inner ear is connected to the cochlea but does not contribute to the sense of hearing.

The semicircular canals are three small fluid-filled loops that help maintain balance by sending information about the position of the head through the vestibular branch of the AUDITORY NERVE to the brain. Infections or other problems in the middle or inner ear may directly or indirectly affect these canals, causing DIZZINESS or VERTIGO. Thus, some deaf children have difficulty with balance and may learn to walk later than a hearing child.

sensorineural acuity level   A way of testing bone conduction hearing by using a bone-conduction vibrator to issue a masking noise at the midline of the skull and noting THRESHOLD shifts caused by the noise in pure-tone air conduction hearing. See also AUDIOMETRY.

sensorineural hearing loss   This form of HEARING LOSS—commonly called nerve deafness—is a general term to describe conditions of the INNER EAR that lead to some measure of deafness, either by injury or malfunction of the inner ear. Sensorineural hearing loss (which results from damage to the hair cells of the inner ear or the nerves that supply it) differs from CONDUCTIVE HEARING LOSS, which is caused by diseases or obstructions in the

outer or MIDDLE EAR. The causes are varied, but many can be treated and others improved with properly adjusted HEARING AIDS.

Every year, about 4,000 U.S. infants are born with nerve deafness from many different causes, including heredity, maternal viral infection during pregnancy and problems during the birth process. Among the elderly, nerve deafness is most often caused by changes in the ear associated with the aging process (also called PRESBYCUSIS).

Still other types of nerve deafness can be caused by injury from stroke or injury to the head that causes irreversible damage to the AUDITORY NERVE and brain. Any tumor that grows close to the auditory nerve or auditory centers in the brain can also cause nerve deafness. Even a loud noise can damage sensory cells and nerve fibers, particularly if the noise occurs over a period of time, such as in constantly listening to loud music or working in a factory or airport. Further, drugs such as aspirin, some antibiotics and diuretics can affect the structure of the inner ear. Diseases that affect the flow of blood to the inner ear can also cause nerve deafness: These include diabetes, emphysema, heart disease, hardening of the arteries and some kidney disorders. Sometimes nerve deafness occurs in the absence of any identifiable condition or injury. Almost always, it is permanent and irreversible (except in the cases of some drug effects) and tends to progressively worsen. In some people, one ear can be affected in a very different way from the other.

The degree of nerve deafness may vary. A mild loss (15–30 dB) will cause a patient to strain to hear; moderate loss (35–55 dB) causes frequent repetition of conversation, much louder TV volume and misunderstood words in conversation. A severe loss (60–90 dB) usually requires a hearing aid, and a person with a profound hearing loss (90 dB or more) hears only very loud sounds, if anything at all.

In general, people with nerve hearing loss have problems understanding speech (also called word discrimination) even when the speech is loud enough to be heard comfortably. Problems in understanding speech usually depend on the frequency (or pitch) at which the hearing loss occurs. For example, if a person can't hear high pitches, he will have problems hearing consonant sounds that do not carry voice (t, p, k, s and so forth). Words such as tea, pea and key will sound alike since, without the consonant, the person hears only the vowel.

Hearing aids that are capable of amplifying some sounds more than others, especially high pitched sounds, can help resolve this problem. SPEECHREADING (lipreading) combined with this type of hearing aid can also be of assistance.

Another problem associated with nerve deafness is RECRUITMENT, that is, an abnormally rapid increase in the perception of sound loudness. Someone with this problem who can hear nothing at one level finds that the slightest increase in loudness causes a painfully loud sound.

Nerve deafness can be diagnosed with a pure tone audiogram to identify the degree to which damage has occurred, although the audiogram will not explain what caused the damage in the first place. A full audiological evaluation and IMPEDANCE measurements by an AUDIOLOGIST will determine the presence of a hearing loss, its type and its degree. This information, with a complete otological exam by an OTOLOGIST, will allow a physician to determine the need for further testing. These other tests could include blood tests, ELECTRONYSTAGMOGRAPHY (a test to determine the presence of damage to the balance system), POLYMOGRAPHY (X rays of the inner ear) and brain scans. See also AUDIOMETRY.

sensory aid   A device that provides sound information to a person with hearing problems through sight or touch. This is distinctive from devices that provide auditory sensation (such as a COCHLEAR IMPLANT).

Bell Laboratories devised the first sensory aid in the 1920s, a vibrating sound analyzer for deaf people, and during World War II, Bell's labs created a visual display of sound called a spectrograph to help unscramble coded voice messages. After the war, the first instant-display spectrograph, the "visible speech translator," was developed for use with deaf people.

Upton Eyeglass Speechreader

The first visual aid that could be worn was the Upton Eyeglass Speechreader, developed by deaf engineer Hubert Upton to improve comprehension beyond speechreading alone. Upton's speechreader features a microphone and analyzer that control separate bars of red light from light-emitting diodes (LED). The LED is mounted in a small projector fitted into the corner of the eyeglass frame, aimed at a reflecting area in the rear surface of the eyeglass lens.

The images of the bar lights appear in the space between the wearer and the speaker. When lighted, each bar indicates a type of sound pattern. Six different bars are assigned by the analyzer to six different types of speech sound patterns as they are picked up by the microphone.

Autocuer

This device also uses a projection display together with a computer that detects vowels and consonants and pairs a consonant with the following vowel to establish a syllable. It then flashes a symbol indicating the category on the eyeglasses of the deaf speechreader, who can decide from the lip and facial movements of the speaker which syllable was spoken.

Computer Speech

Someday, scientists hope they will be able to develop a computer that can recognize spoken sentences and print them on a video screen and translate sentences typed on a keyboard into synthesized speech. While talking computers are now commonplace (for example, the mechanical voice inside your car which reminds you to buckle up)—a device that can *recognize* speech instead of generate it is much more difficult to design.

Theoretically, at least, researchers know how it should work: The interactive speaking computer of the future would convert the sound of a spoken word into a digital code and then search its vocabulary for a word with the same code. When found, the computer would print out the word on paper or on a screen. Most systems today can do this only when the speaker pronounces every word with great clarity and pauses after each one.

The problem is that natural, rapid speech is much more difficult for a computer to recognize. In order for the computer to distinguish between "I scream" and "ice cream," for example, it must be able to discern what the speaker means from the context of the message.

Because of problems like this, scientists predict it will be many years before computers are able to recognize natural speech with any degree of accuracy.

Tactile Speech Aids

Since some people find visual displays distracting, researchers have developed a system that can present sound patterns through vibrations on the skin.

The Boothroyd Portapitch Aid, for example, is worn on the wrist or arm and contains eight vibrators energized by different levels of pitch of the voice received. Other tactile aids have many more stimulators that can respond to various combinations of vowels and consonants.

sensory aphasia   See AUDITORY AGNOSIA.

sensory cells   Located on the surface of the basilar membrane are sensory cells, which together with supporting cells form the ORGAN OF CORTI. Decades ago, it was shown that the production of sensory cells in the ears of mammals stops before birth and that these cells are produced only during embryonic development. This meant that damage to sensory cells later in life was irreparable; it became the basis for considering nerve deafness a permanent condition.

However, recent basic research with animals has shown that under certain conditions sensory cell production can be reactivated in mature damaged ears and that these regenerated cells contribute to recovery of hearing.

Scientists of the NATIONAL INSTITUTE OF DEAFNESS AND OTHER COMMUNICATION DISORDERS believe it is reasonable to expect that within 10 to 20 years progenitors of regenerated sensory cells will be cloned from animals and will aid in the development of ways to recover hearing in humans.

serous otitis media   A middle ear infection that causes thin and watery fluid in the middle ear, reducing hearing acuity by interfering with the movement of the OSSICULAR CHAIN. It has become more common since the use of antibiotics in the treatment of ear infections.

Serous otitis media is the most common cause of hearing problems in children because of the prevalence of ear infections in childhood. Its origin is unclear, although it is believed to be caused by treatment of suppurative otitis media with antibiotics or other drugs without adequate drainage.

After diagnosis of serous otitis media, antibiotics are prescribed and the infection clears. But the fluid, no longer infectious, remains in the middle ear cavity, making the ear more susceptible to further ear infections and reducing hearing acuity. Usually, the person is unaware of the hearing loss until both ears are affected; over time, the fluid can become thickened and glue-like (a condition called "suppurative" otitis media) and can cause a permanent deterioration of the bones of the middle ear.

Other causes of serous otitis media include allergy and viral infection of the middle ear. It can also occur in adults when the EUSTACHIAN TUBE does not function due to a cold or barotrauma (damage to the ear caused by unequal air pressure between the outer and middle ear, as can occur during rapid descent in an airplane).

Physicians recommend that a person recovering from an ear infection have a hearing test each time to make sure healing is complete. Otherwise, if fluid remains in the middle ear, the patient may not know it. Some OTOLOGISTS recommend surgically removing the fluid in the inner ear to prevent permanent damage.

Because some otologists deny there is any inflammation involved, they object to the suffix "itis" and prefer the term "otic transudates." Serous otitis media or glue ear is also called nonsuppurative otitis media, secretory otitis media, middle ear effusion or catarrhal otitis media. See also AERO-OTITIS MEDIA; MUCOUS OTITIS MEDIA; OTITIS MEDIA.

severe-profound hearing loss   Generally considered to be a 70 decibel to 90 dB loss.

short increment sensitivity test   See SISI.

Sicard, Abbé Roch-Ambroise Cucurron (1742–1822)   This pioneer of education for deaf students led the INSTITUT NATIONAL DES JEUNES SOURDS established by ABBÉ CHARLES-MICHEL DE L'EPÉE in 1760.

Sicard was born near Toulouse, France, on September 28, 1742, but little is known of his early life; he was sent to Paris to be trained by de l'Epée because of his educational gifts. After de l'Epée's death, Sicard succeeded him and ran the school with an iron hand for 32 years.

Sicard's early success in educating his prize pupil JEAN MASSIEU assured him fame and the position of headmaster at the Paris institute.

Sicard's educational method was based on a combination of writing and a system of "methodical signs" developed by de l'Epée. This system borrowed some signs from French sign language and invented some others to represent the grammatical structure of French, which represented the first effort at linking a sign and spoken language. Sicard also emphasized extensive grammar drills for his students. In fact, Sicard was widely recognized in France for his excellence as a grammarian, winning him faculty appointments, book contracts and a role as leader of a committee to revise the *Dictionary of the French Language.*

Often dictatorial and unyielding, Sicard's strength and popularity helped him lead his institution through the stormy years of the French Revolution, a time when many clerics were imprisoned as potentially monarchistic.

side-tone   Auditory signal that gives a speaker information about his own speech.

Siglish   Another name for PIDGIN SIGN ENGLISH, Siglish is a form of signing using the vocabulary of AMERICAN SIGN LANGUAGE in English word order along with some FINGERSPELLING and the use of ASL features such as directionality.

signaling devices   These devices add a flashing or vibrating signal to an existing auditory signal and are used for door bells, telephone ring signalers, baby-cry signals, alarm clocks and smoke alarm systems. See Appendix III for information on companies that manufacture and/or distribute these devices.

sign codes   At least four codes for English have been invented, although they all adapt much of their sign vocabulary from AMERICAN SIGN LANGUAGE. Each of these codes tries to duplicate the structure of English in different ways.

Unlike PIDGIN SIGN ENGLISH, these coded English systems use invented signs that correspond directly to English grammar and vocabulary. By matching a sign to a part of English, these systems become codes for English instead of a separate language.

These sign codes were developed in the United States as a way of providing a visual representation of English to improve school performance. Codes include SEEING ESSENTIAL ENGLISH (SEE 1) SIGNING EXACT ENGLISH (SEE 2) and SIGNED ENGLISH.

Developed in the early 1970s, some of these code systems are still used in schools today, although they remain controversial among some deaf people. The invented codes have aroused hostility in the deaf population who believe their native sign languages have not been given dignity and who feel these sign codes create linguistic distortions.

The sign codes now in use are a result of the increasing acceptance of nonoral communication and the wish to teach deaf children the majority oral language by manual means. These codes have been developed as a system, very different from the native and pidgin sign languages that evolved naturally.

Sign codes were developed because it was assumed that oral language can be learned more easily this way rather than by using a native or pidgin sign language. They seem to be easier for parents to learn, since they involve only switching a mode of communication, not learning an entire new language. See also MANUALLY CODED ENGLISH.

Signed English   This is a MANUALLY CODED ENGLISH system used to represent spoken English. Developed in 1973 by GALLAUDET UNIVERSITY educators Harry Bornstein, Karen Saulnier, Lillian Hamilton and Ralph R. Miller Sr., it is considered to be the least complicated of the manual systems. Signed English includes manual gestures signed in the same word order as English, used with speech, to provide a clear language environment for a hard-of-hearing child. It is similar to SEE-1 and SEE-2.

Signed English features two kinds of gestures: sign markers and sign words. A person using Signed English can match each spoken English word with a sign word or with a sign word and a sign marker. Each of the 3,500 sign words matches the meaning of a separate word in English, with all its various meanings. Sign words do not represent any sounds or spelling. The 14 sign markers represent the most frequent grammatical changes (such as singular, plural, possessive). With a vocabulary limited to 3,500 sign words and 14 affixes, it is not possible to represent the whole English language. But by choosing the most-commonly used English words to transcribe into sign words and affixes, the system is complete enough for most general needs. The manual alphabet can be used to supplement vocabulary.

Learning Signed English is facilitated by an extensive series of texts and posters, which include its main reference text, *The Comprehensive Signed English Dictionary,* three other texts, 50 children's books and three posters. The problem with this system and also with SEE-1 and SEE-2 is that they are slow. Although they are easier for hearing people to learn than American Sign Language, they are slower to use because signs usually take twice as long as words to produce. This means that the average idea takes twice as long to express.

Research suggests that most parents and many teachers who are trying to use this system end up leaving out many of the grammatical markers and that many children who are exposed to them end up modifying them to more ASL-like forms.

Sign English   See PIDGIN SIGN ENGLISH.

Signing Exact English (SEE 2)   This manual communication system is one of the most commonly used manually coded English systems in schools. It was developed in 1972 by Gerilee Gustason, a deaf teacher who lost her hearing at age five; Donna Pfetzing, mother of a deaf child; and Esther Zawolkow, daughter of deaf parents.

SEE 2 uses only one sign to represent an English word that may be expressed by several signs in AMERICAN SIGN LANGUAGE, depending on the meaning of the word in context. Hand signs for words, pre-fixes and endings are used to give a clear manual representation of English.

In much the same way as Seeing Essential English (SEE 1), Signing Exact English utilizes the sound-spelling-meaning principle. Although both systems define words either as basic, compound or complex, their definitions of these categories are very different. In Signing Exact English, basic words are words that can have no more taken away and still form a complete word, such as "run" or "trot." Compound words are two or more basic words put together, if the meaning of the words separately is consistent with the meaning of the words together.

Complex words are basic words with an added ending, such as dog*s* and run*ning.* Signing Exact English has signs for about 70 different endings.

According to a 1978–79 survey, the SEE 2 system is the most widely used sign method used in schools and classes for hard-of-hearing students in the United States. Programs have used this system to support spoken English emphasized in a TOTAL COMMUNICATION approach.

Sign Instructors Guidance Network (SIGN)   The original name for the AMERICAN SIGN LANGUAGE TEACHERS ASSOCIATION.

sign language   Sign languages are widely used by deaf people all over the world. Although each country has its own national sign language with its own visual-gestural signs, the sign language does not conform to the grammatical rules and structure of the native language. Within each country there are also different sign language dialects that reflect racial, ethnic or geographical differences. These dialects differ mostly in idiomatic expressions rather than grammar or syntax.

sign language continuum   The range in manual communication, from the completely English representation used in schools to the non-English pattern with its own grammar and syntax used by the deaf community.

sign language interpreter   A person skilled in the ability to translate the meaning of spoken words into sign language as the words are spoken and to translate sign language into English as signs are formed.

Technically, sign language interpretation is only used when describing the communication process between a hearing person and a person using a true sign language, such as AMERICAN SIGN LANGUAGE. A person interpreting to or from a manually coded form of a spoken language (such as SIGNED ENGLISH) is actually "transliterating," not "interpreting."

Sign language interpreters today are trained to practice their skill in a variety of settings: the legal, educational, medical, diplomatic and business areas. They are also trained to translate from either signed to spoken language or from spoken language to sign (also called sign-to-voice or voice-to-sign). Most important, they try to accomplish their communication task without becoming personally involved in the activity and without adding or subtracting any information in either direction.

In addition to standard sign language interpreters, specialized interpreters may at times be necessary. A person who is deaf and blind, for example, may need a specially-trained deaf-blind interpreter. This person can spell words in the deaf person's hand rather than perform traditional sign language. Oral interpreters silently mouth the speaker's words for the deaf person without signing and are skilled in substituting words for words that are difficult to speech-read.

In addition, special settings may require special knowledge or responsibilities on the part of the sign language interpreter. One of the most common places to find an interpreter is in school—from elementary to university. An interpreter is most often needed when the deaf student is mainstreamed and must communicate with many hearing students and teachers.

Interpreters in a medical setting will encounter technical terms and may find medical personnel unfamiliar with the role of an interpreter. Mental health interpreting requires sensitivity in other ways since the importance of accurately communicating in both directions can be of critical importance to treatment success. Legal interpreting also involves extensive technical language in very formal settings.

Due to a range of new legislation and educational opportunities affecting deaf people in the mid-1960s, the demand for qualified sign language interpreters suddenly exceeded the limited supply. At about this time, California State University/Northridge, the NATIONAL TECHNICAL INSTITUTE FOR THE DEAF and three regional technical vocational programs opened their doors to deaf students. In response to a much greater need, these schools also set up programs to train interpreters. At the same time, the national REGISTRY OF INTERPRETERS FOR THE DEAF was established.

Up to that time, it was assumed that if a person could sign, he could interpret; no research had been done into exactly how interpreting was done or the best way to train an interpreter. Because of this, the first interpreter classes focused simply on teaching American Sign Language, which ended up producing people who could converse primarily in PIDGIN SIGN ENGLISH. But in 1973, a federal grant established the Interpreter Training Consortium composed of six colleges charged with developing a curriculum for sign language interpreters.

Eventually, experts realized sign language interpreters must be both bilingual and bicultural; therefore, interpreting training courses must include comparative English/ASL linguistic and cultural analyses; text analysis; consecutive and simultaneous interpreting skills; and an overview of the profession (ethics and business practices). From a six-week course, the education of an interpreter has gradually developed into a formal four-year bachelor degree program of study, which may well progress to a graduate-level program.

All types of interpreters are listed with local and state chapters of the Registry of Interpreters for the Deaf, the only national organization that certifies both oral and sign language interpreters. See also COURT INTERPRETER'S ACT; ORAL INTERPRETERS.

sign-to-voice interpreting Previously called reverse interpreting, sign-to-voice interpretation is now the preferred term for translating from a signed language to speech. Reverse interpreting is no longer used because it is now recognized that one direction of interpretation is not more important than another. See also COURT INTERPRETER'S ACT; ORAL INTERPRETERS; REGISTRY OF INTERPRETERS FOR THE DEAF; SIGN LANGUAGE INTERPRETERS.

sign writing A method of writing down the symbols used in SIGN LANGUAGE. Many ways of sign language writing have been invented by many different researchers for many different reasons.

One of the main problems with sign writing is that the words do not convey the whole message of the sign language sentence. As a way to improve this problem, sign writers write various marks above and below the written word to stand for facial action or body position. But the fact that there is no standard system for these additional descriptors makes sign writing sometimes difficult for everyone to understand.

sim-com See SIMULTANEOUS COMMUNICATION.

simultaneous communication This communication mode combines the use of speech, signs and FINGERSPELLING and is said to offer the benefit of seeing two forms of a message at the same time. The deaf person speechreads what is being spoken and simultaneously reads the signs and fingerspelling of the speaker. In this country, users of simultaneous communication (or sim-com) at times put AMERICAN SIGN LANGUAGE signs in English word order while speaking.

Simultaneous communication is often confused with TOTAL COMMUNICATION since many people use the latter term when they mean speaking and signing at the same time. In the strictest sense, total communication actually refers to a philosophical attitude toward education using all forms of communication; simultaneous communication is one of those forms.

The simultaneous communication method appeared in early 20th-century America following the oral approach as encouraged by ALEXANDER GRAHAM BELL. As educators began to argue over the importance of oral education, more and more classrooms switched from all-manual communication to a combined method using speech, signs and fingerspelling. The combined method meant that part of a student's day might be taught in sign and part in speech and SPEECHREADING. Students might also be divided according to percent of hearing loss; some might be taught orally, others manually.

Eventually, the conviction of the importance of speaking and speechreading grew to the point where most teachers decided they should speak all the time, and by 1950 most elementary school programs were completely oral. Some teachers still believed in the importance of sign, however, and therefore these instructors paired speech with signing.

But by the late 1960s, educators were disappointed with the poor results of oral-only programs and encouraged by the superior performance of offspring of deaf parents who used sign language from birth. Thus the use of simultaneous communication began an upsurge. By the late 1970s, hundreds of programs for deaf students had abandoned the oral-only approach and started to use sim-com, calling it total communication.

Today, sim-com is the most frequently-used method of communication in deaf schools across the country. It is also the standard method of communication at GALLAUDET UNIVERSITY.

Sim-com is also frequently used by a deaf and a hearing person in communication, particularly if the hearing person is not fluent in sign, or in a group of people that includes a person who cannot sign. Deaf people, however, almost never use sim-com among themselves; for many, speech had been forced on them for many years and represents a denial of their own language and culture.

Generally, it is not possible to speak English and sign in American Sign Language, since the word order and structure of ASL is fundamentally different from English. Instead, educators and proponents of sim-com have adapted ASL in order to speak English and sign at the same time. The adaptations include using a form of signing called PIDGIN SIGN ENGLISH, a manual code for English, or an older form of signing modeled after English.

Pidgin Sign English uses signs while relying on English to provide a simplified grammatical structure. The manual codes for English include a range of systems developed in the early 1970s that also use signs and English grammatical structure, together with new signs created to represent English articles, pronouns and affixes (such as -ing, -ed, -s).

These codes include SIGNED ENGLISH, SEEING ESSENTIAL ENGLISH (SEE 1), SIGNING EXACT ENGLISH (SEE 2). Finally, older signers sometimes use modeling English in which the meaning of ASL signs are not changed and English articles or affixes are simply dropped. However, these adaptations are not strictly separated and are often used in combination, because the differences are not well understood by people not fluent in sign.

Simultaneous communication has been controversial because it satisfies neither the proponents of the oral or manual approach. Oralists, who would like to eliminate all signs, believe sim-com doesn't teach good speech skills; those who favor the manual approach counter that the English-linked manual codes usually used in sim-com are pidgin languages.

There are problems with sim-com as well. It is very difficult to speak and sign at the same time and requires such a great deal of concentration that it can inhibit communication. Further, hearing people often do not sign everything they say, which makes it hard for deaf people to follow what they are trying to communicate.

Studies of simultaneous communication have revealed that a person's oral English often deteriorates when speaking and signing; at the same time, the meaning of signs often does not match the meaning of the English words. Further, when speaking and signing together, communication tends to bog down and go much slower than when signing or speaking alone.

Studies of whether simultaneous communication actually helps deaf students learn English have reached conflicting conclusions; it is apparent that these students improve in using a manual code for English but not necessarily in English skills. Studies also do not agree on whether or not deaf students understand and learn better from teachers who use simultaneous communication.

simultaneous interpreting   This form of communicating requires the interpreter to mouth and sign everything that the speaker is saying, as opposed to manual interpreting, in which not everything is mouthed. See also SIGN LANGUAGE INTERPRETERS.

sinus problems and hearing loss   Sinusitis is an inflammation of the linings of the air spaces in the bones of the face around the nose; irritation at the back of the nose may cause swelling around

the EUSTACHIAN TUBE, which can interfere with the normal function of the middle ear, resulting in a temporary hearing loss.

Nasal sprays used to treat sinusitis can aggravate a hearing problem since these sprays can actually increase swelling and irritation around the eustachian tube.

SISI   A type of hearing test (an abbreviation for Short Increment Sensitivity) used by an AUDIOLOGIST to uncover certain types of nerve loss. Because individuals with cochlear lesions often are oversensitive to sound (called RECRUITMENT), a person with recruitment can also detect smaller changes in sound intensity than a person with normal hearing could.

In the test, a steady tone 20 DECIBELS (dB) above the patient's threshold is presented every two minutes. Every five seconds, the intensity is increased one dB, and the patient pushes a button each time a change is heard. A detection percentage is determined by multiplying five times the number of increments out of a maximum of 20 that are perceived. Scores over 60 percent suggest a cochlear disorder. See also AUDIOMETRY.

Smetana, Bedřich (1824–1884)   The creator of the Czech national opera and composer of *My Fatherland*, this Czechoslovakian musician first had hearing problems at the age of 36 and became completely deaf 14 years later as a result of the disintegration of the nervous system caused by SYPHILIS.

Still, he continued to play and compose and completed the last four of his six symphonic poems without being able to hear any of them.

Smith, Erastus (1787–1837)   This Texas folk hero was the chief scout and spy for General Sam Houston, commander in chief of the Texas army.

Erastus "Deaf" Smith was born to a large family near Poughkeepsie, New York. A sickly, solitary child, Smith lost his hearing during early infancy and received little education thereafter.

Nineteen years later he visited what is now Texas, moving there permanently in 1821, where he was known as El Sordo (the Deaf One). After marrying a Spanish woman, he was granted Mexican citizenship and became fluent in Spanish despite his severe hearing problem. The two lived in San Antonio, which at the time was part of Mexico.

A loyal Mexican citizen, he never suspected Texas would one day petition to join the United States. But with the beginning of the Texas Revolution in 1835, Smith's neutrality was soon over; upon returning to his home in San Antonio one day, he found the town occupied by Mexicans and under siege by Texans. When the Mexicans fired on him and refused to let him return to his home, Smith joined General Stephen F. Austin and the Texas forces.

Because he was so familiar with the area, Smith was invaluable to the Texan army, becoming scout to Sam Houston en route to the Alamo. It was Smith who brought back the only two survivors of the massacre there, Mrs. Almeron Dickerson and her baby daughter. It was also Smith's advice to Houston that assured the Texan's victory at San Jacinto, where Santa Anna was captured and Texas gained its independence from Mexico.

Smith died from a lung problem in Richmond on November 30, 1837. Deaf Smith County in Texas is named in his honor.

smoking and hearing loss New research suggests that pregnant women who smoke may triple their child's risk of developing an ear infection, perhaps by interfering with the baby's immune systems. Children of women who smoked during pregnancy were far more likely to suffer middle ear infections or ear surgery by age five than those whose mothers didn't smoke while pregnant.

An Australian study found that children born to women who smoked between one and nine cigarettes each day showed a 60 percent higher risk for ear infection. The children of women who smoked 10 to 19 cigarettes daily showed a 260 percent higher risk, and those who smoked more than 20 cigarettes a day had children with a 330 percent higher risk. The study also found that children born to women who smoked more than a pack a day were three times more likely to undergo ear surgery before their fifth birthday.

social adequacy index (SAI) A measure of the degree to which a patient has problems in hearing and understanding speech. The SAI is computed from the results of speech reception thresholds and speech discrimination tests.

Social Security and hearing loss The Social Security Administration has two benefit programs for people with a hearing loss who meet their state's requirements for "disability": Supplemental Security Income (SSI) and Social Security Disability Insurance (SSDI). Both benefits are awarded to children or adults who meet the criteria for being disabled and—in the case of SSI—for financial need. To be eligible for SSDI, a working adult must have paid Social Security at least five of the last 10 years.

Society of Hearing-Impaired Physicians (SHIP) This organization helps physicians, other health professionals, medical students and prospective medical students whose hearing problem may require different tools and/or approaches to medical practice and training. See also Appendix II.

sociocusis A hearing loss caused by environmental noise.

sound conduction Sound waves move outward in all directions by back and forth movements of molecules through solids, liquids or gases.

Each complete back-and-forth movement (oscillation) is called a cycle, and the number of cycles generated by a sound source every second is known as the frequency. The term *hertz* (abbreviated Hz) represents cycles per second and is named after HEINRICH HERTZ, a famous scientist who studied sound.

Human ears can detect sounds within a frequency range of 20 Hz to 20,000 Hz; the range of speech lies mostly between 100 and 8,000 Hz. The higher the frequency, the higher the pitch or tone; almost all of the sounds we hear are combinations of many frequencies. Sounds used in hearing tests that are only one frequency are called pure tones.

A sound wave's pressure on the surface it contacts is a measure of the sound's intensity, or power.

The greater the intensity of the sound waves on a person's eardrum, the louder the sound that is heard. A sound that is just barely able to be heard is the threshold intensity.

In order to test hearing, it is important to be able to measure the intensity of sounds heard; therefore, an internationally-accepted sound pressure level has been set to correspond approximately to that of a threshold intensity for a sound with a frequency of 1,000 Hz. Other sound pressures are compared to this reference pressure on a scale measured in decibels (dB), a name taken from the inventor of the telephone, ALEXANDER GRAHAM BELL. Sound intensities on this scale increase tenfold for every 20 dB difference in sound pressure.

There are two ways for sound to be conducted through our ears—air and bone conduction. Air conduction occurs when sound moves from the external ear (pinna) to the middle and inner ears. Bone conduction occurs when sound vibrations are transmitted through the skull bones directly to the cochlea.

A blockage in the external or middle ears means an overall reduction in all sound intensities but not a total hearing loss, since sound is also routed through bone. See also AUDIOMETRY.

soundfield testing A hearing test used with young children in which sounds are presented to both ears at once without the use of earphones. See also AUDIOMETRY.

sound spectrograph A device that records the continually changing intensity levels of frequency components in a complex sound wave via a filter analyzer.

sound wave A pressure area produced by vibration moving through air or water, causing reactions in the ear that the brain interprets as sound. See also SOUND CONDUCTION.

Spain This country, which has a deaf population of 120,000, has a deeply-rooted tradition of educating deaf students.

More than 400 years ago, a Spanish monk named PEDRO PONCE DE LEÓN first taught deaf people to speak. Today there is a range of special elementary and secondary schools specializing in deaf education that use a wide variety of approaches. Although some schools favor MAINSTREAMING, this method is opposed by schools who favor the oral approach.

Most deaf children begin school at age four and continue to 18; there are vocational courses open to them but no special university for deaf students. If a deaf student wishes to earn a degree at a regular university, he or she must do so without the use of an interpreter. For this reason, there are not many deaf graduates of Spanish universities.

Deaf Spaniards have a strong community, and communicate in SPANISH SIGN LANGUAGE, although dialects vary from province to province. There are special telephone devices available, but few deaf Spaniards have them in their homes. Television captioning has not yet become available.

Spanish Sign Language The origins of Spanish Sign Language are unknown, but today sign language is used by virtually all Spaniards. It has few dialects, although its grammar is complex and poorly understood by modern linguists.

There seems to be no well-defined subject-verb-object word order in SSL. Verbs are made using one gesture, adding prefixes or suffixes as needed. FINGERSPELLING is rarely used and then only for proper names for when there is no gestural sign.

At present, the teaching of sign language in Spanish schools is under debate; some schools allow SSL and others do not. See also SPAIN.

speech audiometry A measure of hearing spoken words presented at controlled intensity levels. See also AUDIOMETRY.

speech discrimination test A special speech/ hearing test that tries to determine the ability to hear familiar words. See also AUDIOMETRY.

speech frequencies In audiometric testing, these are the pure-tone frequencies that can best predict the level at which speech can be understood (500, 1,000 and 2,000 Hz).

speech-language pathologist A specialist in human communication, its development and its disorders. Also known as a speech pathologist or speech therapist, the speech-language pathologist evaluates and treats persons with communication problems resulting from total or partial hearing loss, brain injury, cleft palate, voice pathology, emotional problems, foreign dialect, development delays, stroke, learning disabilities and so forth. They also provide clinical therapy to help those with speech and language disorders, and help them and their families understand the disorder and develop better communication skills.

In most settings, speech-language pathologists perform screening tests of auditory acuity and tympanometry (a measure of middle ear function). Only a speech-language pathologist is certified to make recommendations for the type of speech language treatment required. Treatment could include a specific program of exercises to improve language ability or speech together with support from the client's family and friends.

To practice speech-language pathology, states require a master's degree in speech-language pathology, more than 300 hours of supervised clinical experience and successful completion of a certifying exam.

speechreading The preferred term for lip-reading, a way of recognizing spoken words by watching the speaker's lips, jaw and tongue movements. Speechreading is the least consistently visible of the communication choices available to deaf people; only about 30 percent of English sounds are visible on the lips, and half are homophonous (that is, they look like other words). For example, the words *kite*, *height* and *night* look almost identical.

The ability to speechread is often contingent on the visibility, shape and configuration of the speaker's mouth. For example, it may be difficult to speechread someone who mumbles, who has a beard or who has no teeth.

Some deaf people become skilled speech-readers, especially if they can supplement what they see with some hearing. Many don't develop much skill at speechreading, but most do speechread to some extent. Because speechreading requires considerable guesswork, very few deaf people rely on speechreading alone when exchanging important information.

One system that has been designed to be used with speechreading is CUED SPEECH, developed by Dr. Orin Cornett of Gallaudet University. Cued speech is a method in which hand movements and location are used to make all of the sounds produced on the lips clear to the speechreader. See also VISEME.

speech reception threshold test A special speech hearing test that determines the softest speech a person can hear. See also AUDIOMETRY.

speech therapist See SPEECH-LANGUAGE PATHOLOGIST.

speech training Teaching speech to profoundly deaf individuals has been the center of a number of controversies in deaf education for hundreds of years. Today, controversy centers on how well deaf people can be taught to speak and the best methods to achieve that goal. Some still question the need to teach speech to deaf students at all.

The wide range of teaching methods vary according to the size of the speech unit taught and the number of senses the student uses in order to learn speech. Those methods that emphasize small units of speech (syllables and speech sounds) are called analytic; methods that teach units of speech no smaller than syllables and stress the importance of connected speech fall into the synthetic category.

speech training aids Devices that display speech electronically to teach those who cannot hear how to use their voice, such as the Matsushita speech system.

With this speech system, which was developed in Japan, a speech therapist and client wear special sensors inside the mouth and on the nose that are linked to a computer. When the therapist pronounces a sound or a word, the computer generates an image on a video screen that illustrates the position of the tongue within the mouth, the vibration of the nose and the intensity of the voice. The student learns to pronounce the sound or word by trying to produce the same pattern on the screen.

Originally used in Japan, the school is testing it for use with American English-speaking students and are helping develop English language software for deaf individuals in the United States.

Other devices have been developed including a computer-based system for children with displays that resemble video games and a laryngograph, which monitors the action of the larynx from two plates held against the throat, displaying voice pitch coordination with other movements and voice quality.

stapedectomy   The removal of the STAPES and its replacement with a prosthesis. The purpose of this operation is to treat hearing loss caused by OTOSCLE-ROSIS, a familial form of deafness that is curable only by surgery. Otosclerosis causes the base of the stapes (stirrup), the innermost of the three bones in the middle ear, to become fixed to the opening of the inner ear by an overgrowth of spongy bone. This interferes with the stapes' ability to transmit sound to the inner ear.

While the patient is under a local or general anesthetic, a surgeon using laser and microscopic techniques opens the ear canal and folds the eardrum forward. All (or most) of the stapes is removed, and a plastic or metal prosthesis is inserted into the entrance to the inner ear; the other end is attached to the incus. The eardrum is then repaired.

Sound now travels from the eardrum to the two normal ear bones, then through the prosthesis and a vein graft to the hearing nerve.

Antibiotics are usually used up to five days after surgery to prevent infection; packing and sutures are removed about a week after surgery. Hearing shows improvement within two weeks and continues to get better over the next three months.

Good candidates for a stapedectomy are patients who have fixed stapes from otosclerosis and a CON-DUCTIVE HEARING LOSS of at least 20 dB with a speech discrimination score of at least 60 percent. Patients with a severe hearing loss might still profit from a stapedectomy, if only to bring their hearing up to a level where a hearing aid could be of help.

The operation improves hearing in more than 90 percent of cases, although about 1 percent of patients experience loss of hearing from damage to the COCHLEA. Because of this risk, a stapedectomy is normally done on one ear at a time, although oto-sclerosis usually affects both ears. It is almost never used on a patient with hearing in only one ear.

Other less common complications from the surgery include change in taste from damage to the chorda tympani nerve, perforated eardrum, vertigo and damage to the ossicular chain. Temporary Bell's palsy (facial nerve paralysis) can occur immediately after the operation. Occasionally, vertigo persists and may require surgery. See also FENESTRATION; STAPES MOBILIZATION.

stapedial footplate   See FOOTPLATE.

stapedial muscle   One of two intra-aural muscles in the middle ear, the stapedial muscle is attached to the top of the stapes and runs behind it.

stapedius   A small muscle in the inner wall of the MIDDLE EAR that inserts into the neck of the STAPES and is responsible for retracting the stapes.

stapes   Commonly called the stirrup, this is the smallest bone in the body and is one of the three tiny bones that make up the OSSICLES in the middle ear. The head of the stapes joins the middle ossicle (anvil). Its base fits into the oval window located in the wall of the inner ear and, as it vibrates, plunges in and out of the oval window.

The condition of OTOSCLEROSIS immobilizes the stapes in the entrance to the inner ear by an over-growth of spongy bone, interfering with the ability of the stapes to move freely and transmit sound to the inner ear, thereby causing deafness. The condition can be helped by a hearing aid but is cured only by surgery (STAPEDECTOMY). Although the oper-ation improves hearing in about 90 percent of patients, about 1 percent of patients actually expe-rience a deterioration of hearing. This is why—although otosclerosis normally affects both ears—a stapedectomy is usually only done on one ear at a time.

stapes mobilization   This operation for OTOSCLE-ROSIS was accidentally discovered during FENESTRA-

TION (an operation creating a new oval window) when the stapes had been accidentally moved too much, loosening the otosclerosis and mobilizing the STAPES. After the operation, the patient had much better hearing than is normal after a simple fenestration.

But although this new type of operation seemed exciting at first, it was discovered that the otosclerosis continued to be active and would again fix the stapes to the OVAL WINDOW, losing all benefits of the mobilization. And for many patients, the otosclerosis had progressed too far and scarred or fixed their stapes too much to be helped with mobilization.

Mobilization today is used primarily for people who were born with problems of the stapes or oval window. In other patients, a STAPEDECTOMY is preferred to treat otosclerosis.

Stenger test A FUNCTIONAL HEARING LOSS test in which both ears are stimulated by the same frequency but at different intensities. This test is used to assess a person's hearing loss in one ear. See also AUDIOMETRY.

stenosis A narrowing of the external ear canal as a result of various disease processes, including chronic OTITIS MEDIA (ear infection), inflammation, allergic reaction, injury or PERICHONDRITIS (an infection primarily of the cartilage covering the pinna).

stirrup See STAPES.

substance abuse The incidence of drug and alcohol abuse among deaf people is similar to the incidence among hearing people. However, deaf abusers historically have faced discrimination in treatment programs and services, with few professionals trained in chemical dependency and deafness, according to the National Information Center on Deafness.

There have been few studies of substance abuse in the deaf community, although it is generally believed that the problem is about the same as substance abuse in the hearing population: one in 10.

Deaf substance abusers generally have few ties with churches, organizations and clubs of the deaf community and live on the fringes of both the deaf and hearing societies. Substance abusers who are deaf high school students follow similar patterns.

Although treatment programs for substance abusers in the United States have proliferated since the 1930s, deaf people have found major barriers to existing treatment facilities. One of the biggest obstacles to treatment may be found in the deaf community itself, which has been reluctant in the past to admit that its members have a problem. Few referrals to substance abuse agencies come from the deaf community.

Further, deaf substance abusers find it difficult to admit to themselves that there is a problem, and self-referrals to treatment are lower in this population than in the general population.

A deaf person seeking treatment for a substance abuse problem, however, faces other hurdles: Most programs have been designed for hearing clients, and counselors lack an understanding of deafness, the deaf community and manual methods of communication. Agencies often cannot afford to hire interpreters, and deafness experts aren't trained in substance abuse rehabilitation.

In 1973 the first treatment center for deaf alcoholics was established in St. Paul, Minnesota, followed a year later by another in San Francisco.

In 1975, the first national conference on substance abuse in the deaf community was held in Cleveland, Ohio. During this time, inpatient treatment for deaf alcoholics, counseling programs and outreach projects were begun. In 1979 the quarterly *AID Bulletin* began to provide updated information to a national membership.

By 1985, alcohol treatment programs had begun in California, Illinois, New York, Ohio, Maryland, Minnesota and Massachusetts. These programs combine an outreach advocacy program run by specialists in substance abuse and deafness.

From the early 1970s on, programs for deaf alcoholics have featured outreach projects directed by substance abuse experts who understand the communication problems of deaf clients. When such treatment is therefore modified, deaf and hearing alcoholics recover at the same rate.

Sweden There are an estimated 530,000 deaf and hard-of-hearing people in Sweden. There are approximately 200 hard-of-hearing babies born each year and of these, about 50 are profoundly deaf. About 87 per 100,000 Swedes are deaf, according to 1930 statistics, one of the higher prevalence rates among developed countries (which range from 300 per 100,000 to 35 per 100,000).

The first school for deaf children in Sweden was opened in Stockholm in 1809, influenced by other European schools and relying on the oral approaches. But unlike many other schools in Europe, Sweden retained an interest in manual education and taught either method to children depending on individual preferences.

Today, deaf Swedes can attend either large state schools for deaf children or local community schools, where many children are mainstreamed.

More than 90 percent of Swedish children go on to a "gymnasium" (higher education) after completing the required nine years of school; although there are no special classes for hard-of-hearing students in these gymnasiums, there is a special gymnasium for deaf students in Orebro, where they may take vocational courses or pre-university studies.

Swedish Sign Language   The language of more than 8,000 Swedish deaf citizens, Swedish Sign Language is unrelated to any other sign language in the world and is not derived from any other sign system.

Still, it shares many characteristics of other sign languages, including a complex structure; signs are made with the hands, while facial expression, body movement and posture are used to indicate clause and sentence type. In addition, lip movements are always used with FINGERSPELLING and may also be used with signs. Sweden's manual alphabet was invented in the early 1800s by Swedish educator Per Aron Borg, who later took this alphabet to Portugal where he established schools for deaf students.

swimmer's ear   Also known as external otitis or otitis externa, this ear problem is an infection of the ear canal that occurs after swimming in dirty or heavily chlorinated water. The risk of getting swimmer's ear increases with the frequency of swimming, the longer the person stays in the water and the more often the head is submerged.

Swimmer's ear usually causes redness and swelling of the ear canal, a discharge and sometimes eczema around the ear opening. Itching may become painful and deafness can occur if pus blocks the ear.

It is treated with drying of the ear followed by antibiotic, antifungal or anti-inflammatory drugs.

For swimmers, this condition can be prevented by putting a few drops of rubbing alcohol in the ear after swimming. Because alcohol evaporates sooner than water, it helps draw water out of the ear. Physicians often recommend that sufferers limit time spent in the water to no longer than one hour with an hour or two wait between dips to allow the ear to dry out. Earplugs are not a good idea since they can irritate the skin of the canal.

Swimmer's ear can also be caused by excessive washing, perspiration, irritation of the ear canal after removal of foreign objects, allergies or a generalized skin disease such as atopic eczema or seborrheic dermatitis.

Swiss Sign Language   Switzerland was traditionally a country that favored the oral approach, but sign language there today is slowly making a comeback in the deaf community.

In a country divided into cultural sections (German, French and Italian), Swiss Sign Language varies widely from strictly sign language to mixtures of sign and spoken language.

Neither the German nor French areas of Switzerland have a manual alphabet. Because of this, the set of handshapes that make up the sign language is more restricted, and there is a tendency to mouth the equivalent word in the spoken language for those ideas that have no sign.

Research suggests that the various dialects of Swiss Sign Language have many similar characteristics in common with other sign languages, including the use of facial expressions, eye gaze and body posture.

In general, sign language is not widely used in the classroom, although both sign language and the pidgin forms of signing are used in the deaf community. There are still an insufficient number of sign language instructors and courses.

Switzerland Life in Switzerland for its 7,200 deaf citizens is a complicated affair since the decentralized country recognizes four languages (German, French, Italian and Romansh) with a bewildering number of dialects, particularly in German and Romansh. Prevalence of deafness is rather high (94 out of 100,000) when compared to other countries, but almost equal to the rate in the United States (100 out of 100,000).

Although education varies among the 23 different cantons (states), in general hard-of-hearing students who use amplification attend regular schools, and deaf students are taught to speechread and speak. Schools are open to deaf students between ages six and 16.

The manual approach is not widespread in Switzerland, but deaf students sign outside of class. Although there are differences among local sign languages, most deaf people can make each other understood across dialects.

sympathetic vibration A vibration in one object produced by vibrations of the same frequency in another object.

syntax The study of the rules of sentence formation. See also LINGUISTICS.

syphilis Whether contracted at birth or later in life, syphilis may cause an inner ear HEARING LOSS. When a pregnant woman becomes infected with the disease, her unborn child usually also contracts the disease; 35 percent of these infants will eventually go on to experience some degree of hearing loss.

This eventual hearing loss from prenatal exposure to syphilis is hard to quantify since the deafness may show up suddenly later in childhood or even in adulthood.

Children tend to experience hearing loss in both ears suddenly, and if it appears before age 10, deafness is usually profound.

Hearing loss in adulthood from syphilis appears more gradually, as either a hearing loss or a fluctuation in intensity.

Treatment with penicillin and steroids is usually given for some months; if hearing improves, the steroids may be continued indefinitely to stave off a recurrent hearing loss. Although some syphilis-caused hearing loss responds immediately to treatment, other cases do not, in spite of continued treatment.

Because syphilis causes a SENSORINEURAL HEARING LOSS, sufferers have a poor understanding of speech even with the use of hearing aids. See also PRENATAL CAUSES OF HEARING LOSS.

syphilitic labyrinthitis See LABYRINTHITIS.

systemic infections and hearing loss Infections such as SCARLET FEVER, typhoid fever, MEASLES and tuberculosis can sometimes cause bilateral SENSORINEURAL HEARING loss.

In particular, scarlet fever can cause a moderate degree of sensorineural deafness with bilateral acute and, later, chronic OTITIS MEDIA.

tactile feedback device   This device provides a substitute for sounds a deaf person cannot hear by converting sounds into a pattern of sensations on the skin. It is generally used in speech therapy, although it may also be used as an aid to speechreading.

One of the more recent devices, the Audiotact (produced by Sevrain-Tech of Madison, Wisconsin), uses 32 electrodes incorporated into a belt worn around the abdomen to stimulate the skin with electrical pulses that feel like finger taps, with different sounds producing different patterns of stimulation. By learning what these sounds "feel" like, a person can learn or pronounce them and eventually put these sounds together in words and sentences.

Unfortunately, it's hard to produce enough distinct patterns with 32 electrodes to represent the large variety of sounds in speech. As a result, the NATIONAL INSTITUTE ON DEAFNESS AND OTHER COMMUNICATION DISORDERS is funding development of a device with 256 electrodes.

tangible reinforcement operant conditioning audiometry (TROCA)   A type of hearing test used for preschool children, which rewards the young patient with positive reinforcement (candy, treats) for appropriate responses to sound See also AUDIOMETRY.

T-coil   See TELECOIL.

TDD   See TELECOMMUNICATIONS DEVICE FOR THE DEAF.

TDD distribution programs   State programs—often established by legislative mandate—that provide eligible deaf and hard-of-hearing people access to telephone communication.

Usually, they are administered by the relevant state agency on deafness, which invites applications from residents who are deaf or hard-of-hearing, or have speech problems. Once applicants are screened for medical and financial eligibility, they may be given a TELECOMMUNICATIONS DEVICE FOR THE DEAF (TDD) at no charge or allowed to buy TDDs at substantially reduced rates.

tectorial membrane   This fine, gelatinous membrane lies on top of the hair cells of the ORGAN OF CORTI, which in turn lies within the full length of the scala media.

When the ear transmits sound, high frequencies stimulate the hair cells at the lower end of the COCHLEA, and low frequencies stimulate hair cells toward the upper end. As the sound waves stimulate the hair cells, the nerves at the base of the cells gather the impulses and send them to the brain.

telecaption adapter   See TELECAPTION DECODER.

TeleCaption decoder   A device once attached to a television set that interpreted closed caption signals broadcast at the same time as the TV program, converting them to typed dialogue across the bottom of the TV screen. Manufactured and distributed by the NATIONAL CAPTIONING INSTITUTE, the devices were compatible with TVs, video cassette recorders (VCRs) and cable hookups.

Since 1993, all TV sets larger than 13 inches must contain built-in closed-caption decoders. See also CAPTION CENTER; CAPTIONED FILMS/VIDEOS FOR THE DEAF; CLOSED CAPTIONS.

telecaptioning   See CLOSED CAPTIONS.

telecoil The telecoil (also called the T-coil and the T-switch) is a tiny electrical component that can sense magnetic forces generated by another coil nearby, such as the speaker coil in a telephone or a loop or wire around the room or around a person's neck. The major use for a telecoil has been with the telephone, allowing clearer sound reception for the hard-of-hearing consumer.

When a hearing aid's control switch is set to the T-switch, the telecoil is connected and the hearing aid's microphone is disconnected. This allows the aid to receive magnetic signals instead of sound, enabling the wearer to hear only the "important" sound coming from the telecoil while screening out annoying background noise.

T-switches have become important with the advent of ASSISTIVE LISTENING DEVICES and assistive listening systems. More and more, public areas (churches, theaters, meeting rooms and so forth) have been fitted with assistive listening systems to help the hearing impaired. Where such an induction loop system is in place, the hearing aid wearer can turn on the T-mode to receive sound through the loop. Or, where certain public places feature FM or infrared systems, the wearer may use a special receiver to connect with the hearing aid in the T-mode.

In much the same way, assistive listening devices use the T-switch to improve hearing of TV and radio.

Not all HEARING AIDS have a telecoil, including most canal or in-the-ear aids. However, many behind-the-ear and all body aids have telecoils. Because there are no regulations or standards regarding telecoils, they can vary as much as 30 decibels in maximum sound output.

Telecommunications Act of 1996 A law enacted by the U.S. Congress that included television captioning requirements. The law requires that video programming be closed captioned, no matter how it is distributed (broadcast, cable, satellite), to ensure access for deaf or hard-of-hearing people. Some exemptions were included to prevent undue economic burdens. To implement the closed captioning requirements included in the act, the U.S. Federal Communications Commission (FCC) established rules and implementation schedules for the captioning of television programming. See also CLOSED CAPTIONS.

telecommunications device for the deaf Known as a TDD, this mechanical/electronic compensatory device allows people to type phone messages over the telephone network. The term *TDD* is generic and replaces the earlier term *TTY*, which refers specifically to teletypewriter machines, although many people still use *TTY*.

Basically a visual typewriter, a TDD connects to a telephone line by a modular plug or acoustic modem. The conversation is displayed on a screen moving from right to left above the keyboard. Some TDDs have a printer, which provides a permanent record on special paper of all messages transmitted and received. A TDD is required at both ends of the phone line in order to communicate.

TDD keyboards follow the typical typewriter's layout, except that most TDDs have three-row keyboards on which the numerals 0 through 9 appear as upper case characters above the letters QWERTYUIOP. Some TDDs have four-row keyboards.

The TDD was invented in 1964 by ROBERT H. WEITBRECHT, a deaf physicist and licensed ham radio operator, together with James Marsters, a deaf orthodontist. The two wanted to investigate the possible ways a hard-of-hearing person might communicate by using a teletypewriter (TTY) with a radio or telephone. Working together in California, the two decided a telephone system would be more logical since many hard-of-hearing and deaf people already had telephones in their homes and a radio system would have required the deaf person to get a license from the Federal Communications Commission.

Weitbrecht developed an acoustic coupler that converted the electrical signals of the teletypewriter into audible tones that could be sent over the telephone network. A deaf person would place a telephone on Weitbrecht's special modem and a modified teleprinter machine. It took Weitbrecht several years to complete his "Weitbrecht Modem." At that same time, the telephone and telegraph companies were replacing their old teletypewriter equipment with newer devices.

Through an agreement between AT&T and the ALEXANDER GRAHAM BELL ASSOCIATION FOR THE DEAF, surplus TTYs were obtained and equipped with acoustic couplers. These devices provided the first way for deaf people to communicate by telephone across the country. Both deaf organizations formed Teletypewriters for the Deaf Distribution Committee in Indianapolis, Indiana (now TELECOMMUNICATIONS FOR THE DEAF, INC.)

In some states, phone companies lend or sell TDDs at subsidized prices, and more and more public agencies are installing them. In addition, relay services are available to connect TDD and voice calls through an interpreter. By law, as of 1991 every state must have in place a TDD RELAY SERVICE.

New Technology

TDDs and computers use different codes for the letters of the alphabet and other characters, and therefore cannot normally communicate. However, it is possible to equip a personal computer with a special modem to make it function as a TDD. (A modem is a device that allows a computer to use a telephone line to transmit information to other computers with compatible modems).

Most TDDs with build-in modems can normally understand only transmissions in the BAUDOT CODE. Personal computers use the ASCII code, and modems designed for use with a computer accommodate only that code. However, there are four modems available that have the ability to communicate in both Baudot and ASCII codes.

Today there are a wide variety of other TDD products for deaf consumers. Some TDDs come in very small, lightweight, portable sizes. Others have built-in answering machines that respond only to TDD calls. For households that require it, there is an answering machine that responds to both voice and TDD calls. However, the Internet and electronic mail have supplanted the popularity of TDDs for everyday communication.

Telecommunications for the Deaf, Inc.
A consumer-oriented organization that sells caption decoders and a directory for deaf people. The group supports legislation and advocates the use of TELECOMMUNICATIONS DEVICES FOR THE DEAF, ASCII code, Emergency Access (911), telecaptioning and visual ALERTING DEVICES in the public, private and government sectors.

Telecommunications for the Disabled Act of 1982
See LEGAL RIGHTS.

Tele-Consumer Hotline
Nonprofit, independent and impartial telephone consumer information service that provides free telephone assistance and publications on special telephone equipment, TDD directories, TDD/voice relay services, choosing a long distance company, selecting a phone, money saving tips and more.

teletext
A form of closed captioning that uses a different decoder than the LINE 21 system TELECAPTION DECODER. The teletext system uses several lines of the vertical blanking interval instead of just one line, as in the line 21 system.

Although similar in appearance to the line 21 system of closed captioning, teletext captioning may also include symbols, or icons, to indicate sound effects and may be quite elaborate. Teletext provides many "pages" of information that can be selected individually, and that don't move up on the screen.

The most well-known teletext system in the United States, the NORTH AMERICAN BASIC TELETEXT SPECIFICATION (NABTS) was adopted by CBS for text services and captioning, which is the only TV network to use the teletext system.

While NABTS decoders have been available since 1984, their use has not been widespread, in part because they require excellent television reception and cannot be used with video recorders. Since 1984 CBS has offered both teletext and line 21 closed captioning. See also CAPTION CENTER; CLOSED CAPTIONS; NATIONAL CAPTIONING INSTITUTE; TELECAPTION DECODER.

Television Decoder Circuitry Act of 1990
As of July 1, 1993, this act required all television sets with screens 13 inches or larger manufactured for sale in the United States to contain built-in closed-caption decoders. In addition to serving as a lifeline for deaf and hard-of-hearing viewers, captioning benefits people learning English as a second language and children and adults learning to read. All decoder-equipped TV sets must now meet the standards issued by the Federal Communications

Commission (FCC). Television manufacturers may also incorporate optional features, such as changeable character colors.

New decoder designs permit captions to appear anywhere on the screen, resulting in more precise positioning of text. (Previously, captions could appear only in the upper- or lower-third of the picture.) This new positioning will more clearly indicate who is speaking, and important parts of the picture will be covered less often. Caption-capable TVs must display italicized characters using either true italics or slanted letters. (Caption agencies often use italics to indicate vital information such as sound effects, narrators and off-screen voices.) Manufacturers may offer other options to denote italics, such as color reversal. The FCC requires the use of a black background (as used in some set-top decoders) to guarantee the legibility of caption characters. Manufacturers may offer other background colors as long as black is available at the user's option.

Beginning January, 1996, new caption-capable TV sets were required to display both lower- and upper-case letters (until 1996, certain televisions were only required to display upper-case letters). Manufacturers must specifically label packing boxes and owner's manuals to inform consumers if the set does not support certain options such as color characters, lower-case characters or "text mode."

temporal bone fracture and hearing loss   Head trauma with skull fracture involving the two temporal bones (which house the structures of the middle and inner ear) often involves the middle ear and causes a CONDUCTIVE HEARING LOSS. A transverse fracture of the temporal bone can also injure the inner ear or internal auditory meatus, causing SENSORINEURAL HEARING LOSS, VERTIGO, TINNITUS and facial nerve paralysis.

temporary hearing loss   A nonpermanent hearing loss that often follows exposure to a loud, explosive NOISE such as a gunshot.

temporomandibular joint syndrome (TMJ)   Severe pain in the jaw, face and head, especially around the ears, that researchers believe is caused by the improper function of the jaw (temporomandibular) joints and their muscles and ligaments.

Other symptoms of TMJ include jaw and ear clicking or popping, "locking" jaws and pain in opening the mouth, and hearing loss.

Clenching and grinding the teeth, which cause the muscles to go into spasm, is the most common cause of TMJ. An incorrect bite, excessive tension, head injury or, rarely, osteoarthritis can also lead to TMJ.

Treatment involves the application of moist heat to relieve the muscle spasm and the use of muscle relaxant medication and pain relievers. In severe cases, joint surgery may be required.

tensor tympani   One of the two intra-aural muscles located in the middle ear. The tensor tympani is attached to the upper portion of the manubrium (the handle of the malleus) and crossed diagonally across the TYMPANUM into the tensor canal. It is supplied by a branch of the TRIGEMINAL NERVE.

threshold   The softest sound or speech a person can hear. See also AUDIOMETRY.

tinnitus   A ringing, buzzing, hissing or whistling noise heard inside the ear when the acoustic nerve transmits impulses to the brain; impulses produced not from outside vibrations but as the result of stimuli produced inside the head. Actually, tinnitus is divided into two different types: tinnitus aurium (ringing in the ear) and tinnitus cerebri (ringing in the head).

Tinnitus is also classified as "vibratory" or "nonvibratory." Vibratory tinnitus originates outside the inner ear and is caused by vibration from any of the middle ear hearing mechanisms, such as a dislocated ossicular chain or wax against the eardrum. It is possible for another person to hear vibratory tinnitus from as far away as several feet.

Nonvibratory tinnitus begins in either the inner ear or the auditory nervous system and is subjective, since only the patient can hear these sounds. Recently, scientists have located the area of the brain that seems to register this ringing sound for some patients, which could be the first step in new treatments for the condition. Studies of a subset of tinnitus patients—those whose ear ringing is linked to the position of the jaw—show that for these patients, the tinnitus does not involve the cochlea but apparently originates within one side of the brain itself.

Tinnitus, which may affect as many as 50 million adults, usually involves almost continuous noise (although the affected person may only be aware of the noise occasionally). Tinnitus does not cause hearing disorders, but it may accompany decreased hearing and other ear symptoms, such as pressure or DIZZINESS, and may be psychologically uncomfortable as well.

Tinnitus often starts after an injury damages some of the sound-sensing hair cells of the inner ear, which lose their sensitivity to sound but still produce activity. Because these impulses travel along the hearing nerve, the brain interprets them as sound.

Tinnitus can be produced by a wide variety of causes, but the most common is extensive exposure to very loud noise for long periods of time, which causes excessive wear of the inner ear. Although tinnitus can occur after a single loud noise, such as a gunshot, it is much more common after continuous noise overexposure, such as from industrial machinery, aircraft engines or loud music.

For example, a person who has worked for many years around mechanical equipment, uses a snowmobile frequently and who spends a lot of time cutting firewood with a power saw would be at much greater risk for developing tinnitus. Some people, however, appear to have a much higher tolerance for similar kinds of excessive noise and do not develop tinnitus under identical circumstances. Researchers as yet do not know why.

After excessive noise, head injury is the next most common cause of tinnitus. Because the delicate mechanisms involved in hearing are buried inside the skull, head injury of almost any kind can produce tinnitus. Even a slap—if it lands directly on the ear—can cause tinnitus, which may show up several days after the injury and then one day simply disappear.

Tinnitus can also be produced by OTOTOXIC DRUGS; aspirin is particularly well-known for a type of tinnitus that disappears after medication is stopped.

On the other hand, quinine can produce a permanent tinnitus. Many of the aminoglycoside antibiotics may also produce tinnitus but only after long-term drug use and after extensive hearing loss has already occurred.

Diseases, such as MÉNIÈRE'S DISEASE, diabetes, thyroid problems, OTOSCLEROSIS, tumor on the hearing nerve, ear infections, or even excess wax against the eardrum, can cause tinnitus. Treatment of some diseases, such as otosclerosis, will also eliminate the tinnitus, but in others (notably, Ménière's disease), the tinnitus symptoms will be altered but not eliminated. Although the tinnitus that sometimes accompanies colds is temporary, people who travel in airplanes while nursing a cold may develop a severe and persistent form of tinnitus.

Physicians tend to consider tinnitus more of a nuisance than a medical condition; however, a person who has tinnitus in only one ear and who has not been exposed to excessive noise that might otherwise explain the tinnitus should immediately see an OTOLOGIST and an AUDIOLOGIST. Unilateral tinnitus can be a symptom of several serious ear diseases, including ACOUSTIC NEUROMA.

There is no cure for tinnitus, but there are ways to relieve the problem. Because the quieter the environment is, the worse tinnitus is, masking techniques that provide background noise will override the tinnitus impulses by keeping the ears busy with nerve signals from actual sounds to pass on to the brain. It takes advantage of a phenomenon called "residual inhibition," which means that following exposure to certain kinds of noise, there is a reduction in the level of tinnitus for a time.

However, not all tinnitus responds to masking; anyone considering buying a masker should first be tested to see if this treatment will bring relief. Playing a radio or tapes of natural sounds (waves or rain forest noises, for example) can often help.

Drug treatment may be effective in some cases, although there have been no definitive studies as yet. Studies have shown that the intravenous use of the local anesthetic lidocaine helps about 87 percent of tinnitus patients. But because the effects are only temporary, it is not practical as a permanent treatment.

The drug Tegretol is effective in about 62 percent of patients who had positive results from lidocaine, but its serious side effects make it a poor choice as a tinnitus treatment. In addition, vasodilators may help improve inner ear circulation and reduce tinnitus.

Because stress can make tinnitus worse, some people have been able to gain control of their tinnitus and suppress symptoms through the use of biofeedback. Biofeedback training helps individuals control some functions of their autonomic nervous system, such as heartbeat, blood pressure, sweating and temperature of hands and feet.

Scientists have found that a direct, positive electrical current can reduce or eliminate tinnitus for up to several weeks, although the time period varies from one person to the next. A transtympanic electrode is used to produce the current, which must be positive (a negative current produces pain or worsens the tinnitus). Although electrical currents can cause tissue damage, researchers hope to lessen the risk by designing stimulation that will lead to long-term suppression of tinnitus symptoms.

Because tinnitus can be psychologically crippling, help can be found through tinnitus support groups. Local hearing associations maintain listings for these groups. The AMERICAN TINNITUS ASSOCIATION sponsors such groups. Counseling may also be helpful in modifying the behavior of tinnitus patients, who sometimes allow their condition to dominate their lives.

The American Academy of Otolaryngology–Head and Neck Surgery suggests that tinnitus patients avoid loud noises and stimulants such as caffeine and nicotine, monitor blood pressure, lower salt intake, exercise, get enough rest and reduce anxiety. It is also a good idea to use an aspirin substitute, such as acetaminophen, since aspirin may worsen tinnitus.

tinnitus masker   Masking is the technique of producing external "white noise" sounds that will mask the TINNITUS (ringing in the ears) and make it less distracting. Masking machines come in both in-the-ear and portable models that produce sounds ranging from random white noise to waterfalls to surf. Hearing aids can also function as maskers by amplifying external sounds. It takes time to find the correct method of treatment and to properly fit and adjust hearing or tinnitus instruments; the first fitting is seldom the final one. At best, masking only provides relief, not a cure.

Otherwise, many people find it helpful to use an electric fan to mask tinnitus, to tune a regular FM radio to an empty frequency to listen to the static. Others who suffer from tinnitus use an audio CD of nature sounds (ocean, jungle, whales or rain) in autorepeat mode before going to bed.

In one recent masking study, 16 percent of patients reported relief using a hearing aid alone, 21 percent reported relief from a tinnitus masker alone and 63 percent reported relief from a combination hearing aid and tinnitus masker. In the latter case, it was important to adjust the hearing aid properly before attempting masking.

It is important for tinnitus patients to visit a tinnitus clinic to test ears for a specific tinnitus sound so that the right "white noise" can be matched up to it.

Simple Maskers

Simple tinnitus maskers generally provide a high frequency band of noise designed to mask the frequency of the tinnitus.

Hearing Aids

Although 90 percent of people with tinnitus also have a hearing problem, only a small percentage have ever used a hearing aid. If the pitch of the tinnitus is low, hearing aids usually help by raising the level of background noise and thereby masking the tinnitus. However, in cases of high-pitched tinnitus, even the highest-frequency hearing aids don't work very well as a masker since environmental noise is not high enough to mask the sound (environmental noise does not usually rise above 4,000 Hz).

Tinnitus Instrument

This is a combination hearing aid and simple masker, used in cases of high-frequency tinnitus and high-frequency hearing loss. It is useful because a simple masker does not work in cases of high-frequency hearing loss since the person cannot hear the frequencies required to mask the tinnitus. There are behind-the-ear and in-the-ear models, and they have independent volume controls.

TMJ   See TEMPOROMANDIBULAR JOINT SYNDROME.

tone control   A special device on a hearing aid that changes the pitch of amplified sound. See also HEARING AIDS.

tone decay test   A test that measures tone decay (auditory fatigue) that can be caused by pressure or damage to the AUDITORY (hearing, or eighth cranial) NERVE. In the test, constant tones are presented at the client's threshold. When it fades, the tone is increased 5 DECIBELS. The amount of decay is determined by subtracting the intensity of the initial signal from the intensity at the end of the test. Clients with a disorder of the auditory nerve will show a difference greater than 10 dB to 15 dB.

topophone   A direction-finder for sound used in the 19th century, this device (worn over the shoulders) helped localize sound because its two ear trumpets were very widely spaced, and therefore one collected more sound than the other. Patented in 1880, it was originally designed for use by sea captains to determine the direction of a whistle in thick fog.

total communication   This philosophy implies an acceptance, exposure and opportunity to use all possible methods of communication to help the deaf child learn to communicate. It is often confused with the SIMULTANEOUS COMMUNICATION (Sim-Com) method, which combines both speech and sign at the same time.

Total communication provides exposure and opportunity to learn all modes of communication and allows the child to use whichever mode is easiest and with which he is best understood.

Rather than focus on one specific training method, parents and teachers who use a total communication approach try to decide which mode is best for a child in any one situation. Options can include SPEECHREADING, speech, SIGN LANGUAGE, auditory training and amplification, writing, audiovisual methods, FINGERSPELLING and graphics.

Total communication was first described by a California teacher and parent of a deaf child, who combined signing and fingerspelling with speech and speechreading. In 1968, the idea was picked up and introduced by the supervisor of a program for deaf students in Santa Ana and then adopted at the Maryland School for the Deaf in the same year.

Within 10 years, two-thirds of schools for deaf students in the United States had begun to use a total communication approach to education. At the same time, the approach was gaining acceptance around the world, and by the 1980s it was widely used to describe a philosophical attitude toward education for deaf students.

Historically, the proponents of particular systems have often disagreed with each other. total communication has provided a compromise, adding to the increasing consensus that whatever system works best for the individual should be used to allow the hard-of-hearing or deaf person access to clear and understandable communication.

Still, schools that embrace total communication usually feature SIMULTANEOUS COMMUNICATION, which combines the manual and oral approaches at the same time. This combination remains controversial since some oral approach proponents claim sim-com does not produce good speech, and manual approach supporters complain about the manual English systems used with sim-com. See also MANUALLY CODED ENGLISH.

toxoplasmosis   A generalized protozoan infection that can be contracted by pregnant women who handle infected cats or their infected litter material. Toxoplasmosis can cause hearing loss in 17 percent of children infected while in the womb. See also PRENATAL CAUSES OF HEARING LOSS.

tragus   A projecting bit of cartilage in the PINNA near the opening of the ear canal.

transliteration   Technically, there are two separate terms for SIGN LANGUAGE interpretation. Transliteration refers to the interpretation process between a hearing person and a person using a manual code of a spoken language (such as SIGNED ENGLISH). Sign language interpretation refers only to the process of interpreting between speech and a true deaf sign language (such as AMERICAN SIGN LANGUAGE). See also SIGN LANGUAGE INTERPRETERS.

trigeminal nerve   The fifth cranial nerve travels from the brain stem and divides into three branches, which supply sensation to the face, scalp, nose, teeth, lining of the mouth, upper eyelid, sinuses and front part of the tongue. The nerve also controls the production of saliva and tears and stimulates contraction of the jaw muscles responsible for chewing.

Abnormalities of the facial nerve branch are often associated with ear malformation. About 60 percent of the population do not have a completely-covered facial nerve canal in the middle ear cavity, which can result in a sensorineural hearing loss. On rare occasions, the facial nerve interrupts the OSSICULAR CHAIN and causes a CONDUCTIVE HEARING LOSS.

TRIPOD   This organization provides a national toll-free hotline for parents and individuals wanting information about raising and educating deaf children. TRIPOD operates a parent/infant/toddler program, a Montessori preschool and an elementary mainstream program for hard-of-hearing students.

T-switch   See TELECOIL.

TTY   See TELECOMMUNICATIONS DEVICES FOR THE DEAF.

tumors of the middle ear   These rare growths can remain undetected until they become quite large and invasive, when both malignant and benign tumors cause a CONDUCTIVE HEARING LOSS by blocking the middle ear and external auditory canal, destroying the ossicles and interfering with the eardrum's movement. Malignant tumors can also cause a SENSORINEURAL HEARING LOSS as the growth protrudes into the inner ear.

Symptoms of both types of tumor include DIZZINESS, bleeding from the ear, deep ear pain, drainage and paralysis of the facial nerve. Middle ear tumors include CHORISTOMA, congenital CHOLESTEATOMA, dermoid cysts, meningioma, facial nerve neuroma, ACOUSTIC NEUROMA, glomus tympanicum and glomus jugulare.

Generally, it is uncommon to find a malignant tumor in the middle ear, but the most common malignant tumor found here is a squamous cell carcinoma or glomus tumor.

Squamous cell carcinoma usually appears in the external ear canal and moves into the middle ear, interfering with sound transmission. It may appear after a chronic suppurative OTITIS MEDIA but can begin to grow for no apparent reason at any age, although it is most common in middle age. Symptoms include a conductive hearing loss, a bloody discharge from the ear and pain in the later stages. Survival rate of this lethal skin cancer, even after treatment with radiation and radical surgery, is only about 30 percent.

A glomus tumor is relatively slow-growing and develops from clusters of nerve cells that regulate body function. These cells are located in either the jugular vein or the back wall of the middle ear. Patients with this type of tumor experience a conductive hearing loss as the tumor grows, filling the middle ear and eroding into the inner ear. More common among women, the symptoms also include a pulselike TINNITUS, which may be followed by a sensorineural hearing loss, DIZZINESS and facial paralysis. Treatment includes radiation and surgery.

tuning forks   An instrument developed in the 19th century and used today by a specialist to determine the presence of a hearing loss. Because it emits a remarkably pure tone as it vibrates, the tuning fork has been a basic tool for people trying to learn how the mind interprets sound. The standard frequencies of tuning forks include 128, 512, 1024 and 2048 Hertz. Four tuning fork tests used most often today are the WEBER, RINNE and SCHWABACH.

While the tuning fork has been replaced by electronic sound makers in some tests, forks are still used to support results of more formal audiological testing. Still, the usefulness of tuning forks is limited for a number of reasons: There is no way to accurately measure the intensity of tone; sound is distorted if the fork is struck too hard; there are problems in isolating response of the ear; and they are hard to use with young children. See also AUDIOMETRY.

tympanic cavity   An air-filled space containing the OSSICULAR CHAIN, this cavity is located in the temporal bone. It is linked to the nasopharynx via the eustachian tube.

tympanic membrane   See EARDRUM.

tympanic plexus   A group of nerves formed by branches of the facial and glossopharyngeal nerves and located on the mound between the round and oval windows. The tympanic plexus supplies sensation to the middle ear.

tympanogram   The graphic representation of ACOUSTIC IMPEDANCE as a function of ear canal pressure. See also AUDIOMETRY; TYMPANOMETRY.

tympanometry   The measure of ACOUSTIC IMMITTANCE in the ear canal as a function of air pressure in the canal. The TYMPANOGRAM is the graphic representation of acoustic admittance or ACOUSTIC IMPEDANCE as a function of this air pressure.

In a person with normal hearing, the acoustic impedance (opposition to air flow) is least when the air pressure is close to 0 (atmospheric level). As the air pressure changes from this level, acoustic impedance increases and acoustic immittance decreases. The air pressure changes stiffen the eardrum and ossicles, reducing energy transfer through the middle ear.

In a patient with a middle ear disorder, acoustic-immittance measures are different and the specific disease can be diagnosed depending on the tympanogram configuration. For example, SEROUS OTITIS MEDIA with fluid results in a flat tympanogram; on the other hand, a disrupted ossicular chain will produce a tympanogram with an abnormally sharp peak. See also AUDIOMETRY.

tympanoplasty   Surgery performed to repair the EARDRUM and/or OSSICLES (tiny bones in the middle ear). It is usually performed to treat CONDUCTIVE HEARING LOSS, provided that the COCHLEA and AUDITORY NERVE can benefit from the improved conductive function.

Normally, sound waves move from the eardrum to the inner ear by the three bones called the ossicles (hammer, stirrup and anvil). Chronic OTITIS MEDIA can erode or fuse these bones, causing some degree of conductive hearing loss. Tympanoplasty is the only way to restore some of the lost hearing.

One form of tympanoplasty (also called MYRINGOPLASTY) involves the repair of a perforated eardrum in order to prevent recurring infections and improve hearing. The hole is closed with a graft (usually taken from the patient's own body)—which is usually a piece of connective tissue from the surface of the temporalis muscle adjacent to the ear or the outer, thin covering of the cartilage from the tragus.

OSSICULOPLASTY is the surgical repair of a defect in the transmission of sound by the middle ear ossicles, usually as a result of chronic ear infection (otitis media), CHOLESTEATOMA or temporal bone fracture. Under general anesthesia, an incision is made next to the eardrum. Using a microscope, the surgeon repairs the ossicles by reshaping the bones or replacing them with either a plastic, cartilage or donor ossicle. The bones are reset, and the eardrum is repaired.

Although the operation often improves hearing, there is no guarantee of success, which depends on the complexity of the problem. If the malleus or stapes is missing, for example, the solution is less predictable.

tympanosclerosis   A MIDDLE EAR problem caused by a chronic middle ear infection. Often seen as a white area in the EARDRUM, it is caused when new bone is formed by calcification of the tissue in the lining of the middle ear. See also OTITIS MEDIA.

tympanum   The main part of the MIDDLE EAR cavity that lies between the tympanic membrane and the lateral bony wall of the internal ear.

typhoid fever   An infectious disease contracted through food or water contaminated with the bacteria *Salmonella typhosa* and sometimes resulting in HEARING LOSS. The infection is found in the feces of an infected person and can be spread by drinking water contaminated by sewage, by flies carrying the bacteria from infected feces to food or by food handling by typhoid carriers.

The bacteria pass from the intestines into the blood, then to the spleen and liver, eventually accumulating in the gallbladder until they are released into the intestine. People who recover from typhoid fever can continue to have typhoid bacteria in the gallbladder, which can be released into the intestine for years.

Epidemics still occur in developing countries, and immunization against the disease is recommended for anyone traveling to these countries. The vaccine is given in two doses with a booster shot after two or three years. Even so, the vaccine does not provide complete protection, and tourists should drink only boiled water when traveling outside developed countries.

Typhoid fever symptoms can take up to two weeks to develop after infection, and the disease can vary from a mild infection to a life-threatening illness. Symptoms begin with a mild headache, fever, loss of appetite and malaise, often followed by delirium. Constipation gives way to diarrhea, and during the second week of the illness, a rash breaks out on the chest and abdomen. The illness usually resolves within one month, but if treatment is delayed, fatal complications can develop.

Treatment with antibiotics can usually control the disease in a few days, although very ill patients may also require corticosteroid drugs. People who recover from typhoid fever have permanent immunity, although failure to take antibiotics correctly can lead to relapses.

umbo   The most inferior point where the MALLEUS is attached to the EARDRUM, the umbo is a prominent landmark for evaluating the normalcy of the eardrum during OTOSCOPY.

unisensory-auditory method   See AUDITORY-ORAL METHOD.

United Kingdom   The prevalence rate for profound prelingual deafness in the United Kingdom is estimated to be between .8 and 1.5 per 1,000 live births. About 62,000 people over age 16 have very severe hearing problems, and about 2.3 million have some degree of hearing difficulties. Approximately 30,000 people use BRITISH SIGN LANGUAGE as their main method of communication.

Early diagnosis (before age one) is emphasized in the United Kingdom; screening and subsequent diagnostic tests are free, as are HEARING AIDS, EARMOLDS, maintenance and batteries. Although only certain types of hearing aids are given to adults, children may be provided with any type of aid available. Once a child has been diagnosed, the family is placed in a home-based parent guidance program.

Education

The Royal Commission of 1889 recommended that every child who is deaf should be educated with the oral approach; consequently, schools throughout the United Kingdom adopted this method. It was not until 1968 that, concerned about the results of the oral approach, the government decided that, while oralism was still desirable, research into the manual approach should be conducted.

In 1982, the British Association of Teachers of the Deaf issued a proclamation promoting the oral approach but recognized that some children might benefit from additional help in other types of communication.

There are both residential and day schools available in the United Kingdom, and since 1979 the trend has been leading away from residential schools and toward placing children in regular schools with special help.

Many special schools for deaf children arrange for their students to attend technical colleges or other types of further education, and some schools offer advanced education specifically for people who are hard-of-hearing. The National Study Group on Further and Higher Education for the Hearing impaired in the United Kingdom publishes directories of available further education courses.

A few deaf students also go on to university or polytechnic schools, and specific facilities for deaf students are available at Sussex University and at the Colleges of St. Hilda and St. Bede of the University of Durham.

Continuing education for adult deaf people is also available through the Centre for the Deaf at the City Literary Institute in London.

Communication Services

Telephone communications are available for deaf people in the United Kingdom through a portable keyboard telephone known as Vistel, replacing earlier teletypewriters. Vistel has an acoustic coupler to which any normal telephone handset may be attached. The message is typed on a conventional typewriter keyboard, displayed on a traveling display on the top of the equipment and sent over the phone lines to the receiver, who can read the same message on his or her own display.

In addition, deaf people in the United Kingdom can have access to Prestel, an interactive terminal

with a large database of commercial and public service information. It provides thousands of pages of
information with a TV, a Prestel decoder and a telephone.

Also available to deaf TV viewers is "teletext," a
method of coding information in digital form in the
unused lines of a TV picture. Teletext also offers the
option to broadcast optional subtitles on ordinary
TV programs at the press of a button.

In addition, special programs for deaf people are
made available through the British Broadcasting
system, called *See Hear*, a show including news
and light entertainment in simultaneous speech,
sign language and open subtitles. Other special BBC
shows for deaf consumers include subtitles of daily
news headlines, a news roundup and a series of
educational programs in British Sign Language. In
addition, some companies are producing special
programs for deaf people in certain regional areas.

U.S. Deaf Skiers Association   This group works
with deaf members of U.S. ski teams involved in
international competition and promotes recreational skiing for hard-of-hearing people.

Usher syndrome   A genetic disorder characterized
by hearing loss and a type of progressive vision loss
called retinitis pigmentosa. Some individuals also
have balance problems. There are three types of
Usher syndrome:

- *Type I:* Profound hearing loss, early onset of
retinitis pigmentosa and balance problems.

- *Type II:* Moderate to severe hearing loss, delayed
retinitis pigmentosa and no balance problems.

- *Type III:* Hearing loss and retinitis pigmentosa
that worsens over time together with the possibility of balance problems.

Symptoms

Individuals with Type I Usher syndrome have a
profound hearing loss in all frequencies at birth.
Many people with this type of Usher syndrome say
they get little or no benefit from HEARING AIDS. Those
few children who have had COCHLEAR IMPLANTS can
distinguish some sounds (even those related to
speech) but still don't understand speech clearly.

The vast majority use sign language as their primary mode of communication and are culturally
deaf.

Children with Type II Usher syndrome are born
with a moderate hearing loss in the lower frequencies; in the higher frequencies, the loss is
severe or profound. However, hearing loss does
not worsen as the person ages. Only a small
amount of additional loss (about 10 decibels)
occurs over several decades in adulthood. Even
within a family, however, there may be some difference in severity from person to person. With
hearing aids, these children do well in regular
classrooms, usually with preferential seating in
the front of the class. These children most commonly use oral speech and language and are culturally hearing, though a few have moderate to
profound hearing loss and have gone to schools
for the deaf. When vision deteriorates, they lose
the ability to read speech from the lips. Because
the hearing aid does not fully correct the hearing
loss, they may become functionally deaf-blind,
particularly in noisy dark environments such as in
restaurants or bars in the evening, at dances or at
other social events. They may then choose to use
FM systems, avoid such environments or converse
in sign language.

Children with Type III Usher syndrome are born
with a progressive hearing loss which gets significantly worse with time. Type III has not been as
well defined as the other two types; only a handful
of reports have appeared in the medical literature,
and most of the documented Type III cases are in
Finland. The primary distinguishing feature in Type
III is that the hearing loss steadily worsens over the
years so that hard-of-hearing teens become deaf in
mid-to-late adulthood.

All children born with any type of Usher syndrome also have retinitis pigmentosa, an eye disease that causes gradual loss of vision. In the
beginning, the eye becomes less able to adjust to
low light, resulting in night blindness. As RP progresses, the field of vision narrows until only central vision remains ("tunnel vision"). Many people
with Usher syndrome will retain at least some central vision for a long time. In Usher's syndrome
Type II, onset of RP is typically delayed until the 20s
or 30s.

Humans need to use three senses to keep themselves balanced—vision, proprioception (feeling the position of bodies and limbs) and a vestibular sense (feeling changes in speed and direction). Children with Type I have a vestibular system that doesn't work; they can't feel changes in speed or direction, and as their vision decreases, their visual balance system becomes less reliable. Those with Type II have a normal vestibular system, but their visual system also becomes less reliable as their vision decreases. Scientists don't know much about the vestibular system of persons with Type III. As more information on Type III becomes available, a more clear picture of vestibular function will emerge.

Originally described in 1959, Usher's syndrome accounts for about 10 percent of all cases of congenital deafness. The condition is one of the rarer autosomal recessive genetic conditions, in which both parents must carry an abnormal gene at the same point on the chromosome for a child to be born with the disease. Because each parent carries only one recessive abnormal gene and one dominant healthy gene, they both have normal hearing because the dominant healthy gene on the paired chromosome counteracts the abnormal recessive one.

The presence of the abnormal gene is revealed when one-fourth of the children of a couple with these recessive abnormal genes inherit both abnormal genes and are born with Usher's syndrome. If a child inherits only one Usher-causing gene (the other gene of the pair cannot cause Usher), that person will not have Usher syndrome, but, like the parents, that child will be a carrier. If a person who has Usher syndrome marries a person who is not a carrier, none of their children will have Usher syndrome but all of their children will be carriers. If a person who carries Usher syndrome marries a person who does not, none of their children will have Usher syndrome, but there is a one in two chance that each child will be a carrier. All of the children born to parents with Usher syndrome caused by the same gene will have Usher syndrome. Scientists have identified genes causing all three types of Usher syndrome on five different places on the chromosomes.

Treatment

Although there is no treatment for this condition, regular exams by an ophthalmologist are recommended for all deaf children, which can help identify Usher's syndrome early (usually before age six).

There are a number of conditions that may be confused with Usher syndrome. Rubella (German measles) used to be one of the most commonly suspected conditions. Other syndromes are characterized by eye symptoms or hearing loss patterns which are different from those in Usher syndrome as well as abnormalities of other body parts.

utricle   A small sac in the VESTIBULE of the inner ear.

vertigo   A feeling of dizziness together with a sensation of movement and—most important—a feeling of rotating in space. It is this sense of rotation (either of the individual or the surroundings) that is an essential ingredient of true vertigo and distinguishes it from simple dizziness.

Vertigo is caused by a disturbance of the SEMICIRCULAR CANALS in the inner ear or the nerve tracts leading from them. It can occur in anyone when sailing or on an amusement ride, while watching a movie, or simply by looking down from a height. It also may be set off by motion sickness, brain disease, drugs (such as streptomycin) or damage to the AUDITORY NERVE.

However, there are more severe forms of vertigo caused by disease: LABYRINTHITIS causes sudden vertigo accompanied by severe vomiting and unsteadiness in conjunction with an ear infection. MÉNIÈRE'S DISEASE is also characterized by vertigo, sometimes severe enough to cause collapse. Sudden attacks of vertigo are usually assumed to be associated with labyrinthitis and are treated with bed rest and antihistamine drugs.

vestibular disorders   A condition characterized by dizziness or balance problems that can be as mild as the momentary imbalance after a whirling carnival ride—or disruptive and debilitating. Dizziness, or vertigo, is among the 25 most common reasons Americans visit the doctor, and U.S. physicians report a total of more than 5 million dizziness or vertigo visits a year.

In many cases, the underlying cause of a vestibular disorder can't be determined. Otherwise, head trauma often causes vestibular disorders among people under age 50. Ear infections such as OTITIS MEDIA and inflammation of the inner ear (LABYRINTHITIS) may also cause damage to the vestibular and hearing structures of the inner ear. Viruses may cause some vestibular disorders. High doses or long-term use of certain antibiotics can also cause permanent damage to the inner ear. Other drugs, such as aspirin, caffeine, alcohol, nicotine, sedatives and tranquilizers (as well as many illegal drugs) can cause temporary dizziness but not permanent damage to the vestibular system. If the flow of blood to the inner ear or the brain is reduced or blocked (as in the case of a stroke), damage to the vestibular system can result. Rarely, a slow-growing tumor on the nerve that leads from the inner ear to the brain (an ACOUSTIC NEUROMA) may interfere with the normal function of the vestibular system.

The most frequently reported symptoms of vestibular disorders are dizziness, unsteadiness or imbalance when walking, vertigo and nausea. These symptoms may be quite mild or extremely severe, resulting in total disability. Because the vestibular system interacts with many other parts of the nervous system, symptoms may also be experienced as problems with vision, muscles, and thinking, and memory.

In addition, people with vestibular disorders may suffer headache and muscular aches in the neck and back, increased tendency to suffer from motion sickness and increased sensitivity to noise and bright lights. Patients with vestibular disorders often report fatigue and loss of stamina and an inability to concentrate. Difficulty with reading and speech may occur during times of fatigue. When these symptoms are constant and disabling, they may be accompanied by irritability, loss of self-esteem, and/or depression.

Tests developed since 1984 enable physicians to diagnose some vestibular disorders that previously could not be documented. Modern diagnostic techniques for vestibular disorders rely on a combination of tests and a careful history of the problem. First, a doctor must complete a physical examination to rule out other causes of dizziness caused by heart or central nervous system disorders. Then the patient will be referred to a specialist (an OTOLARYNGOLOGIST or neuro-otologist) for vestibular testing. Because the vestibular system is close to the hearing apparatus, vestibular testing includes hearing tests. Eye movements often hold clues to vestibular dysfunction, so to record eye movements, doctors use a technique called ELECTRONYSTAGMOGRAPHY. Balance is an essential component of vestibular functioning. During balance testing, patients may be asked to stand on special platforms that record the movement of the body. This kind of testing is called moving platform posturography.

Treatment for vestibular disorders varies according to the diagnosis. In mild cases, the symptoms may disappear their own as the vestibular apparatus heals or the nervous system learns to compensate for the disorder. If symptoms persist, some patients can be cured completely, but for others, symptoms can only be controlled and not eliminated entirely. Treatments may consist of drugs, diets, physical therapy or, in severe cases, surgery.

Although most vestibular disorders are treatable, some people with the disorders find they are temporarily or permanently unable to work or carry on normal activities. Social Security disability as well as many employee disability plans cover chronic, severe disability caused by vestibular disorders, but such payments can be received only if doctors attest to the disabling effects of the disorder.

Anyone troubled by symptoms of dizziness or imbalance should see a doctor; if vestibular disorders are suspected, the family doctor or the VESTIBULAR DISORDERS ASSOCIATION can recommend experts who specialize in diseases of the inner ear and who can perform the necessary tests.

Vestibular Disorders Association A nonprofit organization established in 1983 to provide information and support to people suffering from inner-ear balance disorders (VESTIBULAR DISORDERS), including LABYRINTHITIS and MÉNIÈRE'S DISEASE. The Vestibular Disorders Association helps patients find knowledgeable doctors, distributes information about these disorders and provides videotapes, booklets, a quarterly newsletter and other materials about the problem. See also Appendix II.

vestibular Ménière's disease An atypical form of MÉNIÈRE'S DISEASE in which the sufferer experiences all the symptoms of classical Ménière's (VERTIGO, TINNITUS, nausea) except HEARING LOSS. See also COCHLEAR MÉNIÈRE'S DISEASE; VESTIBULAR SYSTEM.

vestibular nerve section A surgical procedure that replaces LABYRINTHECTOMY (surgical excision of the entire inner ear) for incapacitating VERTIGO in patients with usable hearing in the diseased ear. The selective vestibular nerve section with preservation of hearing evolved from the earlier practice of severing the entire eighth cranial nerve.

vestibular system This system—with its primary receptors located in the inner ear (the cristae of the three semicircular canals and the maculae of the utricle and saccule)—is responsible for the sense of orientation in space, for maintaining an upright balance and posture and for the ability to keep moving objects in focus.

There are five separate vestibular detectors, whose connections in the central nervous system allow the brain to integrate information from a variety of receptors in the eyes, the skin, muscles and joints. The vestibular receptor organs deal with the forces associated with head accelerations and changes in head position. As a result, nerves send messages to the brain centers that use these signals to develop a sense of orientation and to activate muscles that control automatic movements of the eyes, movement and posture.

Many of the vestibular pathways in the central nervous system are organized into reflex pathways, called the vestibular reflex systems, that stabilize and coordinate movements of the eyes, head and body.

Vestibular Development

Although the basic receptors and brain structures of the vestibular system are determined genetically, the development of vestibular function is a process that depends on use and interaction with the environment throughout life. These reflexes must be constantly adjusted in order to adapt to physical changes in the body's growing muscles and bones and to compensate for diseases or changes in the environment.

Research into the workings of the vestibular system is difficult because the fluid-filled receptor organs that detect motion and head position are encased in bone and therefore hard to study.

Vestibular Disorder Symptoms

The vestibular system is complex and highly interactive, capable of continual adaptations to changes in the body and the environment. Because it has many different parts, there are many separate symptoms when things go wrong, ranging from mild discomfort to total incapacitation.

These symptoms may seem unrelated to the ears but result from the complex interactions of different sensory modes that contribute to vestibular function and balance. The symptoms of balance disorders also vary depending on cause, location (one or both ears), age of the patient and so forth. To make things more complicated, the type of symptom—DIZZINESS versus imbalance, for example—may depend on the type of movement the patient is making at the time.

Primary symptoms of a vestibular system gone awry include: VERTIGO, sensation of falling, imbalance, lightheadedness, disorientation, giddiness and visual blurring. Secondary symptoms include nausea and vomiting, faintness, drowsiness, fatigue and depression.

Vestibular Diseases

Because vestibular signals interact with all of the major sensory systems and involve major brain centers, a large number of diseases can impair balance, especially among the elderly.

More than 90 million Americans have experienced dizziness or balance problems, and each year there are an estimated 97,000 new cases of MÉNIÈRE'S DISEASE, a disorder that affects the inner ear and causes episodes of vertigo, fluctuating hearing loss and TINNITUS.

There are many kinds of balance disorders, and motion sickness, with certain stimuli, can occur even in healthy people. Special environments (div-ing, high-speed flying and space travel) are situations for which humans are not genetically programmed, and therefore these reflexes must be overcome or reconditioned if humans are to be able to function in them.

vestibule   A portion of the labyrinth of the inner ear located between the cochlea and the semicircular canals. See also INNER EAR; LABYRINTH.

viral labyrinthitis   See LABYRINTHITIS.

viruses and hearing loss   Viruses are common causes of high-frequency HEARING LOSS. Among the viruses, herpes zoster has been known to cause a sudden severe deafness in one ear.

viseme   A group of speech movements or shapes of the lips that are generally indistinguishable from one another. For example, one consonant category of visemes are the *p*, *b* and *m* sounds. These three consonants make up one viseme and are said to be homophonous.

However, researchers have not categorized vowels into visemes since no two vowels are produced with exactly the same movements. This does not mean, of course, that it is not possible to confuse the vowels when SPEECHREADING, as many do look similar.

visible speech   A system of sound writing (or phonetic transcription) that describes oral sounds through written symbols. Developed by Alexander Melville Bell, it was the first attempt to systematize speech training. Although the system did seem to work for Bell and his sons, it was too intricate for other scientists and was not enthusiastically endorsed.

Bell's system included 29 symbols, with 52 consonants, 26 vowels and 12 diphthongs (a complex sound made by gliding from the position for one vowel to another; for example in "boil" or "house") that, Bell claimed, could be used to represent all of the distinctive sounds of speech (and therefore, all languages) by expressing the movements of the articulators for individual speech sounds.

The elder Bell considered his system to be a way to improve elocution and did not originally design the method to be used for teaching deaf students, although educator GARDINER GREENE HUBBARD saw the possibilities for use with deaf students and arranged lectures for Bell to discuss his system. But it was ALEXANDER GRAHAM BELL who first really developed the system as a way to teach deaf students.

Because his first experience in teaching deaf students with visible speech seemed promising, the younger Bell accepted an invitation to teach the method in Boston. In 1871, Bell introduced the system in the United States at the Horace Mann School in Boston and at the Clarke School for the Deaf in Northampton, Massachusetts, where it was taught for 10 years before it was discarded.

voice reflex test See LOMBARD TEST.

voice-to-sign interpreting Interpretation from a spoken language to a signed language. See also SIGN LANGUAGE INTERPRETERS.

Volta Bureau The headquarters of the ALEXANDER GRAHAM BELL ASSOCIATION FOR THE DEAF, this bureau houses the association's extensive library containing literature on deafness.

The bureau was created and endowed by ALEXANDER GRAHAM BELL from money he received from the Republic of France, which had awarded him its Volta Prize for his inventions. Bell envisioned the bureau as the best way to increase and publicize information about deafness and presented the bureau to the association in 1909.

Much of the archival collection belonging to the association is still housed at the Volta Bureau.

Waardenburg's syndrome A rare genetic syndrome that affects hearing, skin and eye color, and facial structure. About half of all patients with this disorder have a nonprogressive SENSORINEURAL HEARING LOSS ranging from mild to severe in one or both ears, although only a slight few will be profoundly deaf in both ears. There is a great deal of variation in the sensorineural hearing loss among people with the syndrome; at least half of those with the gene have no hearing problems at all. Only about one out of five have a hearing loss severe enough to require hearing aids. Some with the gene are totally deaf; others are deaf in one ear, yet have completely normal hearing in the other ear.

The disorder is genetically transmitted to offspring in a dominant manner (only one gene is needed to cause the syndrome). There is a 50 percent risk that siblings will be born with a variation of the syndrome. Still, only a few people who have this abnormal form of the gene show all the features of the syndrome, and only a very small number have profound deafness in both ears.

A Dutch eye doctor, P. J. Waardenburg, was the first to notice that some people with two different-colored eyes often had hearing problems. Dr. Waardenburg went on to study other characteristics of the syndrome that now carries his name.

Researchers believe there may be some connection between hearing and the development of pigmentation during fetal development.

Other symptoms include two different-colored eyes—usually, one eye is brown and the other is bright blue, but occasionally, patches of brown and blue are mixed in the same eye. As with the hearing loss, not everyone who carries the gene has two different-colored eyes; in fact, in some large families there may be only one or two such individuals. In addition to the distinctive eye coloring, those with the gene may also have a white forelock (a patch of white hair starting at the front of the head and extending backwards). In addition, gene carriers become gray prematurely in their twenties or thirties, but not all gene carriers have these distinctive markings.

In addition, people with the syndrome appear to have eyes more widely spaced than average. Eyebrows that grow together in the center are also sometimes a feature. In addition, there may be cleft lip or cleft palate or a colon problem (Hirschprung disease). These last two features are less common than the primary characteristics of the disease. Other than the hearing loss, most people with WS do not have any particular medical problems.

Because WS is inherited in a dominant fashion, families typically have several generations with one or more of the features. Many of these family members are unaware that they have the gene because the symptoms can be so mild. It's possible that WS may be much more common in the population than previously believed; as many as two to three out of every 100 children in schools for the deaf may have WS. Because most people with the gene have little or no hearing loss, for every child with WS and a severe hearing loss, there are four to five family members who have relatively normal hearing but also have the gene. See also GENETICS AND HEARING LOSS.

wake-up alarms Audio alarms, such as ordinary clock radios or electronic alarms, that have been adapted to flash one or several lights or to turn on a small vibrator under the mattress or pillow. See also ALERTING DEVICES; Appendix III.

Washoe See NONHUMAN SIGNING.

wavelength One of three measurements that describe a SOUND WAVE (the other two are amplitude and frequency). The wavelength is the longitudinal distance between the crests of two successive waves; the longer the wavelength of a sound, the lower its frequency.

Weber test This test determines which ear (if either) hears a TUNING FORK better by BONE CONDUCTION. The base of the vibrating fork is held on the center of the forehead or upper front teeth, and the patient is asked in which ear the fork sounds louder. If hearing isn't the same in both ears, the fork's tone will be heard in only one ear, or appear to be displaced to one side of the head.

A patient complaining of hearing loss in one ear who can hear the fork in the good ear may have a sensorineural hearing loss. If the sound is lateralized to the poor ear, then a conductive loss is suspected.

A mixture of both types of hearing loss will not be accurately revealed by the Weber test.

Weitbrecht, Robert H. (1920–1983) The inventor of the teletypewriter (TTY) for deaf people, which is the forerunner of the present-day TELECOMMUNICATIONS DEVICE FOR THE DEAF (TDD).

Weitbrecht was a deaf physicist who adapted a teletype model so it could be used to communicate over a telephone line with another teletype machine. Weitbrecht's modification was also called a TTY.

Because Weitbrecht's teletype was a surplus machine contributed by AT&T and there were only a limited number of these extra machines, only 25 TTYs were in use by deaf people by 1968. In that year, however, AT&T decided to donate surplus TTYs to deaf people and within several years had distributed several thousand.

white noise A blend of audible frequencies over a wide range that can be used to convert disturbing silence into controlled quiet or to mask distracting noises. Often compared to the sound of escaping steam, white noise basically serves the same purpose as background music in restaurants. White noise has been used by dentists to mask the noise

of the drill, which helps ease tension and pain. See TINNITUS MASKER.

Whitestone, Heather (1973–) See MCCALLUM, HEATHER WHITESTONE.

Wing's symbols One of the first printed systems to help deaf children learn to speak, read and write syntactically correct sentences. Devised in 1883 by a deaf teacher named George Wing, it used numbers and letters to represent the different parts of speech in written language.

Specifically, Wing placed number and letter symbols over words, phrases or clauses. The symbols were grouped into the "essentials," "modifying forms," "correctives" and "special symbols." There were eight "essential" symbols: subject, transitive verb, intransitive verb, passive verb, object, adjective complement, noun and pronoun complement.

word deafness See AUDITORY AGNOSIA.

word recognition test Another name for speech discrimination test. See also AUDIOMETRY.

World Federation of the Deaf This organization, formed by conference members during the 1951 World Congress of the Deaf, provides international visibility for deaf people and serves as an information exchange for deaf experts from around the world. Its main function is to hold international conferences, to help attain full citizenship for deaf people in all countries. To that end, it has represented their interests before various international groups.

One of the interesting developments contributed by this group is the creation of the first international sign language. Born out of the problem of communication presented by members from 57 different nations with many different sign languages and dialects, the federation first adopted French and English as its official languages. Since 1959, members have been trying to develop a true international sign language that can be understandable by all.

Its efforts resulted in GESTUNO, a sign language made up of 1,470 signs appropriated from existing sign languages that were the most easily-produced and the most natural referents.

The federation, which hopes to have gestuno accepted in other settings in addition to the annual congresses of the federation, now uses three sign languages at its plenary sessions: French and English sign language and gestuno. See also Appendix II.

World Games for the Deaf The deaf athlete's Olympics. The World Summer and Winter Games for the Deaf have been held every four years since they began in Paris in 1924. The games are administered by the COMITÉ INTERNATIONAL DES SPORTS DES SOURDS (CISS), a group recognized by the International Olympic Committee.

In 1924, Belgium, Czechoslovakia, France, Great Britain, the Netherlands and Poland met at Pershing Stadium in Paris for the first World Games, where deaf athletes competed in track, swimming, soccer, shooting and cycling. Since then, the World Games have grown in size and number of events.

Today, the summer games are held one year after the Olympic Games followed by the winter games two years later. Host countries are chosen by a majority vote at the Comité six years in advance.

To be eligible, athletes who wish to complete in the games must have an average hearing level for speech greater than 55 decibels in the better ear, documented by audiogram submitted in advance. In addition, an AUDIOLOGIST makes spot checks of competitors and retests all event winners. Hearing aids cannot be worn during competition.

Summer game competitions include badminton, basketball, cycling, shooting, soccer, swimming, table tennis, team handball, tennis, track, volleyball, water polo and wrestling. Both male and female athletes may compete, although women are barred from wrestling, cycling, soccer and water polo. Gold, silver and bronze medals are given to the first three winners, and diplomas are awarded to the next six finishers.

Winter games consist of alpine and nordic ski events and speed skating.

Competitions are conducted under the same rules as the Olympic Games, although some modifications are used to make auditory cues visible. The games are opened with a parade of athletes and raising of the CISS flag. Although the Olympic torch is not used, the International Olympic Committee allows the Olympic flag to be flown.

In 1966, the International Olympic Committee awarded its Olympic Cup in recognition of CISS' service to the cause of sports and the Olympic spirit. The 2007 Winter Games will be held in Park City, Utah.

xylitol   A type of wood sugar that can be made from the cell walls of most plants, refined from a naturally occurring substance called xylan, found most often in straw, corncobs, oat hulls, cottonseed hulls and wood. Some experts suspect it may help to prevent ear infections.

Xylitol is a common food sweetener, but unlike other sugars that boost bacterial growth, xylitol has been proven to inhibit the growth of bacteria. In particular it has been shown to be effective in preventing dental cavities by inhibiting *Streptococcus mutans*. Because the major cause of ear infections is *S. pneumococcus,* a species of bacteria closely related to *S. mutans,* some scientists suspect that xylitol might prove effective in preventing ear infections.

In a 1996 Finnish study published in the November 1996 issue of the *British Medical Journal,* scientists studied 306 children with a history of ear infections. Half chewed xylitol-sweetened gum (two pieces, five times a day—after all meals and snacks); the other half chewed the same amount of ordinary gum. During the two months of the study, 21 percent of the regular gum chewers, but only 12 percent of the xylitol group, had one or more ear infections. Most children in the xylitol group had no side effects, but two of them developed diarrhea (a known side effect of xylitol and other sweeteners). A small number of children (almost all of them of Jewish descent) have a congenital enzyme defect making them unable to digest xylitol. This harmless condition is called pentosuria.

Y-cord   A special cord found on a body-type hearing aid that carries amplified sound to two receivers.

Youth Leadership Program   The Youth Leadership Program is a unique training program for grassroots leaders and is jointly developed and sponsored by the NATIONAL ASSOCIATION OF THE DEAF and GALLAUDET UNIVERSITY.

The program provides participants with opportunities to sharpen leadership skills and learn new techniques that will help their home communities. The national program is offered biennially in odd-numbered years.

APPENDIXES

I. Statewide Services

II. General Organizations and Resources

III. Devices for People with Hearing Loss

IV. Genetics and Deafness Information

V. Health Care Delivery and Special Services

VI. Performance Groups

VII. Periodicals of Interest to Deaf People

VIII. Religious Ministries and Organizations for Deaf People

IX. Residential Programs for Deaf/Emotionally Disturbed Children

X. Summer Camps for Deaf and Hard-of-Hearing Children

XI. Training Centers for Hearing Ear Dogs

XII. Where to Learn Communication Skills

XIII. Books of Interest on Deafness

XIV. Sign Language Dictionaries

APPENDIX I
STATEWIDE SERVICES

ALABAMA

Department of Rehabilitation Services
2129 East South Boulevard
P.O. Box 11586
Montgomery AL 36111-0586
334-281-8780 (V); (334) 613-2249 (TDD); (800) 441-7607 (V/TTY in AL)
www.rehab.state.al.us

ALASKA

Alaska Division of Vocational Rehabilitation
801 West 10th Street, Suite 200
Juneau AK 99801-1894
907-561-4466 (V/TTY)
http://edu.state.ak.us/vocrehab/home.html

ARIZONA

Arizona Commission for the Deaf and Hard of Hearing
1400 West Washington Street, Room 126
Phoenix AZ 85007
602-542-3323 V/TTY; 800-352-8161 (V/TTY)
http://www.achi.state.az.us

ARKANSAS

Office of the Deaf and Hearing Impaired
1616 Brookwood
P.O. Box 3781
Little Rock AR 72203
501-296-1635 V; 501-296-1669 (TTY)
www.state.ar.us/ars/odhi.html

CALIFORNIA

State Office of Deaf Access
Department of Social Services
744 P Street, MS 19-91
Sacramento CA 95814
916-653-8320 (V)
916-653-7651 (TTY)

COLORADO

Colorado Vocational Rehabilitation Services
600 Grant Street, Suite 302
Denver CO 80203
303-894-2515, ext. 222
303-937-0561 (V/TTY)

CONNECTICUT

Connecticut Commission on the Deaf and Hearing Impaired
1245 Farmington Avenue
West Hartford CT 06107
860-561-0196 (V/TTY)

DELAWARE

Delaware Office for the Deaf and Hard-of-Hearing
Division of Vocational Rehabilitation
Department of Labor Building
4425 North Market Street, Third Floor
P.O. Box 9969
Wilmington DE 19809-0969
302-577-2850 (V/TTY)

DISTRICT OF COLUMBIA

Rehabilitation Services Administration
800 Ninth Street SW, Fourth Floor
Washington DC 20024
202-727-0981 (V/TDD)
www.ed.gov/offices/OSERS/RSA/rsa.html

FLORIDA

Deaf & Hard of Hearing Services Program
Division of Vocational Rehabilitation
2002 Old St. Augustine Road, Building A
Tallahassee FL 32399-0696
904-488-2867 (V/TDD)

GEORGIA

Georgia Department of Human Resources
Division of Rehabilitation Services
2 Peachtree Street Northwest
35-414
Atlanta GA 30303-3166
404-657-3073 (V/TDD)
www2.state.ga.us/Departments/DHR/

HAWAII

Hawaii State Coordinating Council on Deafness
919 Ala Moana Boulevard, Room 101
Honolulu HI 96814
808-586-8131 (V/TDD);
808-586-8130 TTY
www.hawaii.gov/health/cpd_indx.htm

IDAHO

Idaho Council for the Deaf and Hard-of-Hearing
1720 Westgate Drive
Boise ID 83704
208-334-0879 (v); 208-334-0803 (TDD) 800-433-1323 (V in ID)
800-433-1361 (TTY in ID)
www2.state.id.us/cdhh/cdhh1.htm

ILLINOIS

Division of Services for Persons who are Deaf or Hard-of-Hearing

Department of Rehabilitation
  Services
100 West Randolph Street,
  Suite 8-100
Chicago IL 60601
312-814-2939 (V); 312-814-3040
  (TDD)
www.dors.state.il.us/programs/
  dsdhh.htm

INDIANA

Deaf and Hard of Hearing Services

402 West Washington Street
Room W-453
P.O. Box 7083
Indianapolis IN 46207-7083
317-232-1143 (V/TDD);
  800-962-8408 (V/TDD in IN)

IOWA

Deaf Services Commission of Iowa

Iowa Department of Human Rights
Lucas State Office Building
Des Moines IA 50319-0090
515-281-3164 (V/TDD)
www.state.ia.us/government/dhr/
  #deaf

Division of Vocational Rehabilitation Services

510 East 12th Street
Des Moines IA 50319
515-281-4151 (V);
  800-532-1486 (V/TDD)

KANSAS

Kansas Commission for the Deaf and Hard-of-Hearing

3640 South Topeka Boulevard,
  Suite 150
Topeka KS 666011
913-296-2874 (V/TDD);
  800-432-0698 (V/TDD in KS)

Rehabilitation Services

Department of Social and
  Rehabilitative Services
3640 South Topeka Boulevard,
  Suite 100
Topeka KS 66611

785-267-5301 (V);
  785-267-5352 (TDD)

KENTUCKY

Kentucky Commission on the Deaf and Hard-of-Hearing

632 Versailles Road
Frankfort KY 40601
502-573-2604 (V/TDD);
  800-372-2907 (V/TDD in KY)
http://www.state.ky.us/agencies/
  kcdhh

LOUISIANA

Louisiana Commission for the Deaf

8225 Florida Boulevard
Baton Rouge LA 70806
(504) 925-4178 Voice
(800) 256-1523 (V); (800) 543-
  2099 (TDD)

MAINE

Division of Deafness

Office of Rehabilitation Services
35 Anthony Avenue
Augusta ME 04333-0150
State Coordinator: Alice C. Johnson
207-624-5318 (V);
  207-624-5322 (TDD);
  800-332-1003 (V/TDD in ME)

MARYLAND

Maryland Division of Rehabilitation Services

2301 Argonne Drive
Baltimore MD 21218
(410) 554-9404 (V/TTY)
www.dors.state.md.us/

MASSACHUSETTS

Massachusetts Commission for the Deaf and Hard-of-Hearing

210 South Street, 5th Floor
Boston MA 02111
617-727-5106 (V/TTY in MA)

MICHIGAN

Division on Deafness

Michigan Department of Labor
350 North Washington Square,
  Suite 250
Box 30659
Lansing MI 48909

517-373-0378 (V/TDD);
  800-729-2253
www.mfia.state.mi.us/mcdc/
  dod.htm

MINNESOTA

Minnesota Commission Serving Deaf and Hard-of-Hearing People

Human Services Building
444 Lafayette Road
St. Paul MN 55155-3814
612-297-7305 (V/TDD)

MISSISSIPPI

Department of Vocational Rehabilitation Services

P.O. Box 1698
Jackson MS 39215
601-853-5310 (V/TDD);
  800-443-1000 (V/TDD in MS)
www.mdrs.state.ms.us/

MISSOURI

Missouri Commission for the Deaf

1103 Rear Southwest Boulevard
Jefferson City MO 65101
573-526-5205 (V/TDD);
  800-796-6499 (V/TDD)
www.oa.state.mo.us/deaf/mcd/shtml

MONTANA

Montana Vocational Rehabilitation

1818 10th Avenue South, Suite 5
Great Falls MT 59405
406-727-7740

NEBRASKA

Nebraska Commission for the Hearing Impaired

4600 Valley Road, Suite 420
Lincoln NE 68510
402-471-3593 (V/TDD);
  800-545-6244 (in NE)
www.nol.org/home/NCDHH/

NEVADA

Rehabilitation Division

2810 West Charleston Boulevard,
  Suite H-79
Las Vegas NV 89102
702-259-3894 (TDD); 775-687-4452

(v, toll-free); 888-337-3839, ext. 4452 (V in NV)

NEW HAMPSHIRE

Program for the Deaf and Hard-of-Hearing
Division of Vocational
  Rehabilitation
78 Regional Drive, Building 2
Concord NH 03301
603-271-3471 (V/TDD);
  800-299-1647 (in NH)

NEW JERSEY

Division of the Deaf and Hard-of-Hearing
New Jersey Department of Human
  Services
P.O. Box 074
Trenton NJ 08625-0074
609-984-7281 (V/TDD);
  800-792-8339 (V/TDD in NJ)

NEW MEXICO

New Mexico Commission for the Deaf and Hard-of-Hearing
1435 St. Francis Drive
Santa Fe NM 87501
505-827-7584 (V/TDD);
  505-827-7588 (TDD);
  800-489-8536 (V/TDD in NM)
www.nmcdhh.org

NEW YORK

Office of Vocational and Educational Services for Individuals with Disabilities
One Commerce Plaza, Room 1601
Albany NY 12234
518-486-3733 (V/TDD);
  800-222-5627 (V/TDD)
www.regents.nysed.gov/
  monthres.html

NORTH CAROLINA

Division of Services for the Deaf and Hard-of-Hearing
Department of Human Resources
319 Chapanoke Road, Suite 108
Raleigh NC 27603
919-773-2963 (V);
  919-773-2966 (TDD)

NORTH DAKOTA

Office of Vocational Rehabilitation
Department of Human Services
600 South Second Street, Suite 1B
Bismarck ND 58504-5729
701-328-3999 (V); 701-328-3975
  (TDD); 800-755-2745 (V in ND)

OHIO

Rehabilitation Services Commission
400 East Campus View Boulevard
Columbus OH 43235-4604
614-438-1325 (V/TTY);
  800-438-1325 (V); 800-282-4536
  (V/TDD in OH)
www.state.oh.us/rsc

OKLAHOMA

Services to the Deaf and Hard-of-Hearing
Department of Rehabilitation
  Services
5813 South Robinson
Oklahoma City OK 73109
405-634-9937 (V/TDD);
  800-833-8973 (V/TDD in OK)

OREGON

Deaf and Hearing Impaired Access Program
Oregon Disabilities Commission
1257 Ferry Street, SE
Salem OR 97310
503-378-3142 (V/TDD);
  800-358-3117 (V/TDD in OR)

PENNSYLVANIA

Office for the Deaf and Hearing Impaired
1110 Labor and Industry Building
Seventh and Forster Streets
Harrisburg PA 17120-0019
717-783-4912 (V/TDD);
  800-233-3008 (V/TDD in PA)

PUERTO RICO

Vocational Rehabilitation Administration
Department of the Family
Box 924
Guaynabo PR 00970
809-782-0011 (V/TDD)

RHODE ISLAND

Commission on the Deaf and Hard-of-Hearing
One Capitol Hill, Ground Level
Providence RI 02908-5850
401-277-1204 (V);
  401-277-1205 (TDD)
www.state.ri.us/ricdhh

SOUTH CAROLINA

Vocational Rehabilitation Department
P.O. Box 15
West Columbia SC 29171
803-896-6630 (V);
  803-896-6635/6636 (TDD)

SOUTH DAKOTA

Communication Services for the Deaf
102 North Krohn Place
Sioux Falls SD 57103
605-361-5760 (V/TDD);
  800-640-6410 (V/TDD in SD)

TENNESSEE

Tennessee Council for the Hearing Impaired and Tennessee Division of Rehabilitation Services
400 Deaderick Street, 11th Floor
Nashville TN 37248-6300
615-313-4913 (V/TDD);
  615-313-5695 TDD
  (answering machine)

TEXAS

Texas Commission for the Deaf and Hard-of-Hearing
P.O. Box 12904
Austin TX 78711
(512) 451-8494
link.tsl.state.tx.us/tx/TCDHH/

UTAH

Utah Community Center for the Deaf
Utah State Office of Rehabilitation
5709 South 1500 West
Salt Lake City UT 84123
801-263-4860 (V/TDD);
  800-860-4860 (V/TDD in UT)
www.usor.state.ut.us/dsdhh/

VERMONT

Division of Vocational Rehabilitation
Department of Aging and Disabilities
103 South Main Street
Waterbury VT 05671-2303
802-241-2186 (V/TDD)

VIRGINIA

Department for the Deaf and Hard-of-Hearing
Ratcliffe Building
1602 Rolling Hills Drive
Richmond VA 23229-5012
804-225-2570 (V/TDD);
    800-552-7917 (V/TDD in VA)
www.state.va.us/hhr/vddhh

WASHINGTON

Office of Deaf and Hard-of-Hearing Services
P.O. Box 45300
Olympia WA 98504-5300
360-753-0703 (V/TDD)

WEST VIRGINIA

West Virginia Commission for the Hearing Impaired
4190 Washington Street West
Charleston WV 25313
304-558-2175 (V/TDD);
    304-558-0026 (TDD)

WISCONSIN

Office for the Deaf and Hard-of-Hearing

Department of Health and Family Services
2917 International Lane
P.O. Box 7852
Madison WI 53707-7852
608-243-5625 (V);
    608-243-5635 (TDD)

WYOMING

Division of Vocational Rehabilitation
Central Office
1100 Herschler Building
Cheyenne WY 82002
307-856-2393 (V/TDD)
www.state.wy.us/governor/boards/
    veterans/page11.html

APPENDIX II
GENERAL ORGANIZATIONS AND RESOURCES

Academy of Dispensing Audiologists
3008 Millwood Avenue
Columbia SC 29205
803-252-5646
800-445-8629
www.audiologist.org

Acoustic Neuroma Association
600 Peachtree Parkway, Suite 108
Cumming GA 30041
770-205-8211
www.anausa.org

Alexander Graham Bell Association for the Deaf
3417 Volta Place NW
Washington DC 20007-2737
202-337-5220 (V)
202-337-5221 (TTY)
www.agbell.org

American Academy of Audiology
8201 Greensboro Drive, Suite 300
McLean VA 22102
703-790-8466 (V)
703-610-9022 (TDD)
800-AAA-2336
www.audiology.org

American Academy of Otolaryngology—Head and Neck Surgery
One Prince Street
Alexandria VA 22314
703-836-4444 (V)
www.entnet.org

American Association of the Deaf-Blind
814 Thayer Avenue, Suite 302
Silver Spring MD 20910-4500
301-495-4402
301-495-4403
www.aadb.org

American Deafness and Rehabilitation Association
P.O. Box 6956
San Mateo CA 94403
501-663-7074 (V/TDD)
www.adara.org

American Hearing Research Foundation
8 South Michigan Avenue, Suite 814
Chicago IL 60603-4539
312-726-9670 (V)
www.american-hearing.org

American Laryngological, Rhinological and Otological Society
555 North 30th Street
Omaha NE 68131
402-446-5500

American Otological Society
2720 Tartan Way
Springfield IL 62707
217-483-6966
itsa.ucsf.edu/~ajo/AOS/AOS.html

American Society for Deaf Children
P.O. Box 3355
Gettysburg PA 17325
717-334-7922
www.deafchildren.org

American Speech-Language-Hearing Association
10801 Rockville Pike
Rockville MD 20852
800-638-8255
www.asha.org

American Tinnitus Association
P.O. Box 5
Portland OR 97207-0005
503-248-9985 (V)
www.ata.org

ASL Access
4217 Adrienne Drive
Alexandria, VA 22309
www.aslaccess.org

Association of Late-Deafened Adults
1131 Lake Street #204
Oak Park IL 60301
877-907-1738 (V)
708-358-0135 (TTY)
www.alda.org

Beginnings for Parents of Children who are Deaf or Hard-of-Hearing
P.O. Box 17646
Raleigh NC 27619
919-571-4843 (V)
919-571-4843 (TDD)
800-541-4327
www.beginningssvcs.com/

Better Hearing Institute
515 King Street, Suite 420
Alexandria VA 22314
800-EAR-WELL (V)
703-684-3391 (V)
www.betterhearing.org

The Caption Center
125 Western Avenue
Boston MA 02134
617-300-3600 (V/TDD)
www.wgbh.org/caption

Captioned Media Program
1447 East Main Street
Spartanburg SC 29307
http://www.cfr.org
864-585-1778 (V)
864-585-2617 (TDD)

Children of Deaf Adults
P.O. Box 30715
Santa Barbara CA 93130
www.coda-international.org

Cochlear Implant Association
5335 Wisconsin Avenue NW, Suite 440
Washington DC 20015
202-895-2781 (V)
202-895-2782 (TDD)
www.cici.org

Conference of Educational Administrators of the Schools and Programs for the Deaf
P.O. Box 1778
St. Augustine FL 32085
904-810-5200 (V/TDD)
www.ceasd.org

Council of American Instructors of the Deaf
P.O. Box 377
Bedford TX 76095
817-354-8414
www.caid.org

Council on Education of the Deaf
Department of Education
Gallaudet University
800 Florida Avenue, NE
Washington DC 20002
202-651-5530 (V/TDD)
www.educ.kent.edu/deafed/hane.htm

D.E.A.F., Inc.
215 Brighton Avenue
Allston MA 02134
617-254-4041 (V/TDD)
www.deafinconline.tripod.com

Deafness Research Foundation
1050 17th St. NW, Suite 701
Washington D.C. 20036
202-289-5850

DEAFPRIDE, Inc.
800 Florida Avenue NE
Washington DC 20003-3660
202-675-6700 (V/TDD)

Deaf Women United
215 Brighton Avenue
Allston MA 02134
617-254-4041 (V/TDD)
www.dwu.org

The Ear Foundation
1817 Patterson Street
Nashville TN 37203
800-545-HEAR (V/TDD)
www.earfoundation.org

Gallaudet Research Institute
Hall Memorial Building,
    Fourth Floor, South Wing
800 Florida Avenue, NE
Washington DC 20002
202-651-5400
800-451-8834
gri.gallaudet.edu

Genetic Services Center
Gallaudet Research Institute
Gallaudet University
800 Florida Avenue, NE
Washington DC 20002
202-651-5258 (V/TDD)
800-672-6720, ext. 5258 (V/TDD)
gri.gallaudet.edu

Hard of Hearing Advocates
245 Prospect Street
Framingham MA 01701
508-875-8662 (V)
hohadvocates.org

Hearing Education and Awareness for Rockers (H.E.A.R.)
50 Oak Street, Suite 101
San Francisco CA 94102
415-431-3277 (V)
www.hearnet.com

Hearing Industries Association
515 King Street, Suite 420
Alexandria VA 22314
703-684-6048 (fax)
www.hearing.org

Hear Now
9745 E. Hampden Avenue, Suite 300
Denver CO 80231
800-648-HEAR (V/TDD)

Helen Keller National Center for Deaf-Blind Youths and Adults
111 Middle Neck Road
Port Washington NY 11050
516-944-8900 (V)
516-944-8637 (TTY)
www.helenkeller.org

House Ear Institute
2100 West Third Street
Los Angeles CA 90057
213-483-9930 (V)
213-483-5706 (TDD)
www.hei.org

Hyperacusis Network
444 Edgewood Drive
Green Bay WI 54302
920-486-4667 (V)
www.hyperacusis.net

Institut National des Jeunes Sords
254 Rue Saint Jacques
75005 Paris, France
33-1-435-48280

International Deaf/Tek and DEAFTEK.USA
P.O. Box 2431
Framingham MA 01701-0404
508-620-1777 (V)
508-620-1777 (TDD)
www.deaftek.org

International Hearing Society
16880 Middlebelt Road,
    Suite 4
Livonia MI 48152
734-522-7200 (V)
800-521-5247 (helpline)
www.ihsinfo.org

Jewish Deaf Congress, Inc.
8400 Jeb Stuart Road
Potomac, MD 20854

Job Accommodation Network
P.O. Box 6080
Morgantown, WV 26506-6080
800-526-7234 (V/TTY) or
    800-ADA-WORK (V/TTY)
www.jan.wvu.edu

Junior National Association of the Deaf Youth Programs
207 North San Marco Avenue
St. Augustine FL 32084
904-827-2540 (V/TDD)
nad.org/jmad.htm

League for the Hard-of-Hearing
71 West 23rd Street
New York NY 10010
917-305-7800 (V)
917-305-7888 (TDD)
www.lhh.org

NAD Law Center
Gallaudet University
800 Florida Avenue NE
Washington DC 20002
202-651-5373 (V/TDD)
www.NAD.org/openhouse/
    programs/LawCenter.html

National Association of the Deaf (NAD)
814 Thayer Avenue
Silver Spring MD 20910
301-587-1788 (V)
301-587-1789 (TTY)
www.nad.org

National Black Association for Speech-Language and Hearing
P.O. Box 50605
Washington DC 20091
202-274-6162

National Board for Certification in Hearing Instrument Sciences
16880 Middlebelt Road, Suite 3
Livonia MI 48154
(734) 522-2900
www.hearingnbc.org

National Captioning Institute, Inc.
1900 Gallows Road, Suite 3000
Vienna VA 22182
703-917-7600 (V/TTY)
www.nciap.org

National Cued Speech Association
23970 Hermitage Road
Shaker Heights OH 44122
800-459-3529
www.cuedspeech.org

National Deaf Education Center
Gallaudet College
800 Florida Avenue NE
Washington DC 20002
202-651-5399 (TTY)
www.clerccenter.gallaudet.edu

National Family Association for Deaf-Blind
111 Middle Neck Road
Sands Point NY 11050
800-255-0411
www.nfadb.org

National Fraternal Society of the Deaf
1118 South 6th Street
Springfield IL 62703
217-789-7429 (V)
217-789-7438 (TDD)
www.nfsd.com

National Hearing Conservation Association
9101 East Kenyon Avenue, Suite 3000
Denver CO 80237
303-224-9022
www.hearingconservation.org

National Information Center for Children and Youth with Disabilities
P.O. Box 1492
Washington DC 20013
800-695-0285 (V/TDD)
www.nichcy.org

National Information Clearinghouse on Children who are Deaf-Blind
345 North Monmouth Avenue
Monmouth OR 97361
800-854-7013 (TDD);
800-438-9376 (v)
www.tr.wou.edu/dblink

National Institute for Hearing Instruments Studies
20361 Middlebelt Road
Livonia, MI 48152
800-521-5247

National Institute on Deafness and Other Communication Disorders
31 Center Drive, MSC 2320
Bethesda MD 20892
301-496-7243 (V)
301-402-0252 (TDD)
www.nidcid.nih.gov

National Organization for the Advancement of the Deaf, Inc. (NOAD)
18719 Set Point Lane
Humble TX 77346
281-812-2174
281-812-2174 (TDD)

National Rehabilitation Information Center
4200 Forbes Boulevard #202
Latham, MD 20706
301-459-5900; (V/TDD)
800-346-2742
www.naric.com

National Technical Institute for the Deaf
52 Lomb Memorial Drive
Rochester NY 14623-5604

716-475-6906 (V)
716-475-6906 (TDD)
http://ntidweb.rit.edu

National Temporal Bone, Hearing and Balance Pathology Resource Registry
Massachusetts Eye and Ear Infirmary
243 Charles Street
Boston, MA 02114-3096
(800) 822-1327 (V);
(888) 561-3277 (TTY)
www.tbregistry.org

The National Theatre of the Deaf
55 Van Dyke Avenue, Suite 312
Hartford CT 06106
860-724-5179 (V)
800-300-5179 (V/TTY)
www.ntd.org

Noise Pollution Clearinghouse
P.O. Box 1137
Montpelier VT 05601
888-200-8332
http://nonoise.org

Quota International, Inc.
1420 21st Street NW
Washington DC 20036-5901
202-331-9694 (V/TDD)
www.quota.org

Rainbow Alliance of the Deaf
c/o Karen L. Rosenthal
2424 South Cottonwood Lane, Lot #10
Tucson, AZ 85713
www.rad.org

Registry of Interpreters for the Deaf, Inc.
333 Commerce Street
Alexandria VA 22314
703-838-0030 (V)
708-838-0459 (TTY)
www.rid.org

The S.E.E. Center for the Advancement of Deaf Children
P.O. Box 1181
Los Alamitos CA 90720
562-430-1467

Self Help for Hard-of-Hearing People, Inc.
7910 Woodmont Avenue, Suite 1200
Bethesda MD 20814

301-657-2248 (V)
301-657-2249 (TTY)
www.shhh.org

Sign Instructors Guidance Network (SIGN)
814 Thayer Avenue, #252
Silver Spring MD 20910
301-587-1788

Society of Hearing-Impaired Physicians
2287 Mowry Avenue, Suite F
Fremont CA 94538
510-797-2939

Society of Otorhinolaryngology and Head-Neck Nurses, Inc.
116 Canal Street, Suite A
New Smyrna Beach FL 32168
386-428-1695
www.sohnnurse.com

Telecommunications for the Deaf, Inc.
8630 Fenton Street, Suite 604
Silver Spring MD 20910
301-589-3786 (V)
301-589-3006 (TTY)
http://www.tdi-online.org

Tele-Consumer Hotline
1910 K Street NW, Suite 610
Washington DC 20006
202-223-4371 (V/TDD)
800-332-1124 (V/TDD)
   (outside D.C.)
http://idi.net/hotline

TRIPOD
1727 W. Burbank Boulevard
Burbank CA 91506
818-972-2080 (V/TDD)
www.tripod.org

Vestibular Disorders Association
P.O. Box 4467
Portland OR 97208-4467
503-229-7705
800-837-8428
www.vestibular.org

World Federation of the Deaf
PO Box 65
00401 Helsinki,
Finland
www.wfdnews.org

APPENDIX III
DEVICES FOR PEOPLE WITH HEARING LOSS*

ASSISTIVE LISTENING DEVICES

AT&T National Special Needs Center
2001 Route 46, #310
Parsippany NJ 07054
800-233-1222 (V)
800-833-3232 (TDD)

Tele-Consumer Hotline
1910 K Street NW, Suite 610
Washington DC 20006
202-223-4371 (V/TDD)
800-332-1244
idi.net/hotline

HEARING AID INFORMATION

Consumer Reports
P.O. Box 1949
Marion OH 43305
How to Buy a Hearing Aid (reprint)
www.consumerreports.org

Council of Better Business Bureaus, Inc.
4200 Wilson Boulevard
Arlington, VA 22203-1800
Facts about Hearing and Hearing Aids
15-page pamphlet, one copy free
www.bbb.org

FDA—Office of Consumer Communication
5600 Fishers Lane
Rockville MD 29857
Tuning in on Hearing Aids
(one copy free)

Superintendent of Documents
U.S. Government Printing Office
Washington DC 20402

(*Note: Inclusion does not indicate endorsement; exclusion does not indicate disapproval.)

Facts about Hearing and Hearing Aids
31-page pamphlet;
order #SN 003-003-02024-9
Hearing Aids
order #SN 003-003-00751-0
www.access.gpo.gov/

SIGNALING DEVICES

Nationwide Flashing Signal Systems
8120 Fenton Street
Silver Spring MD 20910
301-589-6670 (TDD)
301-589-6671 (V)
301-589-5153 (FAX)
Burglar alarms, baby criers, doorbell signalers, fire/smoke alarms, answering machines, pagers, phone signalers, telecaption decoders, bed vibrators, wake-up alarms

AT&T National Special Needs Center
2001 Route 46, #310
Parsippany NJ 07054
800-233-1222 (V)
800-833-3232 (TDD)
phone amplifiers, doorbell and phone signalers, answering machines, telecaption decoders

TELECAPTION DECODERS

National Captioning Institute
1900 Gallows Road, Suite 3000
Vienna VA 22182-3865
800-845-1992 (V)
800-321-8337 (TDD)
www.us.nciap.org

AT&T National Special Needs Center
2001 Route 46, #310

Parsippany NJ 07054
800-233-1222 (V)
800-833-3232 (TDD)

TELECOMMUNICATIONS DEVICES FOR THE DEAF (TDD)

GENERAL INFORMATION

AT&T National Special Needs Center
2001 Route 46, #310
Parsippany NJ 07054
800-233-1222 (V)
800-833-3232 (TDD)

National Information Center on Deafness
Gallaudet University
800 Florida Avenue NE
Washington DC 20002
202-651-5109 (V)
202-651-5976 (TDD)
www.gallaudet.edu

NTID
Department of Public Affairs
One Lomb Memorial Drive
Rochester NY 14623
What You Should Know about TDDs
www.rit.edu/~490www/pubs.html

Self Help for Hard of Hearing People, Inc.
7910 Woodmont Avenue, Suite 1200
Bethesda MD 20814
301-657-2248 (V)
301-657-2249 (TDD)
Beyond the Hearing Aid with Assistive Devices
SHHH Information Series #251
www.aoa.dhhs.gov/aoa/dir/216.html

Telecommunications for the Deaf, Inc.
8630 Fenton Street, Suite 604
Silver Spring MD 20910-3803

800-735-2258 (Maryland Relay
    Service)
301-589-3006 (TDD)
*International Telephone Directory of
the Deaf*
www.teleport.com/~scheffel/
    tdi-online.org

Tele-Consumer Hotline
1910 K Street NW, Suite 610
Washington DC 20006
800-332-1124 (V/TDD)
202-223-4371 (V/TDD)

TDD Relay Center comparison
    chart
www.teleconsumer.org/hotline

TDD/VOICE ANSWERING
MACHINE DISTRIBUTORS

**Deaf Communications of
    Cincinnati**
550 Palmerston Drive
Cincinnati OH 45238

513-451-3722 (V/TDD)
    Brand: Mirac

**AT&T Information Products and
    Systems**
60 Columbia Turnpike, Room
    A-A210
Morristown NJ 07960
800-233-1222 (V)
800-833-3232 (TDD)

APPENDIX IV
GENETICS AND DEAFNESS INFORMATION

In addition, many large universities and hospitals have clinical genetic services. Ask your doctor or local health department for a list of genetic service providers.

American Society of Human Genetics
American Board of Medical Genetics
9650 Rockville Pike
Bethesda MD 20814-3998
301-634-7300
www.faseb.org

Genetic Services Center
Gallaudet University
800 Florida Avenue NE
Washington DC 20002-3695
202-651-5258 (V/TDD)
800-451-8834, ext. 5258 (V/TDD)

202-651-5000
www.gri.gallaudet.edu

March of Dimes Birth Defects Foundation
1275 Mamaroneck Avenue
White Plains NY 10605
888-663-4637
www.modimes.org

National Society of Genetic Counselors
233 Canterbury Drive
Wallingford PA 19086-6617
610-872-7608
www.nsgc.org

APPENDIX V
HEALTH CARE DELIVERY AND SPECIAL SERVICES

Association of Medical Professionals with Hearing Losses
Frank Hochman, M.D.
2287 Mowry Avenue, Suite F
Fremont CA 94538
www.amphil.org

One of the primary aims of this association is to encourage and assist deaf students to enter medicine as a profession.

Promoting Awareness in Health Care, Medical & Deaf (P.A.H., M.D.)
Medical College of Virginia Chapter of AMSA
1008 West Avenue, #2
Richmond VA 23220
http://views.vcu.edu/amsa/pahmd.html

This on-line discussion group is a network of people dedicated to bridging the gap between the medical community and the deaf community. Physicians, nurses, social workers and others interested in health care among deaf persons participate.

SHHH Hospital Program
SHHH (Self Help for Hard of Hearing People, Inc.)
7910 Woodmont Avenue, Suite 1200
Bethesda MD 20814
www.shhh.org/

This is a complete guide to enable hospitals to provide services for people with hearing loss in health care settings and to comply with the Americans with Disabilities Act (ADA). The program includes a 56-page guidebook (*People with Hearing Loss and Health Care Facilities*), a staff training video (*I Only Hear You When I See Your Face*), one "Patient with Hearing Loss" brochure, 10 "Tips for Communication" cards, two "Tips for Staff" posters, and stickers of the International Symbol of Access for Hearing Loss (50 1"x1" stickers; 5 5$\frac{1}{2}$"x7" stickers). The complete Hospital Program is $70 for members and $80 for nonmembers. Components may be purchased separately from SHHH at the address above.

CALIFORNIA

Health Care Partnership and Access Program for the Deaf
Greater Los Angeles Council on Deafness, Inc. (GLAD)
2222 Laverna Avenue
Los Angeles CA 90041
323-478-8000 (TDD/V)
www.gladinc.org

GLAD provides outreach programs to deaf people, including education on AIDS, family planning, sexually transmitted diseases and substance abuse. LIFE SIGNS, a 24-hour medical sign language interpreter referral service, assists in any situations where an individual requires immediate medical care in an emergency room, emergency admittance to a hospital, urgent care center or any emergency matters with law-enforcement personnel.

Special Task Interpreters for the Deaf, Inc. (STID, Inc.)
P.O. Box 482
Atwood CA 92811
800-STIDVIP (784-3847) (V/TTY)
714-996-3774 (V/TTY, in California)
www.stid.org

STID provides trained interpreter/medical aides for medical office visits, 24-hour emergency room and urgent care centers, surgery, recovery, childbirth classes, labor, delivery and all diagnostic testing procedures. STID provides information, advocacy and assistance in medical situations as well as referrals for further support. STID provides continuity of care—the same interpreter is provided for all scheduled medical office visits and hospital procedures.

FLORIDA

Crystal Oaks of Pinellas
Health Care and Rehabilitation Center for the Deaf and Hard-of-Hearing

6767 86th Avenue North
Pinellas Park FL 33782
813-548-5566 (V/TTY)

ILLINOIS

Silent Care
2711 West Howard Street
Chicago IL 60645
773-275-2378 (V/TTY)

A specialized nursing home program responding to the needs of elderly deaf persons at certain long-term care facilities throughout Illinois, providing comprehensive long-term care services to members of the deaf community in a homelike environment. Two sites are currently under development: Lincoln Park Terrace, 2732 N. Hampden Court, Chicago IL and Plaza Terrace, 3249 W. 147th Street, Midlothian IL.

KANSAS

Hear for You
Olathe Medical Center
20333 West 151st Street
Olathe KS 66061
913-791-4311
www.omci.com/omci/hearforyou.html

Hear for You provides 24-hour interpreter services to deaf and hard-of-hearing patients and their families.

KENTUCKY

Heritage Hospice
337 West Broadway
P.O. Box 1213
Danville KY 40422
606-236-3367 (V/TTY)
800-718-7708 (V/TTY)

Heritage Hospice, a four-county rural hospice, is accessible to deaf patients and their families. HOSPICE provides health care in the home under the direction of the patient's doctor.
www.mednexus.com/adverts/heritage/

MARYLAND

Deaf Services Program
Highlandtown Community Health Center
3509 Eastern Avenue
Baltimore MD 21224
410-342-8309 (V)
410-522-9528 (TTY)

The Deaf Services Program makes all services of the Baltimore Medical System accessible to deaf patients through full-time sign language interpreters, health care coordination and health education in sign language, including childbirth education and prenatal care. The Deaf Services Program assists with arranging medical referrals and special tests, advocating for an interpreter at the facility of referral, and also provides information and referral to resources for nonmedical services.

MASSACHUSETTS

Deaf Family Clinic (DFC)
Department of Pediatrics
New England Medical Center
Boston MA
E-mail: defdoc@aol.com

The Deaf Family Clinic acts partly as an advocacy agency for deaf and hard-of-hearing children.

MINNESOTA

Health & Wellness Program Serving Deaf and Hard of Hearing People
St. Paul-Ramsey Medical Center
640 Jackson Street
St. Paul MN 55101-2595
612-221-2719 (V)
612-221-3258 (TTY)

The Health and Wellness Program provides numerous services to deaf and hard-of-hearing people, including interpreting; sexual health and family planning; prenatal and parent education; sexual assault advocacy; and child abuse education, treatment and prevention. Mental health and community education services for deaf, hard-of-hearing and deaf-blind people are provided under the direction of Ramsey's Psychiatric Department.

NEW YORK

Jacob Perlow Hospice-Deaf Services Project
Beth Israel Medical Center
New York NY
212-420-4129 (TTY)
212-420-4543 (V)
www.whitmore.org/hospicedeaf.html

The Jacob Perlow Hospice-Deaf Services Project provides specialized care to patients with end-stage disease and can assist deaf patients with deaf or hearing families and hearing patients with deaf family members. This culturally sensitive and linguistically appropriate hospice program provides communication access to physicians, nurses, social workers, special therapists and chaplains through qualified and specially trained interpreters. Trained volunteers from the deaf, hard-of-hearing and adjoining American Sign Language community provide additional support.

APPENDIX VI
PERFORMANCE GROUPS

The following list of performance groups of and for deaf people are both professional and amateur, some touring locally, some nationally.

Cleveland Signstage Theatre
8500 Euclid Avenue
Cleveland OH 44106
216-229-2838 (V);
  216-229-0431 (TTY)
www.signstage.org

Deaf West Theatre
5112 Lankershim Boulevard
North Hollywood CA 91601
818-762-2998 (TTY)
818-762-2782 (V)
www.deafwest.com

Deafywood
14431 Ventura Boulevard,
  Suite 173
Sherman Oaks CA 91423
818-760-0164 (TTY)
818-760-0165 F
www.deafywood.com

Expression
Southwest Collegiate Institute for
  the Deaf
3200 Avenue C
Big Spring TX 79720
915-264-3700 (V/TDD)
www.hc.cc.tx.us/swcid/swadl.htm

**Florissant Valley Theatre of
the Deaf**
St. Louis Community College
Florissant Valley
3400 Pershall Road
Ferguson MO 63135
314-595-4477 (V)
314-595-2255 (TDD)
www.stlcc.cc.mo.us/fv/theater/

Gallaudet Dance Company
Physical Education Department
800 Florida Avenue NE
Washington DC 20002
202-651-5493 (V/TTY)
202-651-5591 (TTY/V)
www.gallaudet.edu/dance

**Gallaudet University Theatre
Arts**
800 Florida Avenue NE
Washington DC 20002
202-651-5501 (V)
202-651-5502 (TDD)
www.gallaudet.edu/theatre

**Illuminations. . . Theatre with
The Deaf**
1475 West Gray
Houston TX 77019
713-529-6909 (TTY)
713-529-6910 (V/F)

**InterAct Children's Theatre For
The Deaf**
1626 LeConte Drive
Maryville TN 37803
865-609-1646 (TTY/V)
web.utk.edu/~jdaniels/interact.
  html

Invisible Hands, Inc.
6213 Springhill Court #302
Greenbelt MD 20770
301-982-5640 (T)
813-685-2565 (V)

Lenoir-Rhyne Sign Troupe
Box 7483, Lenoir-Rhyne College
Hickory NC 28603

(828) 328-7347 (TTY)
(828) 328-7298 (V)
www.lrc.edu

National Theatre of the Deaf
55 Van Dyke Avenue, Suite 312
Hartford CT 06106
860-724-5179 (V/TTY)
860-300-5179 (T/V)
www.ntd.org

New York Deaf Theatre, Ltd
138 South Oxford St. #4F
Brooklyn NY 11217
718-398-5227 (T)
718-398-6794 (F)

**Northwest Theatre of
the Deaf**
P.O. Box 6435
Portland OR 97228-6435
www.idwiz.com/nwtd

Robert F. Panara Theatre
NTID Performing Arts at
  Rochester Institute of Technology
52 Lomb Memorial Drive
Rochester NY 14623-5604
716-475-6251 (T/V)
716-475-6787 (F)
www.rit.edu/~423www

Theatre of Silence
819 South Grand Avenue
Bozeman MT 59717
406-586-9201 (V/TTY)

APPENDIX VII

PERIODICALS OF INTEREST TO DEAF PEOPLE

AAAD Bulletin
American Athletic Association of the Deaf
1052 Darling Street
Ogden UT 84403
www.aaad.org

ALDA News
Association of Late-Deafened Adults
1145 Watgate Street, Suite 206
Oak Park IL 60301
www.alda.org

American Annals of the Deaf
Gallaudet University
409 Fowler Hall
800 Florida Avenue NE
Washington DC 20002
www.gallaudet.edu
    (Scholarly journal of research related to deaf
    education; published five times a year; $50/year)

ASHA
10801 Rockville Pike
Rockville MD 20852
www.asha.org

The Broadcaster
814 Draper Avenue
Silver Spring MD 20910-4500
www.nad.org/bcads.html
    (Published by the National Association of the Deaf)

CODA Connection
P.O. Box 681
Medford MA 02155
    (*Children of Deaf Adults* published quarterly)

The Communicator
P.O. Box 10076
Beaumont TX 77710
    (National Association for the Advancement of the Deaf)

Cued Speech Journal
Journal of the National Cued Speech Association
4245 East Avenue
Rochester NY 14618

Cued Speech News
Grate Media

1715 Eighth Street East
Menononie WI 54751
    (Published quarterly; $6/year)

The Deaf American **Monograph Series**
814 Thayer Avenue
Silver Spring MD 20910
    (Published by the National Association of the Deaf;
    $20/year, free to members of NAD)

The Deaf Catholic
814 Thayer Avenue
Silver Spring MD 20910
    (International Catholic Deaf Association)

The Deaf Episcopalian
1616 Calle Santiago
Pleasanton CA 94566
    (Episcopal Conference of the Deaf)

Deaf Life
c/o MSM Productions, Ltd.
P.O. Box 23380
Rochester NY 14692
    (Published monthly; $30/year; Special interest stories
    in the deaf community)

The Deaf Lutheran
1333 South Kirkwood Road
St. Louis MO 63122
www.rit.edu/~txecpm/ilda/deafluth.html

Deaf Nation
P.O. Box 3521
Grand Rapids MI 49544
www.icdri.org.deafnation.html
    (Monthly Newspaper $19.95/yr)

Deaf USA
Eye Festival Training Center
North Hollywood CA 91607
    (Published monthly; $20/year; general community
    news of interest to the deaf community)

The Endeavor
The American Society for Deaf Children
1820 Tribute Road, Suite A
Sacramento CA 93815
    (Organization newsletter for parents of deaf children;
    published bimonthly; $30/year; fee includes
    membership)

The Frat
National Fraternal Society of the Deaf
118 South 6th Street
Springfield IL 62705
www.nfsd.com
　(Published bimonthly; $8/year; insurance information
　and news about members)

Gallaudet Media Distribution Catalog
Gallaudet Media Distribution
Gallaudet University Library
Gallaudet University
800 Florida Avenue NE
Washington DC 20002
　(Published once every 18 months; deaf awareness and
　sign language instructional audiovisual resources
　available for free loan and for sale)

Gallaudet Research Institute Newsletter
Gallaudet Research Institute
Fay House
Gallaudet University
800 Florida Avenue NE
Washington DC 20002
　(Biannual; highlights work of the GRI.)

Gallaudet Today
The National Center for Law and the Deaf
Gallaudet University
800 Florida Avenue NE
Washington DC 20002
　(Published quarterly; $10/year. Special issues on
　deafness-related topics)

Gallaudet University Bookstore Catalog
Gallaudet University Bookstore
Gallaudet University
800 Florida Avenue NE
Washington DC 20002
　(Annual with periodic flyers; list of popular books on
　deafness and sign language; gift items and electronic
　devices for the deaf)

Gallaudet University Extension Catalog
Office of Extension and Summer Programs
College for Continuing Education
Gallaudet University
800 Florida Avenue NE
Washington DC 20002
　(Information on graduate credit courses, workshops
　and training sessions that can be offered throughout
　the country on request)

Gallaudet University Press Catalog
Gallaudet University Press
Gallaudet University
800 Florida Avenue NE
Washington DC 20002
　(Annual periodic flyers; catalog of books on deafness
　from scholarly works to children's materials)

GA-SK
Telecommunications for the Deaf, Inc.
c/o American Association of Deaf
8630 Fenton Street, Suite 604
Silver Spring MD 20910-3803
　(Published quarterly; $15/year; publication for
　telecommunication users)

Hearing Aid Journal
205 Benson Building
Sioux City IA 51101
　(Monthly commercial trade magazine; $5/year)

Hearing Health
P.O. Box V
Ingleside TX 78362
www.hearinghealthmag.com/homehtm
　(Published 6 times/year ($15) for deaf individuals and
　health professionals)

Hearing Heart Magazine
The American Ministries to the Deaf
PMB #173
7150 Hamilton Boulevard
P.O. Box G
Trexlertown PA 18087

The Hearing Instrument
1 East First Street
Duluth MN 55802
　(Monthly commercial trade magazine; $10/year)

HiP magazine
1563 Solano Avenue 137
Berkeley CA 94707
　(Nonprofit magazine for deaf/hard-of-hearing
　Children 8-14; published six times/year;
　$14.95/year)

International Perspectives
International Center on Deafness
Gallaudet University
800 Florida Avenue NE
Washington DC 20062
　(Three to five times yearly; highlights international
　activities relating to deafness and deaf education)

JADARA
P.O. Box 27
Roland AR 72135
　(Published 3 times yearly, $60/year; for professionals
　working with deaf people)

Journal of Deaf Studies and Deaf Education
Oxford University Press
2001 Evans Road
Cary NC 27513
　(Scholarly journal for research relating to deafness;
　four issues a year: $42/year; individuals; $120/year;
　institutions; $24/year students.)

Junior NAD Newsletter
Junior National Association of the Deaf
Branch Office
445 North Pennsylvania Street, Suite 804
Indianapolis IN 46204
   (Published nine times a year from September through
   May; $8/year; for young people who are members of
   Junior NAD)

Listening
The National Catholic Office of the Deaf
7202 Buchanan Street
Landover Hills MD 20784

The Nat-Cent News
The Helen Keller National Center for Deaf-Blind Youths
   and Adults
111 Middle Neck Road
Sands Point NY 11050
www.helenkeller.org

Newsounds
Alexander Graham Bell Association for the Deaf, Inc.
3417 Volta Place NW
Washington DC 20007
www.agbell.org/
   (See *Volta Review*)

Newswaves for Deaf and Hard-of-Hearing People
302 North Goodman Street, Suite 205-A
Rochester NY 14607-1149
   (A monthly general-interest national newspaper for
   people with hearing impairments and those who live
   and work with them; $18/yr.)

NTID Focus
National Technical Institute for the Deaf
52 Lomb Memorial Drive
Rochester NY 14623-5604
www.rit.edu/nyipwww/new/NTID.html
   (Published quarterly; free; NTID technical and
   professional education programs)

On Cue
The National Cued Speech Association
P.O. Box 31345
Raleigh NC 27622

Otolaryngology—Head and Neck Surgery
1 Prince Street
Alexandria VA 22316
   (Journal of the American Academy of
   Otolaryngology—Head/Neck Surgery)
www.entnet.org

OTO Review
House Ear Institute
2100 West Third Street
Los Angeles CA 90057
www.hei.org/welcome.htm

Our Kids Magazine
Alexander Graham Bell Association for the Deaf
3417 Volta Place NW
Washington DC 20007
www.agbell.org

The Quotarian
Quota International, Inc.
1420 21st Street NW
Washington DC 20036

The Receiver
Deafness Research Foundation
9 East 38th Street
New York NY 10016

SHHH Journal
Self Help for Hard of Hearing People, Inc.
7800 Wisconsin Avenue
Bethesda MD 20814
www.shhh.org/journal/hearloss.htm
   (Published six times a year; $25/year; educational
   journal about hearing loss for hard-of-hearing people)

Silent News
135 Gaither Drive Suite F
Mount Laurel NJ 08054
www.silentrew.org
   (Published monthly; $20/year; newspaper devoted to
   current events in the deaf community)

Tattler
Rainbow Alliance of the Deaf
P.O. Box 14182
Washington DC 20044
www.rad.org

Tinnitus Today
American Tinnitus Assoc.
P.O. Box 5
Portland OR 97207
www.ata.org

Transaction
100 17th Street NW
Washington DC 20036
   (Bimonthly published by the American Academy of
   Ophthalmology and Otolaryngology)

The Voice
11931 North Central Expressway, #11
Dallas TX 75243
   (Published nine times annually; $10/year; for deaf
   and hard-of-hearing people, health care professionals,
   libraries, agencies, schools and organizations)

Volta Review
Alexander Graham Bell Association for the Deaf
3417 Volta Place NW
Washington DC 20007
www.agbell.org/publications/periodicals.html

(*Newsounds* published 10 times, *Volta Review* five times yearly; $50/year membership includes both; promotes the association's goals of teaching speech and speechreading and the use of residual hearing)

Volta Voices
Alexander Graham Bell Association for the Deaf
3417 Volta Place NW
Washington DC 20007
www.agbell.org/publications/periodicals.html
(Magazine highlights inspirational stories from parents of children who are deaf and hard-of-hearing, legislative news, technology, updates and stories pertaining to speech, speechreading and the use of residual hearing. Published 6 times per year:

$50/year; $30/year for students/retirees. Fee includes membership and subscription to *Volta Review*)

Washington Sounds
National Association for Hearing and Speech Action
814 Thayer Avenue
Silver Spring MD 20910

The World Around You
Gallaudet University
800 Florida Avenue NE
Washington DC 20002
800-526-9105 (V/TTY)
(Published three times a year; $10/year; magazine for deaf and hard-of-hearing junior and senior high schoolers)

APPENDIX VIII
RELIGIOUS MINISTRIES AND ORGANIZATIONS FOR DEAF PEOPLE

Baptist Sunday School Board Special Ministries
127 Ninth Avenue N
Nashville TN 37234
800-436-3869

Catholic Deaf Apostolate
243 Steele Road
West Hartford CT 06117
203-523-7530 (V/TDD)

Cave Spring United Methodist Church
Ministries to Deaf Children
P.O. Box 305
Cave Spring GA 30124
404-777-8624 (V/TDD)

Central Bible College
3000 North Grant Street
Springfield MO 65803
417-833-2551 (V)
www.cbcag.edu

Christian Record Services
Division for the Deaf
4444 South 52nd Street
P.O. Box 6097
Lincoln NE 68516-1302
402-488-0981 (V)
402-488-1902 (TDD)

Deaf Missions
21199 Greenview Road
Council Bluffs, IA 51503

712-322-5493 (V/TDD)
www.deafmissions.com

Episcopal Conference of the Deaf
P.O. Box 27069
Philadelphia PA 19118
215-449-1602 (V);
   315-449-1602 (TDD)
www.open.org/~ecdhilda

General Council of the Assemblies of God
1445 Boonville Avenue
Springfield MO 65802-1805
417-862-2781 ext. 3258 (V)
417-862-1217 (TDD)

International Lutheran Deaf Association
1333 South Kirkwood Road
St. Louis MO 63122
800-433-3954 (V)
888-899-5031 (TTY)
http://www.rit.edu/~texpm/ilda/

Jewish Advocates for Deaf Education
5800 Park Heights Avenue
Baltimore MD 21215

Lutheran Church Missouri Synod
Mission to the Deaf and Blind
1333 South Kirkwood Road

St. Louis MO 63122
314-965-9917, ext. 321 (V/TDD)
888-843-5267
www.lcms.org/

Mennonite Board of Missions
Office of Deaf Ministries
P.O. Box 370
500 South Main Street
Elkhart IN 46516
219-294-7523, ext. 254 (V/TDD)

Mill Neck Foundation
Lutheran Friends of the Deaf
P.O. Box 100 Frost Mill Road
Mill Neck NY 11765
800-264-0662 (V/TDD)

National Catholic Office for Persons with Disabilities
415 Michigan Avenue NE,
   Suite 240
Washington DC 20017
202-529-2933 (V)
202-529-2934 (TDD)

Presbyterian Church USA
Education and Congregational
   Nurture
100 Witherspoon
Louisville KY 40202
502-569-5000 (V)
800-872-3283
www.pcusa.org

APPENDIX IX
RESIDENTIAL PROGRAMS FOR DEAF/ EMOTIONALLY DISTURBED CHILDREN

ALABAMA

The Learning Tree, Inc.
P.O. Box 908
Jacksonville AL 36265
205-447-9349 (V/TDD)

CONNECTICUT

PACES Program
American School for the Deaf
139 North Main Street
West Hartford CT 06107
860-570-2220 (V/TDD)
http://www.asd-1817.org

FLORIDA

National Deaf Academy
19650 U.S. Highway 441
Mt. Dora FL 32757
800-752-7345 (V/TDD)
www.nationaldeafacademy.com

Tampa Bay Academy
The Charter School of Tampa Bay
   Academy
12012 Boyette Road
Riverview FL 33569
800-678-3838 (TTY)
866-678-3838 (V)
813-677-6700 (in Tampa: V)
813-677-2502 (in Tampa: TTY)
www.tampabay-academy.com
www.deafprogram.com

ILLINOIS

Center on Deafness
Centerview Therapeutic School
3444 Dundee Road
Northbrook IL 60062
847-559-0110 (V/TDD)

MASSACHUSETTS

Special Needs Department
Beverly School for the Deaf

6 Echo Avenue
Beverly MA 01915
978-927-7070 (V/TDD)
www.beverlyschoolforthedeaf.org

Walden House
The Learning Center for Deaf
   Children
848 Central Street
Framingham MA 01701-4815
(508) 626-8581 (V/TDD)
(508) 875-9203 (Fax)
www.geocities.com/tlcdeaf/

NEW JERSEY

**Marie H. Katzenbach School for
   the Deaf**
P.L.U.S Program
P.O. Box 535
Trenton NJ 08625-0535
(609) 530-3196 (V/TTY)
www.mksd.org/plus/plus.htm

**Pressley Ridge Schools–Western
   Pennsylvania School for the
   Deaf Collaborative**
300 Swissvale Avenue
Pittsburgh PA 15218
412-371-7000 (V)
412-371-2233 (TDD)
412-244-4223 (Fax)

NEW YORK

The Lake Grove School
P.O. Box 712
Moriches Road
Lake Grove NY 11755
516-585-8776 (V/TTY)

Hillside Children's Center
RTF-Ely College
1183 Monroe Avenue
Rochester NY 14620

716-265-7757 (V/TDD)
www.cayuganet.org/hsc/hillside.
   html

OHIO

Buckeye Boy's Ranch
5665 Hoover Road
Grove City OH 43123
614-875-2371 (V)
614-875-6066 (TDD)
www.buckeyeranch.org

PENNSYLVANIA

Elwyn, Inc.
Program for Deaf and Hearing
   Impaired
111 Elwyn Road
Elwyn PA 19063
215-895-5500
610-895-5595 (TDD)
www.elwyn.org

WASHINGTON

Children's Hospital
Deaf Services Program
4800 Sand Point Way NE
Seattle WA 98105
206-527-3886 (V)
206-528-5028 (TDD)

WYOMING

Cathedral Home for Children
P.O. Box 520
Laramie WY 82073
800-676-1909
307-745-8997
307-745-0797 (TTY)
www.cathedralhome.org

APPENDIX X
SUMMER CAMPS FOR DEAF AND HARD-OF-HEARING CHILDREN

ALABAMA

Camp Shocco for the Deaf
Shocco Springs AL
800-264-1225 ext. 220
www.alsbom/org/campshocco

Space Camp and Aviation Challenge
For the Deaf and Hard of Hearing
Huntsville AL
412-371-7000 (T/V)
412-224-4223 (F)
www.spacecam.com

Summer Enrichment Camp
Alabama School for the Deaf
P.O. Box 698
Talladega AL 35161-2057
256-761-3222 (V/TTY)
256-761-3278 (F)

ALASKA

Camp Aurora
Adventure Camp for Deaf and
  H/H Youth
The Arc of Anchorage
2211 Arca Drive
Anchorage AK 99508
907-258-2232 (TTY)
800-770-3456 (TTY/V)

ARIZONA

Lions Camp Tatiyee
P.O. Box 6910
Mesa AZ 85216
480-380-4254 (V)
www.geocities.com/lionscampt

CALIFORNIA

Deaf Kid's Kamp
Sproul Ranch, Inc.

45446 Seventh Street East,
  Suite 21
Lancaster CA 93535

Camp Grizzly Youth Leadership Camp
Norcal Center on Deafness, Inc.
4708 Roseville Road, Suite 112
North Highlands CA 95660
916-349-7500 (TTY/V)

Deaf Camp 2003
California Lions Camp
P.O. Box 577663
Modesto CA 95357

Lions Wilderness Camp for Deaf Children
North Camp—Sylvester at Pinecrest,
  CA
South Camp—Teresita Pines,
  Wrightwood CA
P.O. Box 61
Mt. Eden CA 94557
888-613-1557 (toll-free: TTY/V)
877-896-1598 (toll-free: TTY/V)
www.lionswildcamp.org

COLORADO

Aspen Camp School for the Deaf
Box 1494
Aspen CO 81612
970-923-2511 (V)
970-923-6609 (TDD)
www.acsd.org/

CONNECTICUT

Camp Isola Bella
American School for the Deaf
139 North Main Street
West Hartford CT 06107
860-727-1300 (V)
860-727-1422 (TDD)

Camp Washington
190 Kenyon Road
Lakeside CT 06758
860-567-9623
860-567-3037 (F)
www.campwashington.org/

DELAWARE

Children's Beach House, Inc.
1800 Bay Avenue
Lewes DE 19958
302-645-9184 (V)
302-645-9467 (F)
www.cbhinc.org

DISTRICT OF COLUMBIA

Basketball Camp
Gallaudet University
800 Florida Avenue NE
Washington DC 20002-3695
212-651-5603
www.gallaudet.edu

Gallaudet University Sports Camp
800 Florida Avenue NE
Washington DC 20002-3695
202-651-5047 (TTY)
202-651-5603 (TTY/V)
http://athletics.gallaudet.edu/sports_
  camps.htm

Leadership Opportunities for Teens (LOFT)
at St Joseph Institute for the Deaf,
  St. Louis MO
3417 Volta Place NW
Washington DC 20007
202-337-5221 (TTY)
202-337-5220 (V)

"Let's Go Underwater and Visit Sea Life"
Gallaudet University

Child Development Center
800 Florida Avenue NE
Washington DC 20002-3695
202-651-5130 (TTY/V)

FLORIDA

Camp Endeavor, Inc.
P.O. Box 910
Dundee FL 33838
813-439-1300

Camp FSD for Hearing Impaired Campers
Camp Florida School for the Deaf and Blind
207 North San Marco Avenue
St Augustine FL 32084
904-827-2383 (TTY/V)

GEORGIA

Camp Best Friends
Hearing Impaired Camps at South Bend and Adams Park
675 Ponce de Leon Avenue, CH-E
Atlanta GA 30308
404-658-6381

IDAHO

Idaho Summer Camp for the Deaf at Camp Sawtooth
Idaho School for the Deaf and Blind
1450 Main Street
Gooding ID 83330
208-934-4457 (V/TDD)

ILLINOIS

Camp Sign
Chicago Hearing Society
2001 North Clybourn Avenue
Chicago IL 60614
773-248-9174 (TTY)
773-248-9121 (V)
www.chicagohearingsociety.org

Reynoldswood Camp
2814 Dekalb Avenue
Sycamore IL 60178
815-748-9088 (TTY)
815-756-5633 (V)

INDIANA

Indiana Deaf Camps Foundation, Inc.

100 West 86th Street
Indianapolis IN 46260
317-571-4258 (TTY)
317-251-3404, ext. 305 (V)
www.deafcamps.org

IOWA

Bible Camp for the Deaf
Deaf Missions 2003
21199 Greenview Road
Council Bluffs IA 51503
712-322-5493 (TTY/V)
www.deafmissions.com

Camp Albrecht Acres of the Midwest
P.O. Box 50
Sherrill IA 52073
563-552-1711
www.albrechtacres.org

KENTUCKY

DTQuest Summer Camp for Deaf Teens
1806 Addington Avenue
Louisville KY 40220
www.dtquest.org

Kentucky Lions Youth Camp
Lions Camp Crescendo, Lebanon Junction KY
626 Colonial Terrace
Frankfort KY 40501-1329
502-223-8514 (V)

Kentucky School for the Deaf
303 South Second Street, Box 27
Danville KY 40423-0027
859-236-7017, ext. 2333 (V/TDD)

MAINE

Cue Camp Mechuwana
Cue Camp Maine
13 Keith Street
Chelsea ME 04330

Hidden Valley Camp
RR1, Box 2360
Freedom ME 04941
207-342-5177 (V)
800-922-6737
http://www.hiddenvalleycamp.com

MARYLAND

Lions Camp Merrick

P.O. Box 56
Nanjemoy MD 20662
301-870-5858
www.lionscampmerrick.org

MASSACHUSETTS

Camp Paul
39 Concord Road
P.O. Box 53
Chelmsford MA 01824
508-256-4396 (V)

Clarke Camp
Round Hill Road
Northhampton MA 01060
413-584-3450 (V/TDD)
www.clarkeschool.org

Camp Joy Program
Horace Mann School for the Deaf and Hard of Hearing
40 Armington Street
Allston MA 02134
617-635-5041 (TTY)
617-635-4920 (V)
boston.k12.ma.us/mann/

SIGNS of Summer
Worcester Public Schools
Deaf and Hard of Hearing Programs
20 Irving Street
Worcester MA 01609
508-799-3026 (TTY)
508-799-3056 (V)

MICHIGAN

Camp Chris Williams
2929 Covington Court, Suite 200
Lansing MI 48912-4939
800-YOUR-EAR (TTY/V)
517-487-0202 (TTY)
517-487-0066 (V)
517-487-2586 (F)
madhs.us.net/training/chris.shtml

MINNESOTA

Courage North
37569 North Courage Drive
P.O. Box 1626
Lake George MN 55406
218-266-3658
www.couragecamps.org

MISSOURI

Camp Barnabas
Route 2, Box 131
Purdy MO 65734
417-476-2565 (V)

NEW JERSEY

Happy Hands Summer Day Camp
Camden County College
P.O. Box 200 College Drive
Blackwood NJ 08012
856-374-4855 (TTY)
845-227-7200, ext. 4255 (V)

NEW MEXICO

Apache Creek Deaf and Youth Ranch
Deaf Camp
P.O. Box 260
Reserve NM 87830-0260
505-533-6969 (V/F)
www.gilanet.com/apachecreek/
    deafcamp.html

NEW YORK

Children's Aid Society
Wagon Road Camp
105 East 22nd Street
New York NY 10010-5413
914-238-4761 (V)

Explore Your Future Camp
National Technical Institute for
    the Deaf
52 Lomb Memorial Drive
Rochester NY 14623
585-475-6705 (V/TDD)

OREGON

Camp Taloali
P.O. Box 4758
Salem OR 97383
503-679-6415 (TTY/V)
www.taloali.com

Meadowood Springs Speech and Hearing Camp
P.O. Box 1025
Pendleton OR 97801-0030
541-276-2752 V
www.meadowoodsprings.com

PENNSYLVANIA

PA Lions Beacon Lodge Camp
114 State Road 103 S
Mount Union PA 17066-0000
717-242-1113 (V)
http://www.columbiapa.org/
    coalition/agencies/lions.beacon.
    html

Camp H.E.R.O.
(Here Everyone Really Is One!)
at Camp Victory, Millville, PA
Bloomsburg University
Navy Hall Office 16B
Bloomsburg PA 17815
570-389-5131 (V)

Camp Overbrook: In Sign 2003
St. Charles Borromeo Seminary
Wynnewood PA
215-587-0510 (TTY)

Camp Ramah
The Pavilion Suite 734
261 Old York Road
Jenkintown PA 19046
610-924-9531 (TTY)
215-885-8556 (V)

Lions Camp Kirby
1735 Narrows Hill Road
Upper Black Eddy PA 18972
610-982-5731
215-249-3710
lionscampkirby.org

SOUTH CAROLINA

Reach for the Stars Camp
South Carolina School for the Deaf
    and the Blind
355 Cedar Springs Road
Spartanburg SC 29302
864-577-7640 (TTY/V)
888-447-2732 (toll free)

SOUTH DAKOTA

National Middlers Leadership and Literacy Camp (NMLLC)
Camp Lakodia, Madison, SD
102 North Krohn Place
Sioux Falls SD 57103
866-273-3323 T (TTY, toll free)
800-642-6410 (V)
www.c-s-d.org

TENNESSEE

Deaf Camps at Bill Rice Ranch
627 Bill Rice Ranch Road
Murfreesboro TN 37128-4255
800-253-7423 (V/TDD)
www.billriceranch.org/deafweeks.
    htm

Camp SummerSign
Brentwood Baptist Deaf Church
7777 Concord Road
Brentwood TN 37027
615-373-9574 (TTY)
615-850-3194 (V)
www.brentwoodbaptist.com

TEXAS

Isaiah's Place
231 HRC 1207
Whitney TX 76692
254-694-7771 (V)
www.isaiahsplace.org

VERMONT

Austine Green Mountain Lions Camp
60 Austine Drive
Brattleboro VT 05301
802-258-9502 (TTY/V)
www.state.vt.us/schools/aus/

WASHINGTON

Camp Sealth
8511 15th Avenue NE
Seattle WA 98115
206-524-8550 (V)

Camp Don Bosco
CYO Outdoor Ministries
Archdiocese of Seattle
910 Marion Street
Seattle WA 98104
206-382-4851 (V)

WISCONSIN

Wisconsin Lions Camp
3834 County Road A
Rosholt WI 54473
715-677-4761 (V/TDD)
www.wi-net.com/~lioncamp/
    index.html

APPENDIX XI
TRAINING CENTERS FOR HEARING EAR DOGS

NATIONAL PROGRAMS

American Humane Association
9725 East Hampden Avenue
Denver CO 80231
303-695-0811
www.americanhumane.org

Canine Companions for Independence
P.O. Box 446
Santa Rosa CA 95402
800-572-2275
www.caninecompanions.org

Canine Helpers for the Handicapped, Inc.
5699-5705 Ridge Road
Lockport NY 14094
716-433-4035 (V/TDD)
caninehelpers.netfirms.com

Dogs for the Deaf, Inc.
10175 Wheeler Road
Central Point OR 97502-9360
541-826-9220
www.dogsforthedeaf.org

International Hearing Dogs, Inc.
5901 East 89th Avenue
Henderson CO 80640
303-287-3277 (V/TDD)

National Education for Assistance Dog Services
P.O. Box 213
West Boylston MA 01583
978-422-9064 (V/TDD)

National Hearing Dog Center
1116 South Main
Athol MA 01331-2108
508-249-9264 (V)

REGIONAL PROGRAMS

CALIFORNIA

Companion Animal Program for the Deaf
Riverside Humane Society
5791 Fremont Street
Riverside CA 92504
909-688-4340 (V)

San Francisco SPCA
Hearing Dog Program
2500 16th Street
San Francisco CA 94103
415-554-3020 (V)
415-554-3022 (TDD)
www.sfpca.org

CONNECTICUT

Connecticut Hearing Dog Program
239 Maple Hill Avenue
Newington CT 02504
203-666-4648 (TDD/V)

MARYLAND

Canine Companions
14238 Briarwood Terrace
Rockville MD 20853
301-460-3040 (V/TDD)
www.caninecompanions.org

MICHIGAN

Ears for the Deaf, Inc.
1235 100th Street SE
Byron Center MI 49302
616-698-0688 (V/TDD)

Paws with a Cause
4646 South Division
Wayland MI 49348
616-877-PAWS (V/TDD)
800-253-PAWS (V/TDD)
www.pawswithacause.org

MINNESOTA

Hearing Dog Program of Minnesota
2223 East 35th Street
Minneapolis MN 55407
612-729-5986 (V)
612-729-5914 (TDD)

OHIO

Hearing Dogs of Columbus, Inc.
290 North Hamilton Road
Columbus OH 43230-2606
614-471-7397 (V/TDD)

SOUTH CAROLINA

Southeastern Assistance Dogs (SEAD)
Speech, Hearing and Learning Center
811 Pendleton Street
9-11 Medical Court
Greenville SC 29601
803-235-6065 (V/TDD)

APPENDIX XII

WHERE TO LEARN COMMUNICATION SKILLS

AUDITORY TRAINING CLASSES

Auditory training classes and instruction in listening skills help hard-of-hearing people learn to use their remaining hearing. For more information, call:

**American Speech-Language-
Hearing Association Helpline**
800-638-8255 (V/TDD)

CUED SPEECH

**National Cued Speech
Association**
23970 Hermitage Road
Shaker Heights OH 44122
800-459-3529
www.cuedspeech.org

Cue Speech Discovery
23970 Hermitage Road
Cleveland OH 44122
216-292-6213
www.isl.net/~cuedspmn

**West Coast Cued Speech
Programs**
348 Cernon Street
Vacaville CA 95688
707-448-4060

SIGN LANGUAGE

The best way to learn sign is with a teacher in a class. Contact the following:

- local school system, community college or university extension program
- state or county department of public instruction, education or special education
- county vocational rehabilitation services (many states have a coordinator of services for the deaf)
- United Way
- recreation and community centers (YWCA, YMCA)
- adult education/continuing education centers
- religious organizations
- libraries
- deafness-related organizations or groups (see Appendixes I and II)
- state school for the deaf
- state office/commission or state association for the deaf (see Appendixes I and II)

In addition, each April the *American Annals of the Deaf* includes a comprehensive list of services, schools and classes for deaf students. These would be good contacts for information on the availability of sign language.

If there are no classes available, text and tape materials are available. Check your local library.

SPEECHREADING

For more information, contact:

**American Speech-Language-
Hearing Association Helpline**
800-638-8255 (V/TDD)
www.asha.org/index.htm

**Alexander Graham Bell
Association for the Deaf**
3417 Volta Place NW
Washington DC 20007
202-337-5220 (V/TDD)
www.agbell.org

APPENDIX XIII
BOOKS OF INTEREST ON DEAFNESS

Chute, Patricia M., and Nevins, Mary Ellen. *The Parent's Guide to Cochlear Implants.* Washington D.C.: Gallaudet University Press, 2002.
A straightforward, thorough, and highly accessible guide written especially for the parents of deaf children detailing everything there is to know about cochlear implants, including a no-nonsense discussion of their pros and cons.

Cohen, Leah Hagar. *Train Go Sorry: Inside a Deaf World.* Boston: Houghton Mifflin Company, 1994
A good introductory book for grades 9 through early college that discusses the author's experiences as the daughter of the principal for Lexington School for the Deaf and as a member of the deaf community.

Groce, Nora Ellen. *Everyone Here Spoke Sign Language: Hereditary Deafness on Martha's Vineyard.* Cambridge, Mass.: Harvard University Press, 1985.
A study of hereditary deafness on Martha's Vineyard. Since almost everyone on the island knew someone who was deaf, most people spoke sign language and there was not much social differentiation between the deaf and nondeaf.

Kisor, Henry. *What's That Pig Outdoors?: A Memoir of Deafness.* New York: Penguin Books, 1990.
Kisor's book from the oral perspective about his experiences as a deaf person offers a different point of view from books discussing the cultural deaf position.

Lane, Harlan. *When the Mind Hears: A History of the Deaf.* New York: Random House, 1976.
One of the first real histories of the U.S. deaf community. Written in the first person.

———. *The Mask of Benevolence: Disabling the Deaf Community.* New York: Knopf, 1992.
This widely acclaimed book discusses oralism and the history of oppression of the deaf community, although it does avoid differences within the deaf community.

Lowell, Gloria Roth, and Brooks, Karen Strormer. *Elana's Ears, or How I Became the Best Big Sister in the World.* Washington, D.C.: American Psychological Association, 2000.

A funny, informative picture book for ages four to eight about deafness and pets.

Luczak, Raymond. *Eyes of Desire: A Deaf Gay & Lesbian Reader.* Boston: Alyson Publications, 1993.
A collection of short autobiographical stories by gay and lesbian deaf individuals.

Medwid, Daria, and Weston, Denise Chapman. *Kid-Friendly Parenting With Dear and Hard of Hearing Children: A Treasury of Fun Activities Toward Better Behavior.* Washington, D.C.: Clerc, 2002.
A child-friendly, deaf-friendly, parent-friendly guide that focuses on parenting and dealing with childhood behaviors.

Padden, Carol, and Humphries, Tom. *Deaf in America: Voices from a Culture.* Cambridge, Mass.: Harvard University Press, 1988.
This book stresses the cultural aspects of the U.S. deaf community.

Preston, Paul Michael. *Mother Father Deaf: Living Between Sound and Silence.* Cambridge, Mass.: Harvard University Press, 1994.
This book discusses the difficulties experienced by children of deaf adults (CODAs) and tries to evaluate how to overcome the linguistic and cultural barriers between the deaf and hearing people.

Schwartz, Sue. *Choices in Deafness: A Parents' Guide to Communication Options.* Bethesda: Woodbine House, 2003.
A straightforward, comprehensive discussion of various methodologies of teaching communication to deaf children.

Van Cleve, John Vickrey, and Crouch, Barry A. *A Place of Their Own: Creating the Deaf Community in America.* Washington, D.C.: Gallaudet University Press, 1989.
A major text on the deaf community

Walker, Lou Ann. *Hand, Heart, and Mind: The Story of the Education of America's Deaf People.* New York: Dial Books, 1994.
An excellent children's book on deaf culture, it is designed to help grade-schoolers better understand the deaf community.

Wrigley, Owen. *The Politics of Deafness.* Washington, D.C.: Gallaudet Press, 1997.
An interesting academic text on the politics of deafness.

SUGGESTED READINGS FOR CHILDREN AND PARENTS

For Children:

Arthur, Catherine. *My Sister's Silent World.* Chicago: Children's Press, 1979.

Blatchford, Claire. *Yes, I Wear A Hearing Aid.* New York: Lexington School for the Deaf, 1976.

Glazzard, Margaret H. *Meet Camille & Danielle: They Are Special Persons.* Lawrence, Kaus.: H&H Enterprises, 1978.

Hlibok, Bruce. *Silent Dancer.* New York: Messner, 1981.

LaMore, Gregory S. *Now I Understand.* Washington, D.C.: Gallaudet University Press.

Peterson, Jeanne W. *I Have A Sister, My Sister Is Deaf.* New York: Harper & Row, 1977.

Rosenberg, Maxine. *My Friend Leslie: The Story of a Handicapped Child.* New York: Lothrop, Lee & Shepard, 1983.

Scott, Virginia. *Belonging.* Washington, D.C.: Gallaudet University Press, 1986.

Walker, Lou Ann. *Amy, the Story of a Deaf Child.* New York: Lodestar Books/Dutton, 1985.

Wolf, Bernard. *Anna's Silent World.* New York: Lippincott, 1977.

For Parents:

Angus, Jean R. *Watch My Words: An Open Letter to Parents of Young Deaf Children.* Cincinnati, Ohio: Forward Movement Publications, 1974.

Benderly, Beryl L. *Dancing Without Music: Deafness in America.* New York: Anchor Press/Doubleday, 1980.

Featherstone, Helen. *A Difference In The Family, Living With a Disabled Child.* New York: Penguin Books, 1981.

Ferris, Caren. *A Hug Just Isn't Enough.* Washington, D.C.: Gallaudet University Press, 1980.

Forecki, Marcia C. *Speak to Me.* Washington, D.C.: Gallaudet University Press, 1985.

Frederickson, Jeannette. *Life After Deaf.* Silver Spring, Md.: National Association of the Deaf, 1985.

Glick, Ferne P., and D. Pellman. *Breaking Silence: A Family Grows With Deafness.* Scotsdale, Pa.: Herald Press, 1982.

Harris, George. *Broken Ears, Wounded Hearts.* Washington, D.C.: Gallaudet University Press, 1983.

Ling, Daniel, ed. *Early Intervention for Hearing-Impaired Children: Oral Options.* San Diego, Calif.: College Hill Press, 1984.

Luterman, David. *Deafness in the Family.* Boston, Mass.: Little, Brown, 1987.

Meadow, Kathryn P. *Deafness and Child Development.* Berkeley, Calif.: University of California Press, 1980.

Mendelsohn, Jacqueline Z., and Bonnie Fairchild. *Years of Challenge, A Guide For Parents of Hearing Impaired Adolescents.* Silver Spring, Md: National Association of the Deaf, 1982.

Ogden, Paul, and Suzanne Lipsett. *The Silent Garden: Understanding the Hearing Impaired Child.* New York: St. Martin's Press, 1982.

Schwartz, Sue, ed. *Choices in Deafness: A Parents' Guide.* Kensington, Md.: Woodbine House, 1987.

Spradley, Thomas S., and James P. Spradley. *Deaf Like Me.* Washington, D.C.: Gallaudet University Press, 1985.

Tweedie, David, and Edgar Shroyer, eds. *The Multihandicapped Hearing Impaired: Identification and Instruction.* Washington, D.C.: Gallaudet University Press, 1982.

APPENDIX XIV
SIGN LANGUAGE DICTIONARIES

Butterworth, Rod R., and Flodin, Mickey. *The Perigee Visual Dictionary of Signing: An A to Z Guide to Over 1,350 Signs of American Sign Language.* New York: Perigee, 1995.
A comprehensive, alphabetized guide to American Sign Language that includes more than 1,350 signs, accompanying illustrations that show precise hand positions and exact movements, and helpful hints.

Costello, Elaine. *Random House Webster's American Sign Language Medical Dictionary.* New York: Random House, 2000.
This book includes all the important medical terms a patient or doctor needs to communicate in ASL, clearly described and illustrated by the former director and editor in chief of Gallaudet University Press.

——. *Random House American Sign Language Dictionary.* New York: Random House, 1994.
This fairly complete dictionary offers large, clear drawings.

Fant, Lou. *The American Sign Language Phrase Book.* Chicago: Contemporary Books, 1994.
This phrase book is an excellent way to begin understanding American Sign Language's grammatical structure.

Lane, Leonard G., and Skrobisz, Jan. *Gallaudet Survival Guide to Signing.* Washington, D.C.: Gallaudet University Press, 1990.
An affordable, easy-to-understand guide to the basics of sign, and a good choice if you need to find a word in a hurry.

Proctor, Claude O., and McGregor, Tony Landon. *Signing in Fourteen Languages.* New York: Black Dog and Leventhal Publishers, 2000.
Detailed line drawings indicate how to sign each word, accompanied by the same word translated into Arabic, Chinese, Dutch, French, German, Italian, Japanese, Korean, Portuguese, Russian, Spanish, and Swedish. A convenient cross-indexing feature makes it easy to find the appropriate sign language gesture, using any of the languages, without having to translate the word. Fingerspelling charts for both American Sign Language and International Sign Language enable readers to spell out uncommon words and names.

BIBLIOGRAPHY

Abercrombie, D. *Elements of General Phonetics.* Chicago: Aldine, 1967.

Aiello, B. *The Hearing-Impaired Child in the Regular Class.* Washington, D.C.: The AFT Teachers' Network for Education of the Handicapped, 1981.

Akens, David. *Loss of Hearing and You.* Huntsville, Ala.: Strode, 1970.

Albertini, J., B. Meath-Lang, and Caccamise, F. "Sign Language Use: Development of English and Communication Skills." *Audiology* 9 (1984): 111–126.

Allen, J. C., and M. L. Allen. "Discovering and Accepting Hearing Impairment." *Volta Review* 81, no. 5 (1979): 279–285.

Allen, T. E., and T. I. Osborn. "Academic Integration of Hearing-Impaired Students: Demographic, Handicapping and Achievement Factors." *American Annals of the Deaf* 129, no. 2 (1984): 100–113.

———, C. S. White, and M. A. Karchmer. "Issues in the Development of a Special Edition for Hearing-Impaired Students of the Seventh Edition of the Stanford Achievement Test." *American Annals of the Deaf* 128, no. 1 (1983): 34–39.

Altshuler, K. A. "Psychiatric Considerations in the Adult Deaf." *American Annals of the Deaf* 107, no. 5 (1962): 560–561.

———. "The Social and Psychological Development of the Deaf Child: Problems, Their Treatment and Prevention." *American Annals of the Deaf* 119, no. 4 (1974): 365–376.

———, W. E. Deming, and J. Vollenweider. "Impulsivity and Profound Early Deafness." *American Annals of the Deaf* 121, no. 3 (1976): 331–345.

———, and J. Rainer, eds. *Mental Health and the Deaf: Approach and Prospects.* Washington, D.C.: U.S. Department of Health, Education and Welfare, Social and Rehabilitation Services, 1968.

American Society for Deaf Children. *Position Statements on Education, Educational Options, Parental Involvement in Education, Communication, Total Communica-tion.* Silver Spring, Md.: American Society for Deaf Children, 1983.

Angus, Jean Rich. *Watch My Words: An Open Letter to Parents of Young Deaf Children.* Cincinnati, Ohio: Forward Movement Publications, 1974.

Anthony, D., W. Dekkers, and C. Erikson. *Seeing Essential English: Code-breaker.* Boulder, Colo.: Pruett, 1978.

Archbold, S., et al. "Educational Placement of Deaf Children Following Cochlear Implantation." *British Journal of Audiology* 32, no. 5 (October 1998): 295–300.

Arnos, K. S. "The Implications of Genetic Testing for Deafness," *Ear Hear* 24/4 (August 2003): 324–331.

Axon, P. R., et al. "Cochlear Ossification After Meningitis." *American Journal of Otolaryngology* 19, no. 4 (November 1998): 724–729.

Baker, C., and R. Battison. *Sign Language and the Deaf Community.* Silver Spring, Md.: National Association of the Deaf, 1980.

———, and D. Cokely. *American Sign Language: A Teacher's Resource Text on Grammar and Culture.* Silver Spring, Md.: T. J. Publishers, 1980.

Barnett, S. "Clinical and Cultural Issues in Caring for Deaf People." *Family Medicine* 31, no. 1 (January 1999): 17–22. Review.

Battison, Robbin. *Lexical Borrowing in American Sign Language.* Silver Spring, Md.: Linstok Press, 1978.

Beard, Jonathan D. "Magnetic Implants Aid Hearing." *Popular Science* 245 (November 1994): 38.

Beck, B. "Self-Assessment of Selected Interpersonal Abilities in Hard of Hearing and Deaf Adolescents," *International Journal of Rehabilitation Research* 11, no. 4 (1988): 343–349.

Becker, G. *Growing Old in Silence.* Berkeley: University of California Press, 1980.

Bekesy, G. *Experiments in Hearing.* New York: McGraw-Hill, 1960.

Bellugi, Ursula, and D. Newkirk. "Formal Devices for Creating New Signs in American Sign Language." *Sign Language Studies* 30 (1981): 1–35.

Bender, R. *The Conquest of Deafness.* Cleveland, Ohio: Case Western Reserve, 1970.

Benzaia, Diana. "Hold on to Your Hearing." *Saturday Evening Post* 261 (January/February 1989): 40.

———. "Help Your Hearing." *The Saturday Evening Post* 261 (March 1989): 16.

Berendt, R. D., E. Corliss and M. Ojalvo. *Quieting: A Practical Guide to Noise Control.* U.S. Dept. of Commerce, National Bureau of Standards, Washington, D.C., 1976.

Berg, F. S. *Educational Audiology: Hearing and Speech Management.* New York: Grune & Stratton, 1976.

Bergman, M. *Aging and the Perception of Speech.* Baltimore, Md.: University Park Press, 1980.

Beynon, G. J., et al. "'Doctor, Do I Need A Hearing Aid?'" *Practitioner* 242/1587 (June 1998): 421.

Birch, J. *Hearing-Impaired Pupils in the Mainstream of Education.* Reston, Va.: Council for Exceptional Children, 1974.

Blackwell, P. *Teaching Hearing Impaired Children in Regular Classrooms.* Washington, D.C.: Center for Applied Linguistics, 1983.

Block, M., and M. Okrand. "Real-time Closed Captioned Television as an Educational Tool." *American Annals of the Deaf* 128, no. 5 (1983): 636–641.

Bodner-Johnson, B. A. "The Family Environment and Achievement of Deaf Students." *Exceptional Children* 52 (1986): 443–449.

Boettcher, F. A., and R. J. Salvi. "Salicylate Ototoxicity: Review and Synthesis." *American Journal of Otolaryngology* 12 (1991): 33–47.

Bonnickson, K. "A Functional Language Program That Works." *Volta Review* 87, no. 2 (1985): 67–76.

Bornstein, Harry. "A Description of Some Current Systems Designed to Represent English." *American Annals of the Deaf* 118 (1973): 454–464.

———. "Towards a Theory of Use for Signed English: From Birth Through Adulthood." *American Annals of the Deaf* 127, no. 1 (1982): 26–31.

———, and Karen Saulnier. *The Signed English School Book.* Washington, D.C.: Kendall Green Publications, Gallaudet University Press, 1987.

———, K. Saulnier, and Lillian Hamilton, eds. *The Comprehensive Signed English Dictionary.* Washington, D.C.: Gallaudet University Press, 1983.

Bottrill, I. "Diagnosing and Treating Ménière's Disease." *Practitioner* 242, no. 1587 (June 1998): 482–484.

Boughman, J. A., and K. A. Shaver. "Genetic Aspects of Deafness: Understanding the Counseling Process." *American Annals of the Deaf* 127, no. 4 (1982): 393–400.

Braddy, N. *Anne Sullivan Macy: The Story Behind Helen Keller.* New York: Doubleday, 1933.

Brasel, K., and S. P. Quigley. "Influence of Certain Language and Communication Environments in Early Childhood on the Development of Language in Deaf Individuals." *Journal of Speech and Hearing Research* 20 (1977): 95–107.

———. *Mainstreaming the Prelingually Deaf Child.* Washington, D.C.: Gallaudet University Press, 1978.

Brietzke, C. E. "Listen Up!" *The Saturday Evening Post* 265 (September/October 1993): 36.

Brown, Mary Daniels. "The Ears: Your Personal Sound System." *Current Health II* 19 (November 1992): 6–11.

Bruce, Robert. *Alexander Graham Bell and the Conquest of Solitude.* Boston: Little, Brown, 1973.

Buchman, C. A., et al. "Cochlear Implants in the Geriatric Population: Benefits Outweigh Risks." *Ear Nose & Throat Journal* 78, no. 7 (July 1999): 489–494.

Caccamise, F., ed. "Sign Language and Simultaneous Communication: Linguistic, Psychological and Instructional Ramifications." *American Annals of the Deaf,* November 1978.

———, et al., eds. *Introduction to Interpreting for Interpreters/Transliterators, Hearing-Impaired Consumers, Hearing Consumers.* Silver Spring, Md.: Registry of Interpreters for the Deaf, 1980.

———, and D. Hicks, eds. *American Sign Language in a Bilingual Bicultural Context.* Silver Spring, Md.: National Association of the Deaf, 1980.

———, and W. Newell. "A Review of Current Terminology in Deaf Education and Signing." *Journal of the Academy of Rehabilitative Audiology* 17 (1984).

Caldwell, D. "Closed Captioned Television and the Hearing Impaired." *Volta Review* 83, no. 5 (1981): 285–289.

Calvert, D. *A Parent's Guide to Speech and Deafness.* Washington, D.C.: Alexander Graham Bell Association for the Deaf, 1984.

———, and S. R. Silverman. *Speech and Deafness.* Washington, D.C.: Alexander Graham Bell Association for the Deaf, 1983.

Casano, R. A., et al. "Inherited Susceptibility to Aminoglycoside Ototoxicity: Genetic Heterogeneity and Clinical Implications." *American Journal of Otolaryngology* 20, no. 3 (May–June 1999): 151–156.

Catford, J. *Fundamental Problems in Phonetics.* Bloomington: University of Indiana Press, 1966.

Chess, S., and P. Fernandez. "Impulsivity in Rubella Deaf Children: a Longitudinal Study." *American Annals of the Deaf* 125, no. 40 (1980): 505–509.

Chomsky, N. *Language and Mind.* New York: Harcourt Brace Jovanovich, 1968.

Chough, S. K. "Speech Is Not Equivalent to Personality Development." *Social Work* 22, no. 4 (1977): 310–312.

Christiansen, J. B., and D. P. Polakoff. "Characteristics of Social Workers and Social Work Programs at Residential and Day Schools for the Deaf." *American Annals for the Deaf*, June 125, no. 4 (1980): 482–487.

Clarke, B. R., and D. Ling. "The Effects of Using Cued Speech." *Volta Review* 78 (1976): 23–34.

Cohen, O. P. "Deaf Children from Ethnic, Linguistic and Racial Minority Backgrounds: An Overview." *American Annals of the Deaf* 135, no. 2 (1992): 67–93.

———. "At-Risk Deaf Adolescents." *Volta Review* 93, no. 5 (1991): 57–72.

Cokely, D. "When Is a Pidgin Not a Pidgin? An Alternate Analysis of the ASL-English Contact Situation." *Sign Language Studies* 38 (1983): 1–24.

———, and R. Gawlik. "A Position Paper on the Relationship Between Manual English and Sign." *Deaf American*, May 7–11, 1973.

Cole, E., and H. Gregory, eds. *Auditory Learning.* Washington, D.C.: Alexander Graham Bell Association for the Deaf, 1986.

Combs, Alec. *Hearing Loss Help.* Santa Maria, Calif.: Alpenglow Press, 1986.

Compton, Cynthia, and Fred Brandt. *Assistive Listening Devices.* Washington, D.C.: National Information Center on Deafness.

Connor, L., ed. *Speech for the Deaf Child: Knowledge and Use.* Washington, D.C.: Alexander Graham Bell Association for the Deaf, 1971.

Conrad, R. *The Deaf School Child.* London: Harper & Row, 1979.

Consumer Reports Editors. "Hearing aids." *Consumer Reports 1994 Buying Guide* 58 (December 15, 1993): 230–232.

———. "How to Buy a Hearing Aid." *Consumer Reports* 57 (November 1992): 716–721.

Consumer's Digest Editors. "New Generation Hearing Aids." *Consumer's Digest* 32 (September/October 1993): 76.

Corbett, E. E., Jr., and C. J. Jensema. *Teachers of the Deaf: Descriptive Profiles.* Washington, D.C.: Gallaudet University Press, 1981.

Craig, H. B. "Parent-Infant Education in Schools for Deaf Children." *American Annals of the Deaf* 128, no. 21 (1983): 82–98.

Craig, W. "Effects of Pre-School Training on the Development of Reading and Lipreading Skills of Deaf Children." *American Annals of the Deaf* 109, no. 3 (1964): 280–296.

Crammatte, A. B. *Deaf Persons in Professional Employment.* Springfield, Ill.: Thomas, 1968.

———. *Meeting the Challenge: Hearing Impaired Professionals in the Workplace.* Washington, D.C.: Gallaudet University Press, 1987.

———. *Questions and Answers About Employment of Deaf People.* Washington, D.C.: National Information Center on Deafness, 1988.

Crandall, K. E., and N. A. Orlando. "The Use and Learning of Spoken Language Systems." *American Annals of the Deaf* 125, no. 3 (1980): 335–448.

———. "A Comparison of Signs Used By Mothers and Deaf Children During Early Childhood." In *Proceedings of the Convention of American Instructors of the Deaf, 1975.*

Dale, D. M. *Individualized Integration: Studies of Deaf and Partially-Hearing Children and Students in Ordinary Schools and Colleges.* Springfield, Ill.: Thomas, 1984.

Daniloff, R., G. Schuckers, and L. Feth. *The Physiology of Speech and Hearing: An Introduction.* Englewood Cliffs, N.J.: Prentice-Hall, 1980.

Davidson, A., and J. Nuru. "Creating a Culturally Diverse Community: Academic Administrators as Agents for Change." *Gallaudet Today* 21, no. 2 (1990–1991, Winter): 18–23.

Day, P. S. "Deaf Children's Expression of Communication Intentions." *Journal of Communication Disorders* 19, no. 5 (1986): 376–386.

Daya, H., et al. "The Role of a Graded Profile Analysis in Determining Candidacy and Outcome for Cochlear Implantation in Children." *International Journal of Pediatric Otorhinolaryngology* 49, no. 2 (August 5, 1999): 135–142.

Delgado-Gaitan, C. *Literacy for Empowerment: The Role of Parents in Children's Education.* New York: Falmer Press, 1990.

Dichgans, M., et al. "Bacterial Meningitis in Adults: Demonstration of Inner Ear Involvement Using High-Resolution MRI." *Neurology* 52, no. 5 (March 23, 1999): 1,003–1,009.

DiPietro, L. *A Look at Fingerspelling.* Washington, D.C.: The National Academy, Gallaudet University, 1976.

Discover Editors. "Sound: In Your Ear (Philips XP Peritympanic Device)." *Discover* 14 (October 1993): 71.

DuBow, S. "Courts Interpret Mainstreaming: How Residential Schools Can Adapt." *American Annals of the Deaf* 129, no. 2 (1984): 92–94.

Dunan, J. G. "Recent Legislation Affecting Hearing-Impaired Persons." *American Annals of the Deaf* 129, no. 2 (1984): 83–91.

Eisenberg, R. "The Development of Hearing in Man: An Assessment of Current Status." *ASHA* 12 (1970): 119–123.

Erting, C., and R. Meiesegeier, eds. *Social Aspects of Deafness.* Washington, D.C.: Gallaudet University Press, 1982.

Evans, L. *Total Communication: Structure and Strategy.* Washington, D.C.: Gallaudet University Press, 1982.

FDA Consumer Editors. "FDA Approves Marketing of Cochlear Implant for Children." *FDA Consumer* 24 (October 1990): 2–3.

Farrugia, D., and G. F. Austin. "A Study of Social-Emotional Adjustment Patterns of Hearing-Impaired Students in Different Educational Settings." *American Annals of the Deaf* 125, no. 5 (1980): 535–541.

Fasold, R. *The Sociolinguistics of Society.* Oxford, England: Blackwell, 1984.

Fischel-Ghodsian, N. "Mitochondrial Deafness," *Ear Hear* 24/4 (August 2003): 303–13.

Flexer, C. "Audiological Rehabilitation in the Schools," *ASHA* 32, no. 4 (April 1990): 44–45.

Fonseca, S. "Identification of Permanent Hearing Loss in Children: Are the Targets for Outcome Measures Attainable?" *British Journal of Audiology* 33, no. 3 (June 1999): 35–43.

Foster, S., and MacLeod, J. "Deaf People at Work: Assessment of Communication Among Deaf and Hearing Persons in Work Settings," *International Journal of Audiology* 42/Suppl 1 (July 2003): S128–S139.

Franck, Irene, and Brownstone, David. *The Parents' Desk Reference.* New York: Prentice Hall, 1991.

Freeman, Roger D., Clifton F. Carbin, and Robert J. Boese. *Can't Your Child Hear?* Baltimore: University Park Press, 1981.

Friedman, R. A., et al. "Maternally Inherited Nonsyndromic Hearing Loss." *American Journal of Medical Genetics* 84, no. 4 (June 4, 1999): 369–372.

Frishberg, N. "Arbitrariness and Iconicity: Historical Change in American Sign Language." *Language* 51, no. 3 (1975): 696–719.

———. *Interpreting: An Introduction.* Silver Spring, Md.: RID Publications, 1985.

Froehlinger, V. *Today's Hearing Impaired Child: Into the Mainstream of Education.* Washington, D.C.: Alexander Graham Bell Association for the Deaf, 1981.

Funk, B. "Being Ignored Can Be Bliss—How to Use a Sign Language Interpreter." *Deaf American,* 34, no. 6 (1982).

Furth, Hans G. *Thinking Without Language: Psychological Implications of Deafness.* New York: Free Press, 1966.

Galenson, E., and R. Miller, E. Kaplan, A. Rothstein et al. "Assessment of Development in the Deaf Child." *Journal of the American Academy of Child Psychiatry* 18, no. 1 (1979): 128–142.

Gannon, J. *Deaf Heritage: A Narrative History of Deaf Americans.* Silver Spring, Md.: National Association of the Deaf, 1981.

Garcia, W. J., ed. *Medical Sign Language.* Springfield, Ill.: Thomas, 1983.

Gates, G. A. and Miyamoto, R. T. "Cochlear Implants," *New England Journal of Medicine* 349/5(July 31, 2003): 421–423.

Geeslin, Ned. "After Live Aid and Farm Aid, Hearing Aid May be Next for Unwary Victims of Rock." *People Weekly* 31 (January 23, 1989): 95–96.

Gelfland, S. *Hearing: An Introduction to Psychological and Physiological Acoustics.* New York: Dekker, 1981.

Gerkin, K. P. "The High-Risk Register for Deafness." ASHA 26, no. 3 (1984): 17–23.

Gibbs, K. W. "Individual Differences in Cognitive Skills Related to Reading Ability in the Deaf." *American Annals of the Deaf* 134, no. 3 (July 1989): 214–218.

Gilbert, L., ed. "Deafness and Aging in the USA." *Gallaudet Today* 12, no. 2 (Winter 1982).

Glick, F. P., and D. Pellman. *Breaking Silence.* Scottsdale, Ariz.: Herald Press, 1982.

Goldstein, M. H., Jr. and A. Proctor. "Tactile Aids for Profoundly Deaf Children." *Journal of the Acoustical Society of America* 77, no. 11 (1985): 258–265.

Graff, Stewart and Polly Anne. *Helen Keller: Toward the Light.* New York: Dell, 1971.

Gray, R. F., Jones, S. E., and Court, I. "Cochlear implantation for progressive hearing loss," *Archives of Diseases of Childhood.* 88/8(August 2003): 708–711.

Greenberg, M. T. "Family Stress and Child Competence: The Effects of Early Intervention for Families with Deaf Infants." *American Annals of the Deaf* 128, no. 4 (1980): 407–417.

———, and R. Calderon. "Early Intervention for Deaf Children: Outcomes and Issues." *Topics in Early Childhood Special Education* 4 (1984): 1–9.

Gregory, S. *The Deaf Child and His Family.* New York: Wiley, 1976.

Groce, N. *Everyone Here Spoke Sign Language.* Cambridge, Mass.: Harvard University Press, 1985.

Grosjean, F. *Life With Two Languages: An Introduction to Bilingualism.* Cambridge, Mass.: Harvard University Press, 1982.

Gustason, G., E. Pfetzing, and E. Zawolkow. *Signing Exact English.* Silver Spring, Md.: National Association of the Deaf, 1980.

Hagborg, W. J. "A Sociometric Investigation of Sex and Race Peer Preferences Among Deaf Adolescents," *American Annals of the Deaf* 134, no. 4 (October 1989): 265–267.

Hairston, E., and L. Smith. *Black and Deaf in America: Are We That Different?* Silver Spring, Md.: T. J. Publishers, 1983.

Halmagyi, et al. "Gentamicin Toxicity." *Otolaryngology-Head and Neck Surgery* 111 (1994): 571–574.

Hardie, N. A., et al. "Sensorineural Hearing Loss During Development: Morphological and Physiological Response of the Cochlea and Auditory Brainstem." *Hearing Research* 128/1–2 (February 1999): 147–165.

Hardy, R., and J. Cull, eds. *Educational and Psycho-Social Aspects of Deafness.* Springfield, Ill.: Thomas, 1974.

Harner, S. G. et al. "Transtympanic Gentamicin for Ménières Syndrome." *Laryngoscope* 108, no. 10 (October 1998): 1,446–1,449.

Haring, Norris, ed. *Exceptional Children and Youth.* Columbus, Ohio: Merrill, 1981.

Harris, G. *Broken Ears, Wounded Hearts.* Washington, D.C.: Gallaudet University Press, 1983.

Harris, S., M. Casselbrant, A. Ivarsson, and O. Tjernström. "Hearing Threshold Measurement in Ménières Disease." *Audiology* 1984 23(1): 46–52.

Haybach, P. J. "Tuning Into Ototoxicity." *Nursing* 23(6) (1993): 34–40.

Heffner, R. *General Phonetics.* Madison: University of Wisconsin Press, 1960.

Henggeler, S. W., and P. F. Cooper. "Deaf Child-Hearing Mother Interaction." *Journal of Pediatric Psychology* 8 (1983): 83–95.

Hester, T. O., et al. "Stapes Footplate Fistula and Recurrent Meningitis." *Otolaryngology/Head Neck Surgery* 121, no. 3 (September 1999): 289–292.

Higgins, P. *Outsiders in a Hearing World: A Sociology of Deafness.* Beverly Hills, Calif.: Sage Publications, 1980.

Hochberg, I., H. Levitt, and M. J. Osberger, eds. *Speech of the Hearing Impaired: Research, Training and Personnel Preparation.* Baltimore, Md.: University Park Press, 1983.

Holborow, C. "Deafness as a World Problem." *Advances in Oto-Rhino-Laryngology* 29 (1983): 174–182.

Holte L. "Early Childhood Hearing Loss: A Frequently Overlooked Cause of Speech and Language Delay," *Pediatric Annals* 32/7(July 2003): 461–465.

Hughes, Gordon B., M. D., and Lawrence Koegel, M.D. "Ototoxicity." In *Textbook of Clinical Otology.* New York: Thieme-Stratton, 1985.

Hull, R., and K. Dilka, eds. *The Hearing Impaired Child In School.* Orlando, Fla.: Grune & Stratton, 1984.

Jacobs, L. *A Deaf Adult Speaks Out.* Washington, D.C.: Gallaudet University Press, 1980.

———. "The Community of the Adult Deaf." *American Annals of the Deaf* 119, no. 11 (1974): 41–46.

Jamison, S. L., ed. *Signs for Commuting Terminology.* Silver Spring, Md.: National Association of the Deaf, 1983.

Jeffers, J., and M. Barley. *Speechreading (Lipreading).* Springfield, Ill.: Thomas, 1971.

Jensema, C., and J. Mullins. "Onset, Cause, and Additional Handicaps in Hearing-Impaired Children." *American Annals of the Deaf* 119, no. 6 (1974): 701–705.

Johnson, I., et al. "Who Benefits from Cochlear Implantation?" *Practitioner* 242, no. 1587 (June 1998): 434, 437–438, 444.

Kampfe, C. M. "Parental Reaction to a Child's Hearing Impairment," *American Annals of the Deaf* 134, no. 4 (Oct. 1989): 255–259.

Kannapell, B., Lillian Hamilton, and H. Bornstein. *Signs for Instructional Purposes.* Washington, D.C.: Gallaudet University Press, 1969.

Kaplan, H. *Anatomy and Physiology of Speech.* New York: McGraw-Hill, 1971.

Karchmer, M. A., et al. "The Functional Assessment of Deaf and Hard of Hearing Students."

American Annals of the Deaf 144, no. 2 (April 1999): 68–77.

Katsuki, J., et al. "Application of Theory of Signal Detection to Dichotic Listening." *Journal of Speech and Hearing Research* 27 (1984): 444–448.

Kettrick, Catherine. *American Sign Language: A Beginning Course.* Silver Spring, Md.: National Association of the Deaf, 1984.

King, S. "Comparing Two Causal Models of Career Maturity for Hearing-Impaired Adolescents," *American Annals of the Deaf* 135, no. 1 (Spring 1990): 43–49.

Klane, J. "Are Your Workers Protected to Deaf?" *Occupational Health and Safety* 67, no. 10 (October 1998): 90–4, 96.

Klein, Larry. "Progress in Hi-Fi Hearing Aid Design." *Radio-Electronics* 61 (February 1990): 24–25.

Klima, E., and U. Bellugi. *The Signs of Language.* Cambridge, Mass.: Harvard University Press, 1979.

Kluwin, T. N. "The Grammaticality of Manual Representations of English in Classroom Settings." *American Annals of the Deaf* 126 (4) (June 1981): 417–421.

———. "A Rationale for Modifying Classroom Signing Systems." *Sign Language Studies* 23 (1979): 99–136.

Koegel, L. "Ototoxicity: A Contemporary Review of Aminoglycosides, Loop Diuretics, Acetylsalicylic Acid, Quinine, Erythromycin, and Cisplatinum." *American Journal of Otology* 6, no. 2 (1985): 190–198.

Kothman, V. "Classroom Auditory Trainers." *Hearing Aid Journal* Dec. 1981, 8–9, 41–43.

Krebs, D. E., K. M. Gill-Body, P. O. Riley, and Parker, S. W. "Double-Blinded, Placebo-Controlled Trial of Rehabilitation for Bilateral Vestibular Hypofunction: Preliminary Report." *Otolaryngology-Head and Neck Surgery* 109 (1993): 735–741.

Kretschmer, R., and L. Kretschmer. *Language Development and Intervention with the Hearing Impaired.* Baltimore Md.: University Park Press, 1978.

Ladefoged, P. *A Course in Phonetics.* New York: Harcourt Brace Jovanovich, 1975.

Lash, J. *Helen and Teacher: The Story of Helen Keller and Anne Sullivan Macy.* New York: American Foundation for the Blind, 1980.

Lass, N. *Speech and Language: Advances in Basic Research and Practice.* Vol. 8. New York: Academic Press, 1982.

———, *Speech, Language and Hearing.* Philadelphia: Saunders, 1982.

Levine, E. *The Ecology of Early Deafness: Guide to Fashioning Environments and Psychological Assessments.* New York: Columbia University Press, 1981.

———, and E. Wagner. "Personality of Deaf Persons." *Perceptual and Motor Skills* 39 (1974): 1,167–1,236.

Levitt, H. "Hearing Impairment and Sensory Aids." *Journal of Rehabilitation Research and Development* 23, no. 1 (1986): xiii–xviii.

Libbey, S. S., and W. Pronovost. "Communication Practices of Mainstreamed Hearing-Impaired Adolescents." *Volta Review* 82, no. 4 (1980): 197–213.

Liben, L. S., ed. *Deaf Children: Developmental Perspectives.* New York: Academic Press, 1978.

Ling, D. *Early Intervention for Hearing-Impaired Children: Oral Options.* San Diego, Calif.: College-Hill Press, 1984.

———. *Early Intervention for Hearing-Impaired Children: Total Communication Options.* San Diego, Calif.: College-Hill Press, 1984.

———. *Speech and the Hearing Impaired Child.* Washington, D.C.: Alexander Graham Bell Association for the Deaf, 1976.

Liston, S. L. "Beethoven's Deafness." *Laryngoscope* 99, no. 12 (Dec. 1989): 1,301–1,304.

Locke, J. *Phonological Acquisition and Change.* New York: Academic Press, 1984.

Lubinski, R. B. "A Review of Recent Research on Verbal Communication Among the Elderly." *International Journal of Aging and Human Development* 9 (1978–79): 237–245.

Luey, H. S., and M. Per-Lee. *What Should I Do Now: Problems and Adaptations of the Deafened Adult.* Washington, D.C.: Gallaudet University Press, 1983.

Luterman, D., et al. "Identifying Hearing Loss: Parents' Needs." *American Journal of Audiology* 8/1 (June 1999): 13–18.

Luterman, D. M., ed. *Deafness in Perspective.* San Diego, Calif.: College-Hill Press, 1986.

———. *Counseling Parents of Hearing Impaired Children.* Boston: Little, Brown, 1979.

———. *Deafness in the Family.* Boston: Little, Brown, 1987.

Lyxell, B., et al. "Working-Memory Capacity and Phonological Processing in Deafened Adults and Individuals with a Severe Hearing Impairment," *International Journal of Audiology* 42/Suppl 1 (July 2003): S86–S89.

Markowicz, H. "American Sign Language: Fact and Fancy." Washington, D.C.: The National Academy, Gallaudet University, 1977.

Marshall, L. "Auditory Processing in Aging Listeners." *Journal of Speech and Hearing Disorders* 46, no. 3 (August 1981).

Martin, F. N. *Introduction to Audiology.* Englewood Cliffs, N.J.: Prentice-Hall, 1981.

Marschark, M. "Interactions of Language and Cognition in Deaf Learners: From Research to Practice," *International Journal of Audiology* 42/Suppl 1 (July 2003): S41–S48.

McArthur, Shirley H. *Raising Your Hearing-Impaired Child: A Guideline for Parents.* Washington, D.C.: Alexander Graham Bell Association for the Deaf, 1982.

McFarland, W., and B. P. Cox. *Aging and Hearing Loss.* Washington, D.C.: National Information Center on Deafness/American Speech-Language-Hearing Association, 1987.

Meadow, K. P. *Deafness and Child Development.* Berkeley, Calif.: University of California Press, 1980.

———. Greenberg, M. T., and C. Erting. "Attachment Behavior of Deaf Children with Deaf Parents." *Journal of the American Academy of Child Psychiatry* 22 (1983): 23–28.

———, M. T. Greenberg, C. Erting, and H. Carmichael. "Interactions of Deaf Mothers and Deaf Pre-school Children: Comparisons with Three Other Groups of Deaf and Hearing Dyads." *American Annals of the Deaf* 126, no. 4 (1981): 454–468.

Mendelsohn, J. Z., and B. Fairchild. *Years of Challenge, A Guide for Parents of Hearing-Impaired Adolescents.* Silver Spring, Md.: National Association of the Deaf, 1982.

Miller, S. T., et al. "Better Use of Hearing Aids in Hearing-Impaired Adults." *Journal of the American Geriatric Society* 46, no. 9 (September 1998): 168–169.

Mills, J. H., and J. A. Going. "Review of Environmental Factors Affecting Hearing." *Environmental Health Perspectives* 44 (1982): 119–127.

Moeller, M. P. "Parents' use of Signing Exact English: a descriptive analysis," *Journal of Speech and Hearing Disorders* 55, no. 2 (May 1990): 327–337.

Moore, D. R., et al. "Conductive Hearing Loss Produces a Reversible Binaural Hearing Impairment." *Journal of Neuroscience* 19, no. 19 (October 1, 1999): 8,704–8,711.

Moore, B. *An Introduction to the Psychology of Hearing.* 2d ed. New York: Academic Press, 1982.

Moores, D. *Educating the Deaf: Psychology, Principles, and Practices.* 3d ed. Boston: Houghton Mifflin, 1987.

Morlet, T., et al. "Auditory Screening in High-Risk Pre-Term and Full-Term Neonates Using Transient Evoked Otoacoustic Emissions and Brainstem Auditory Evoked Potentials." *International Journal of Pediatric Otorhinolaryngology* 45, no. 1 (September 15, 1998): 31–40.

Murphy, Kate. "Hearing Aids Get Smart—and Better-Looking." *Business Week,* May 8, 1995, p. 116.

Mutton, P. "Early Identification of Deaf Babies." *Lancet* 352/9145 (December 19–26, 1998): 1,951–1,952.

Naiman, D., and J. Schein. *For Parents of Deaf Children.* Silver Spring, Md.: National Association of the Deaf, 1978.

Nash, J., and A. Nash. *Deafness in Society.* Lexington, Mass.: Heath, 1981.

National Center for Law and the Deaf. *Legal Rights of Hearing-Impaired People.* Washington, D.C.: Gallaudet University Press, 1986.

National Information Center on Deafness. *Communicating with Deaf People.* Washington, D.C.: Gallaudet University Press, 1987.

Neisser, A. *The Other Side of Silence: Sign Language and the Deaf Community in America.* New York: Knopf, 1983.

NIH. "Early Identification of Hearing Impairment in Infants and Young Children." *NIH Consensus Statement Online* 11, no. 1 (March 1993): 1–24.

———. "Cochlear Implants in Adults and Children." *NIH Consensus Statement Online* 13, no. 2 (May 15–17, 1995): 1–30.

Nikolopoulos T. P., et al. "Age at Implantation: Its Importance in Pediatric Cochlear Implantation." *Laryngoscope* 109, no. 4 (April 1999): 595–599.

Nix, G. W. "The Right To Be Heard." *Volta Review* 83, no. 4 (1981): 199–205.

———. *Mainstream Education for Hearing Impaired Children and Youth.* New York: Grune & Stratton, 1976.

Norris, C. H. "Drugs Affecting the Inner Ear: A Review of Their Clinical Efficacy, Mechanisms of Action, Toxicity and Place in Therapy." *Drugs* 36 (1988): 754–772.

Northcott, W. H. *The Hearing Impaired Child in a Regular Classroom.* Washington, D.C.: Alexander Graham Bell Association, 1973.

Odkvist, L. M., C. Moller and K. A. Thomas. "Otoneurologic Disturbances Caused by Solvent Pollution." *Otolaryngology-Head and Neck Surgery* 106, no. 6 (1992): 687–692.

O'Donoghue, G. M., et al. "Speech Perception in Children After Cochlear Implantation." *American Journal of Otolaryngology* 19, no. 6 (November 1998): 762–7.

———. "Cochlear Implants in Young Children: The Relationship Between Speech Perception and Speech Intelligibility." *Ear Hear* 20, no. 5 (October 1999): 419–425.

Ogden, P., and S. Lipsett. *The Silent Garden: Understanding the Hearing Impaired Child.* New York: St. Martin's Press, 1982.

Orlans, H. *Adjustment to Adult Hearing Loss.* San Diego, Calif.: College-Hill Press, 1985.

Osberger, M. J. "Audiological Rehabilitation with Cochlear Implants and Tactile Aids." *ASHA* 32, no. 4 (April 1990): 38–43.

Ozdamor, O., N. Kraus, and L. Stein. "Auditory Brainstem Responses in Infants Recovering from Bacterial Meningitis." *Archives of Otolaryngology* 109 (January 1983): 13–18.

Panara, R.F. "Cultural Arts Among the Deaf." *The Deaf American* 32, no. 9 (1980): 9–11.

———, and J. Panara. *Great Deaf Americans.* Silver Spring, Md.: T.J. Publishers, 1983.

Parasnis, I. "Visual Perceptual Skills and Deafness." *Journal of the Academy of Rehabilitative Audiology* 16 (1983): 148–160.

Perrin, E., et al. "Evaluation of Cochlear Implanted Children's Voices." *International Journal of Pediatric Otorhinolaryngology* 47, no. 2 (February 15, 1999): 181–186.

Pimental, A. T. "A Barrier-Free Environment for Deaf People." *The Deaf American* 32, no. 5 (1980): 7–9.

Poizner, H. "Visual and Phonetic Coding of Movement: Evidence from American Sign Language." *Science* 212 (1981): 691–693.

Port, Otis. "They're Bearing the Gift of Sound." *Business Week,* February 6, 1995, p. 152–153.

Porter, A. "Sign-language Interpretation in Psychotherapy with Deaf Patients." *American Journal of Psychotherapy* 53, no. 2 (Spring 1999): 163–176.

Prasher, D., et al. "The Role of Otoacoustic Emissions in Screening and Evaluation of Noise Damage." *International Journal of Occupational Medicine and Environmental Health* 12/2 (1999): 183–192.

Quigley, S. P., and R. E. Kretshmer. *The Education of Deaf Children: Issues, Theory and Practice.* Baltimore, Md.: University Park Press, 1982.

Rainer, J. D., K. Z. Altshuler, and F. J. Kallmann, eds. *Family and Mental Health Problems in a Deaf Population.* Springfield, Ill.: Thomas, 1969.

Ramsdell, D. A. "The Psychology of the Hard of Hearing and Deafened Adult." In *Hearing and Deafness,* 499–510. New York: Rinehart & Winston, 1978.

Reardon, W. "Prevalence, Age of Onset, and Natural History of Thyroid Disease in Pendred Syndrome." *Journal of Medical Genetics* 36, no. 8 (August 1999): 595–598.

Reardon, W. "Sex-linked deafness," *Journal of Medical Genetics* 27, no. 6 (June 1990): 376–379.

Reefhuis, J., et al. "Risk of Bacterial Meningitis in Children with Cochlear Implants," *New England Journal of Medicine* 349/5(July 31, 2003):435–445.

Rezen, Susan, and Carl Hausman. *Coping with Hearing Loss.* New Jersey: Barricade Books, 1993.

Ronnberg, J. "Cognition in the Hearing Impaired and Deaf as a Bridge Between Signal and Dialogue: A Framework and a Model," *International Journal of Audiology* 42/Suppl 1 (July 2003): S68–S76.

Rupp, R. "The Roles of the Audiologist." *Journal of the Academy of Rehabilitation Audiology* 10, no. 1 (1977): 10–17.

Rutman, D. "The Impact and Experience of Adventitious Deafness," *American Annals of the Deaf* 134, no. 5 (Dec. 1989): 305–311.

Rybak, L. P. "Hearing: The Effects of Chemicals." *Otolaryngology–Head and Neck Surgery* 106, no. 6 (1992): 677–686.

Sataloff, Joseph, M.D., and Paul L. Michael, Ph.D. *Hearing Conservation.* Springfield, Ill.: Thomas, 1973.

Sattler, J. *Assessment of Children's Intelligence and Special Abilities.* 2d ed. Boston: Allyn and Bacon, 1982.

Schaeffer, Benson, Arlene Musil, and George Kollinzas. *Total Communication: A Signed Speech Program for Nonverbal Children.* Springfield, Ill.: Research Press, 1980.

Schildroth, A. N., and M. A. Karchmer, eds. *Deaf Children in America.* San Diego, Calif.: College-Hill Press, 1986.

Schleuning, A., R. M. Johnson, and J. A. Vernon. "Masking and Tinnitus." *Ear and Hearing* 6, no. 2 (March–April 1980): 71–72.

Schowe, B. *Identity Crisis in Deafness.* Tempe, Ariz.: Scholars Press, 1979.

Scott, P. M., and M. V. Griffiths. "A Clinical Review of Ototoxicity." *Clinical Otolaryngology* 19 (1994): 3–8.

Scouten, E. L. *Turning Points in the Education of Deaf People.* Danville, Ill.: Interstate, 1984.

Schroedel, J. G., and W. Schiff. "Attitudes Towards Deafness Among Several Deaf and Hearing Populations." *Rehabilitative Psychology* 19 (1972): 59–70.

Solow, S. *Sign Language Interpreting: A Basic Resource Book.* Silver Spring, Md.: National Association of the Deaf, 1981.

Soviero, Marcelle M. "Signal Processing for Ears (Digital Hearing Aid System Developed by Janet Rutledge)." *Popular Science* 239 (July 1991): 30.

Spahn, C., et. al. "A Comparison Between Parents of Children with Cochlear Implants and Parents of Children with Hearing Aids Regarding Parental Distress and Treatment Expectations," *International Journal of Pediatric Otorhinolaryngology* 67/9 (September 2003): 947–955.

Spradley, Thomas S., and James P. Spradley. *Deaf Like Me.* Washington, D.C.: Gallaudet University Press, 1978.

Stone, H. "Hearing Loss and Mental Health." *Shhh* 3, no. 6 (November/December 1982).

Sullivan, P., and M. Vernon. "Psychological Assessment of Hearing-Impaired Children." *School Psychology Review* 8, no. 3 (1979): 271–290.

Switzer, M. E., and B. R. Williams. "Life Problems of Deaf People: Prevention and Treatment." *Archives of Environmental Health* 15 (1967): 249–256.

Tomblin, J. B., et al. "A Comparison of Language Achievement in Children with Cochlear Implants and Children Using Hearing Aids." *Journal of Speech-Language Hearing Research* 42, no. 2 (April 1999): 497–509.

Turkington, Carol A. "Cochlear Implants: Deliver-ing Sound to the Deaf." *The World Book Health and Medical Annual.* Chicago: World Book, Inc., 1996.

———. *The Hearing Loss Sourcebook.* New York: Penguin, 1997.

Turner, C. W., et al. "Speech Audibility for Listeners with High-Frequency Hearing Loss." *American Journal of Audiology* 8, no. 1 (June 1999): 47–56.

Valente, Michael. "Programmable Aids Improve Hearing." *USA Today* 122 (October 1993): 12–13.

Van Cleve, J. V., ed. *Gallaudet Encyclopedia of Deaf People and Deafness.* New York: McGraw-Hill, 1987.

Van Naarden, K., et al. "Relative and Attributable Risks for Moderate to Profound Bilateral Sensorineural Hearing Impairment Associated with Lower Birth Weight in Children 3 to 10 Years Old." *Pediatrics* 104/4 Pt 1 (October 1999): 905–910.

Warner, David. "An Unexpected Phone Bill: Business Phones Must Be Able To Be Used by Persons with Hearing Aids." *Nation's Business* 81 (May 1993): 72.

Wax, Teena, and Loraine DiPietro. *Managing Hearing Loss Later in Life.* Washington, D.C.: National Information Center on Deafness/American Speech-Language-Hearing Association, 1987.

Wilbur, R. *American Sign Language and Sign Systems.* Baltimore, Md.: University Park Press, 1979.

Wilcox, S. A., et al. "Connexin26 Deafness in Several Interconnected Families." *Journal of Medical Genetics* 36, no. 5 (May 1999): 383–385.

Williams, Rebecca. "Enjoy, Protect the Best Ears of Your Life." *FDA Consumer* 26 (May 1992): 25–27.

Williamson, W. D., M. M. Desmond, N. LaFevers, L. H. Taber, F. I. Catlin, and T. G. Weaver. "Symptomatic Congenital Cytomegalovirus: Disorders of Language, Learning and Hearing." *American Journal of Diseases of Children* 136 (1982): 902–905.

Wong, D., et al. "PET Imaging of Cochlear-Implant and Normal-Hearing Subjects Listening To Speech and Nonspeech." *Hearing Research.* 132, nos. 1–2 (June 1999): 34–42.

Woodward, J. "Historical Bases of American Sign Language." In *Understanding Language Through Sign Language Research,* edited by R. Siple. New York: Academic Press, 1978.

Wright, T. "Bacterial Meningitis and Deafness." *Clinical Otolaryngology* 24, no. 5 (September 1999): 385–387.

Yeo, K. L., et al. "Outcomes of Extremely Premature Infants Related to Their Peak Serum Bilirubin Concentrations and Exposure to Phototherapy." *Pediatrics* 102, no. 6 (December 1998): 1,426–1,431.

Yoken, C., ed. *Interpreter Training: The State of the Art.* Washington, D.C.: The National Academy of Gallaudet College, 1980.

Yoshinaga-Itano, C., et al. "The Development of Deaf and Hard of Hearing Children Identified Early Through the High-Risk Registry." *American Annals of the Deaf* 143, no. 5 (December 1998): 416–424.

———. "Identification of Hearing Loss After Age 18 Months Is Not Early Enough." *American Annals of the Deaf* 143/5 (December 1998): 380–387.

Youniss, J. *Parents and Peers in Social Development.* Chicago: University of Chicago Press, 1980.

INDEX

Boldface page numbers indicate major treatment of a subject.

A

AA. *See* arachidonic acid 177–178

AAPTSD. *See* American Association to Promote the Teaching of Speech to the Deaf

ABC television network 42, 43, 48, 124

ABLB. *See* alternate binaural loudness balance test

ABLEDATA **1**

aborigines, Australian 27

ABR. *See* auditory brainstem response test

Academy for the Deaf and Dumb 37–38

Academy of Dispensing Audiologists **1**

ACCD NewsNet (periodical) 10

accessibility requirements 16
under Americans with Disabilities Act 14–15
under Architectural Barriers Act 16
under Rehabilitation Act 122–123

accommodation
Job Accommodation Network **116**
reasonable accommodation standard 14–15

acetaminophen
for chicken pox 45
with hydrocodone 144
for measles 131

acetazolamide mannitol 164

acoupedic method. *See* auditory-oral method

acoustic admittance 1, 23–24

acoustic admittance tests 23–24

acoustical impedance, measurement of 107

Acoustical Society of America **1**
Journal of the Acoustical Society of America 117

acoustic bridge 107

acoustic feedback **79,** 108

acoustic immitance **1,** 23–24

acoustic immitance tests 1

acoustic impedance **1,** 23–24
tympanogram of **209**

acoustic nerve. *See* auditory nerve; eighth cranial nerve

acoustic neuroma **1–4,** 26, 208
tinnitus in 2, 26, 205
vestibular disorders in 215

Acoustic Neuroma Association **4**

acoustic reflex **4**

acoustic reflex test 24

acoustics **4**

acoustic spectrum **4**

acoustic trauma **4**. *See also* noise
in inner ear 152

acquired immundeficiency syndrome. *See under* AIDS

acupuncture **4**

acyclovir, for chickenpox 45

ADA. *See* Americans with Disabilities Act of 1990

ADARA. *See* American Deafness and Rehabilitation Association

adenocarcinoma 137

adenoid cystic carcinoma 137

adenoidectomy **4–5**

adenoids **5**

adhesive otitis media **5,** 137

adults, hearing tests for, frequency of 22

adventitious deafness **5**
organizations for 19

advocacy groups
for African-American deaf persons 145
for communications issues 147, 203

for deaf persons 92, 115, 144, 145

for disabled persons 9–10, 143–144

for families of deaf persons 14

for hearing aid consumers 111

for legal rights 10, 143–144, 145, 146–147

for prevention of deafness 144

aero-otitis media **5,** 76
conductive hearing loss and 100
inner ear and 109
perilymph fistula in 169

affirmative action, for handicapped persons 122

African-American deaf persons
advocacy groups for 145
ASL dialect of 13

agencies, public. *See* governmental agencies

aging
hearing loss in **6–7,** 101, 109, 152, **173**
fear of admitting 97–98
treatment of 91
inner ear and 109
ototoxic drugs and 163
presbycusis 6, **173**
senior citizen services 7

agnosia, auditory **25,** 66

AID Bulletin (periodical) 197

AIDS, and hearing loss **7,** 107

AIDS.Net **7**

AIDS-related complex (ARC), and hearing loss **7**

AIED. *See* autoimmune inner ear disease

air bags and hearing loss **7**

air bone gap **7,** 23

air conduction **7,** 194

air conduction audiometry **7,** 22–23, 46

air conduction test, pure tone **7,** 22–23, 46

airplane flight, ear problems and. *See* aero-otitis media

AKA (alphabet of assisted kinemes) 33

alarms. *See* alerting devices; wake-up alarms

Alberti, Salomon **7**

alcohol
abuse
by deaf persons 197
treatment for 134, 197
fetal alcohol syndrome **80,** 172
ototoxic properties of 163, 172

alerting devices **8**. *See also* signaling devices; wake-up alarms

Alexander Graham Bell Association for the Deaf 7, **8,** 10, 38, 57–58, 158, 202–203, 218

Allen, R. 153–154

allergies
ear canal blockage in 77
external ear canal narrowing in 197
Ménière's disease and 132
middle ear effusion and 141
retracted eardrum in 179

allophones 170

All Souls Church, Philadelphia 76

alphabets, manual. *See* fingerspelling

Alport's disease **8–9,** 109

alternate binaural loudness balance test (ABLB) **9,** 177

alternative listening systems. *See* assistive listening systems

Ambrosi, Gustinus **9**

American Academy of Audiology **9**

American Academy of Otolaryngology–Head and Neck Surgery **9**

American Academy of Pedi-
atrics 68, 150
American Annals of the Deaf
(periodical) **9**
American Association for the
Advancement of Science 105
American Association for the
Hard of Hearing 144
American Association of the
Deaf-Blind **9–10**
American Association to Pro-
mote the Teaching of Speech
to the Deaf (AAPTSD) 8,
10, 35, 105
American Asylum for the
Education and Instruction of
Deaf and Dumb Persons 12,
54–55
American Athletic Association
of the Deaf (AAAD) **10**
American Athletic Union of
the Deaf 10
American Board of Examiners
in Speech Pathology and
Audiology 58
American Board of Otolaryn-
gology 162
American Coalition of Citizens
with Disabilities **10**
American Deafness and Reha-
bilitation Association
(ADARA) **10–11,** 116, 123
American Foundation for the
Blind 119
American Hearing Research
Foundation **11**
American Humane Associa-
tion **11**
American Laryngological, Rhi-
nological and Otological
Society **11**
American manual alphabet.
See fingerspelling
American Ministries to the
Deaf **11**
American National Standards
Institute 16
American Otological Society
11
American School for the Deaf
9, **11–12,** 39, 41, 48, 54–55,
85, 86
American Sign Language
(ASL) **12–13.** *See also* sign-
language interpreters; simul-
taneous communication;
total communication
advocates of 43, 145
in Canada 41

education and 70
English fluency and 72
fingerspelling and 81
history of 82
as language 71
manually coded English
and 128–129
nonhuman use of
153–154
nonmanual behaviors **154**
organizations for information on 17
psychological testing and
135
and simultaneous commu-
nication 135, 191–192
American Sign Language
Teachers Association
(ASLTA) **13–14**
American Society for Deaf
Children (ASDC) **14**
American Speech-Language-
Hearing Association (ASHA)
14, 20, 44, 45–46, 58, 63,
116, 144
American Standard Code for
Information Interchange. *See*
ASCII
Americans with Disabilities
Act of 1990 (ADA) **14–15,**
116
American Tinnitus Association
15, 206
Ameslan. *See* American Sign
Language
amikacin 15, 164, 172
aminoglycosides
hearing loss from, prenatal
172
loop diuretics and 125
ototoxicity of 109, 120,
164
tinnitus in 205
amoxicillin **15**
amplification. *See* assistive listening devices; hearing
aid(s)
amplified telephone. *See* assistive listening devices
amplitude **15**
ampulla **15**
anacusia **15**
anacusis. *See* anacusia
anakusis. *See* anacusia
analgesia, auditory **25**
analytic speech training methods 195
anoxia **15,** 170
Anthony, David 184

antibiotics
for catarrhal deafness 43
hearing loss from **15,** 109,
130, 164, 173, 185
inner ear ototoxicity 109
for malignant otitis
externa 127
for measles 131
for Ménière's disease 133
for meningitis 134
for otitis media 141, 161
for perforated eardrum 67
for serous otitis media 187
in stapedectomy 196
for typhoid fever 210
and vestibular disorders
215
anticancer drugs, ototoxic
effects of 165
antidiscrimination law
122–123
antiemitics, for dizziness 65
antihistimines
for dizziness 65
for labyrinthitis 121, 215
antitragus **16**
Antivert (meclizine) 132, 169
anvil (incus) **16.** *See also*
incus; ossicles; ossicular
chain
apes, sign language use by
153–154
aphasia **16,** 66
auditory, *see* auditory
agnosia
arachidonic acid (AA)
177–178
ARC. *See* AIDS-related complex
architectural acoustics 4
Architectural and Transportation Barriers Compliance
Board 16, **16,** 122
Architectural Barriers Act of
1968 (Public Law 90-480)
16, **16**
Aristotle **17**
arsenic, and encephalitis 75
artherosclerosis, hearing loss
in 101
ASCII (American Standard
Code for Information Interchange) **17,** 31, 203
ASHA. *See* American Speech-
Language-Hearing Associa-
tion
ASHA Reports (periodical) 116
ASL. *See* American Sign Language

ASL Access **17**
ASLTA. *See* American Sign
Language Teachers Association
aspirin
hearing loss from **17,** 163,
165, 173, 185
and tinnitus 17, 205, 206
assessment. *See also* audiometry
psychological, organiza-
tions providing 11
vocational, organizations
providing 11
assistive listening devices
17–19. *See also* speech training aids; tactile feedback
device
autocuer **28,** 59, 186
cochlear implant **51–54,**
98, 105, 130
function of 51–52
in Mondini's dysplasia
139
research on 104
information sources on
99, 100
input methods 17–18
obtaining information on
17
telephone devices 18–19
for televisions 19
T-switches and 202. *See
also* T-switch
assistive listening systems **19**
T-switches and 202
assistive technology products,
database of 1
Association of Late-Deafened
Adults **19**
Asylum for the Education and
Instruction of the Deaf and
Dumb 86
AT&T 202–203
athletics for deaf persons
American Athletic Association of the Deaf **10**
American Athletic Union
of the Deaf 10
Comité International des
Sports des Sourds 10,
55, 221
at Gallaudet University 89
NFS awards 148
U.S. Deaf Skiers Associa-
tion 212
World Games for the Deaf
10, **221**
Ativan, for perilymph fistula
169

North American Basic Teletext Specification (NABTS) **155,** 203

Northampton vowel and consonant charts **155**

North Carolina Research Triangle Institute, Center for Biomedical Engineering 28

Norway, communication in 61

Norwegian Sign Language (NSL) **155**

NSL. *See* Norwegian Sign Language

NTD. *See* National Theatre of the Deaf

NTID. *See* National Technical Institute for the Deaf

O

OAE test. *See* otoacoustic emissions (OAE) test

occupational hearing loss 153, **157**

Occupational Safety and Health Act of 1970 **157**
audiology services and 20
noise control and 153

ODAS. *See* Oral Deaf Adults Section

Office of Education, U.S. 146

Office of Special Education and Rehabilitative Services 63

Olympic Committee, U.S., Handicap in Sports Committee 10

Olympics for deaf persons. *See* World Games for the Deaf

On Cue (periodical) **147**

On Cue News Flash (periodical) **147**

on-the-body hearing aids **36,** 97, 223

open captions 43, **157**

open-set speech recognition **157**

oral approach **158**
debate over 34–35, 38–39, 71–72, 76, 85, 102–103, 110, 119, 135, 158–159
in Denmark 61
education and 128
in France 82–83
history of 37–38
in Israel 112–113
in Italy 113
in Japan 115

in Mexico 136
in Netherlands 150
in New Zealand 151
in Puerto Rico 174
simultaneous communication and 193–194
speech training 195–196
in Sweden 198
in Switzerland 198
in United Kingdom 211

oral-aural method. *See* oral approach

oral contraceptives, ototoxic properties of 163

Oral Deaf Adults Section (ODAS) 8, **158–159**

oral interpreters **159,** 190

organ of Corti 31, 51, 54, 57, 95, 103, **159–160**
aging and 109
in Cogan's syndrome 54
in ear anatomy 183
head injuries and 109
perinatal injury to 15
sensory cells in 187

osseous labyrinth. *See* labyrinth, inner ear

ossicles 136, **160.** *See also* anvil (incus); malleus (hammer); ossicular chain; stapes (stirrup)
and acoustic impedance 1
bypassing of 79–80
conductive hearing loss and 100–101
damage to 136–137
ear massage and 68
in mucous otitis media 140
removal of 130
sound detection and 69
surgical repair of 209

ossicular chain **160**
acoustic reflex and 4
acoustic trauma and 4
disrupted, tympanogram of 209
hearing process and 96
intra-aural muscles and 112
serous otitis media and 187

ossicular interruption **160**

ossiculoplasty **160,** 209

osteitis deformans. *See* Paget's disease

osteogenesis imperfecta **160**

osteoma **160**

otic capsule **160**

otic transudates 187

otitis externa. *See* swimmer's ear

otitis interna. *See* labyrinthitis

otitis media **160–161.** *See also* aero-otitis media; serous otitis media
adenoids and 5
adhesive **5,** 137
AIDS and 7
in children 100, 137, 161
cholesteatoma 47
chronic
cancer and 208
consequences of 209
in Down's syndrome 66
earache in 67
ear canal blockage in 77
ear canal narrowing in 197
in fenestration 80
hearing loss and 6, 45, 46, 100, 160–161
immune system and 107
labyrinthitis in 65, 121
mastoid bone and 129–130
in measles 131
mucous **140**
perinatal 169
serous otitis media and 187
smoking and 193
staphylococcus 83
treatment of 15, 129–130, 141, 161
tympanostomy tube in 133
vaccine for **68**
vestibular disorders in 215

otoacoustic emissions (OAE) test 46, **161**

OtoLAM **161**

otolaryngologist 97, **161–162**

otolaryngology **162**

otolith organs 183

otologist **162**
audiometry and 24–25
hearing aid dispensing 97

otology **162**
organizations for 11, 104

otorhinolaryngologists 75, 161

otorhinolaryngology **162**

otorrhea **162**
in middle ear tumors 208
in swimmer's ear 198

otosclerosis 36, 137, **162–163**
carhart notch in **43**
fluoride and 81

tinnitus in 163, 205
treatment of 79–80, 100–101, 102, 196–197

otoscope 161, **163**

otoscopy **163,** 211

otospongiosis. *See* otosclerosis

ototoxic drugs **163–164**
antibiotics **15**
hearing loss from 109, 130, 164, 173, 185
inner ear ototoxicity 109
diuretics 120, **125,** 163, 164, 185
elderly persons and 173
inner ear and 109
in kidney disease treatment 120
for Ménière's disease 133
narcotics **144**
neonatal hearing loss from 104
nicotine **151,** 163
prenatal hearing loss from 172
tinnitus in 205
and vestibular system 109
and workplace hearing loss 153

ototoxicity **164**

Our Kids Magazine 8

Our Saviour Lutheran Church for the Deaf, Chicago **126**

outer ear (external ear; pinna; auricle) **164–165.** *See also* external auditory canal
cancer of **42**
cauliflower ear **43**
cosmetic surgery on **57**
diseases of **77**
hearing process and 96
infections of 168
tumors of 42, 77

oval window 36, 51, 136, **165.** *See also* fenestra ovalis
hearing process and 96

overtone **165**

P

PACES program 12

Paget, Lady Grace **167**

Paget, Sir Richard **167**

Paget-Gorman sign system (PGSS) **167**

Paget's disease 109, **167**

painful hearing **167.** *See also* recruitment

paracusia willisiana **167**